Clinical
Biochemistry

Clinical Biochemistry

ALISTAIR F. SMITH

MD, FRCPEdin, FRC Path
Senior Lecturer in Clinical Biochemistry
University of Edinburgh

GEOFFREY J. BECKETT

BSc, PhD, MRCPath
Reader in Clinical Biochemistry
University of Edinburgh

SIMON W. WALKER

DM, MB, BS
Senior Lecturer in Clinical Biochemistry
University of Edinburgh

PETER W.H. RAE

PhD, MBChB, MRCP, MRCPath
Consultant Clinical Biochemist
Western General Hospital
Edinburgh

Sixth Edition

Blackwell
Science

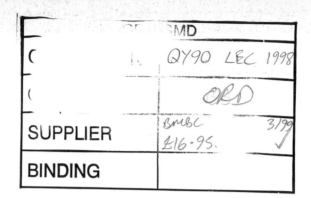

© 1975, 1980, 1984, 1988,
1993, 1998 by
Blackwell Science Ltd
Editorial Offices:
Osney Mead, Oxford OX2 0EL
25 John Street, London, WC1N 2BL
23 Ainslie Place, Edinburgh EH3 6AJ
350 Main Street, Malden
 MA 02148 5018, USA
54 University Street, Carlton
 Victoria 3053, Australia
10, rue Casimir Delavigne
 75006 Paris, France

Other Editorial Offices:
Blackwell Wissenschafts-Verlag GmbH
Kurfürstendamm 57
10707 Berlin, Germany

Blackwell Science KK
MG Kodenmacho Building
7–10 Kodenmacho Nihombashi
Chuo-ku, Tokyo 104, Japan

First published 1975
Revised reprint 1977
Reprinted 1978
Second edition 1980
Third edition 1984
Reprinted 1987
Fourth edition 1988
Reprinted 1989, 1991
Fifth edition 1993
Reprinted 1994, 1996
Sixth edition 1998

Set by Excel Typesetters Co.,
Hong Kong
Printed and bound in the
United Kingdom by the
University Press, Cambridge

A catalogue record for this title
is available from the British Library

ISBN 0-632-04834-4

Library of Congress
Cataloging-in-publication Data

Lecture notes on clinical biochemistry
 /[edited by] Alistair F. Smith.
       p.   cm.
   Includes bibliographical
references and index.
   ISBN 0-632-04834-4
   1. Clinical chemistry.
   2. Clinical biochemistry.   I. Smith,
A. F. (Alistair Fairley)
     [DNLM: 1. Biochemistry.
QU 4 L471 1998]
RB40.L4   1998
616.07'56—dc21
DNLM/DLC
for Library of Congress   97-43308
                        CIP

DISTRIBUTORS

 Marston Book Services Ltd
 PO Box 269
 Abingdon, Oxon OX14 4YN
 (Orders: Tel: 01235 465500
          Fax: 01235 465555)

USA
 Blackwell Science, Inc.
 Commerce Place
 350 Main Street
 Malden, MA 02148 5018
 (Orders: Tel: 800 759 6102
           781 388 8250
           Fax: 781 388 8255)

Canada
 Login Brothers Book Company
 324 Saulteaux Cresent
 Winnipeg, Manitoba R3J 3T2
 (Orders: Tel: 204 224-4068)

Australia
 Blackwell Science Pty Ltd
 54 University Street
 Carlton, Victoria 3053
 (Orders: Tel: 3 9347 0300
           Fax: 3 9347 5001)

Contents

Preface, vii

Abbreviations, viii

1 Requesting and Interpreting Tests, 1

2 Disturbances of Water, Sodium and Potassium Balance, 15

3 Acid–Base Balance and Oxygen Transport, 35

4 Renal Disease, 51

5 Disorders of Calcium, Phosphate and Magnesium Metabolism, 69

6 Abnormalities of Proteins in Plasma, 86

7 Plasma Enzyme Tests in Diagnosis, 101

8 Liver Disease, 110

9 Gastrointestinal Tract Disease, 124

10 Clinical Biochemical Measurements in Nutrition, 136

11 Disorders of Carbohydrate Metabolism, 149

12 Disorders of Plasma Lipids and Lipoproteins, 165

13 Disorders of Iron and Porphyrin Metabolism, 175

14 Disorders of Purine Metabolism, 186

15 Abnormalities of Thyroid Function, 191

16 Disorders of the Adrenal Cortex and Medulla, 205

17 Hypothalamic and Pituitary Hormones, 221

18 Gonadal Function, Steroid Contraceptives and Pregnancy, 230

19 Clinical Biochemistry in Paediatrics and Geriatrics, 246

20 Molecular Biology in Clinical Biochemistry, 263

21 Central Nervous System and Cerebrospinal Fluid, 282

22 Therapeutic Drug Monitoring and Chemical Toxicology, 284

Appendix A: Collection of Specimens, 295

Appendix B: Near-Patient Testing, 298

Appendix C: SI Units and 'Conventional' Units, 302

Reference Books and Further Reading, 305

Index, 307

Preface

Since the last edition of this book, our senior author, Professor Gordon Whitby, has retired and Dr Peter Rae has taken his place as co-author. However, our intended readership remains the same, namely medical students in the clinical phases of the medical curriculum and junior doctors. So far as the content is concerned, we have tried to reflect comments from our readers. We have also recognized the changes now being introduced into undergraduate medical curricula as a result of the recommendations from the General Medical Council.

All of the chapters have been revised and brought up to date to reflect current practice. In general, we have tried to emphasize those aspects of clinical biochemistry which may be regarded as being part of a core medical curriculum. As a result, those chapters which deal with common problems and with investigations that are used frequently have been slightly expanded. On the other hand, chapters dealing with less common disorders have been shortened.

In the last edition of this book, a limited number of case histories were introduced. This feature has been well-received and in this edition the number of cases has been increased.

Overall, our objectives have remained unchanged from those outlined in previous editions. They are to help our readers:

1 to acquire knowledge and understanding of the potential value and the limitations of commonly available chemical investigations, and to be able to ensure their reliable performance and proper interpretation;

2 to develop the ability to select chemical investigations that are appropriate to the diagnosis of disease and for the management of treatment in individual patients, and to be able to interpret the results of these investigations correctly;

3 to maintain a responsible and critical attitude in the use they make of the diagnostic services provided by clinical biochemistry and the other laboratory-based specialties.

In conclusion, first of all, we would like to thank Professor Whitby for the enormous amount of invaluable work which he put into all previous editions of this book. So far as this edition is concerned, we would like to thank Dr Jean Kirk for her help with the paediatric biochemistry section, Dr Danny Simpson for advice on Chapter 22, Dr Sadie Gow for advice on Chapter 18, Dr Cathy Sturgeon for advice on the tumour marker section, Dr Alison Avenell for her critical appraisal of some of the chapters and Dr Steven Morley for his helpful comments on Chapter 20.

Alistair F. Smith
Geoffrey J. Beckett
Simon W. Walker
Peter W. Rae

Abbreviations

The following list consists of abbreviations that are used frequently in this book. Abbreviations are also defined in each chapter when first used.

Concentrations are indicated by means of square brackets. For example, plasma [urea] means 'the concentration of urea in plasma'.

The following *atomic symbols* are used without further explanation in this book:

C	Carbon	K	Potassium
Ca	Calcium	N	Nitrogen
Cl	Chloride	Na	Sodium
Fe	Iron	O	Oxygen
H	Hydrogen	P	Phosphorus
I	Iodine	S	Sulphur

Units of measurement (examples)

Abbreviation	Molar concentration	Prefix to mole
mmol/L	10^{-3}	milli-
μmol/L	10^{-6}	micro-
nmol/L	10^{-9}	nano-
pmol/L	10^{-12}	pico-

The same applies to units of mass concentration (e.g. g/L, mg/L, etc.), international units (IU/L, mIU/L, etc.), and certain other units (e.g. U/L, mU/L, etc.).

A	angiotensin (AI–AIII)
ABP	androgen-binding protein
ACE	angiotensin-converting enzyme
ACTH	adrenocorticotrophic hormone
ADH	antidiuretic hormone
A&E	accident and emergency
AFP	α_1-fetoprotein
ALA	aminolaevulinic acid
ALP	alkaline phosphatase
ALT	alanine aminotransferase
AMP	adenosine monophosphate
ANP	atrial natriuretic peptide
API	α_1-protease inhibitor
apoB	apolipoprotein B
APRT	adenine phosphoribosyltransferase
ARMS	amplification-refractory mutation system
AST	aspartate aminotransferase
ATP	adenosine triphosphate
ATPase	adenosine triphosphatase
BAC	bacterial artificial chromosome
BMI	body mass index
BMR	basal metabolic rate
BT-PABA	N-benzoyl-L-tyrosyl p-aminobenzoic acid
CAH	congenital adrenal hyperplasia
cal	calorie
cAMP	cyclic adenosine monophosphate
CBG	cortisol-binding globulin
CCK-PZ	cholecystokinin-pancreozymin
cDNA	copy deoxyribonucleic acid
CDT	carbohydrate-deficient transferrin
CEA	carcinoembryonic antigen
CF	cystic fibrosis
ChE	cholinesterase
CK	creatine kinase
CNS	central nervous system
CoA	coenzyme A
COHb	carboxyhaemoglobin
CRH	corticotrophin-releasing hormone
CRP	C-reactive protein
CSF	cerebrospinal fluid

CT	computed tomography	HGPRT	hypoxanthine guanine phosphoribosyltransferase
Da	dalton (a measure of molecular mass)	5-HIAA	5-hydroxyindoleacetic acid
DDAVP	1-deamino-8-D-arginine vasopressin	HIV	human immunodeficiency virus
		HLA	human leucocyte antigen
DHCC	dihydrocholecalciferol	HMG-CoA	β-hydroxy-β-methylglutaryl-coenzyme A
DHAS	dehydroepiandrosterone sulphate	HMMA	4-hydroxy-3-methoxymandelic acid
DHT	dihydrotestosterone		
DIT	di-iodotyrosine	HPA	hypothalamic–pituitary–adrenal (axis)
DN	dibucaine number		
DNA	deoxyribonucleic acid	HPGRT	hypoxanthine-guanine phosphoribosyltransferase
DXM	dexamethasone		
ECF	extracellular fluid	hPL	human placental lactogen
ECG	electocardiography, electrocardiogram	HPLC	high-performance liquid chromatography
EcoRI	*Escherichia coli* restriction endonuclease I	HRT	hormone replacement therapy
		HSD	hydoxysteroid dehydrogenase
EDTA	ethylenediamine tetraacetic acid	5-HT	5-hydroxytryptamine
		5-HTP	5-hydroxytryptophan
ERCP	endoscopic retrograde cholangiopancreatography	HVA	homovanillic acid
		ICF	intracellular fluid
ESR	erythrocyte sedimentation rate	IDDM	insulin-dependent diabetes mellitus
FAD	flavin-adenine dinucleotide		
FHH	familial hypocalciuric hypercalcaemia	IDL	intermediate-density lipoproteins
FSH	follicle-stimulating hormone	Ig	immunoglobulin (the class is often specified, e.g. IgG, IgM)
g	gram		
Gal-1-PUT	galactose-1-phosphate uridylyltransferase	IRT	immunoreactive trypsin
		IU	international unit
GC-MS	gas chromatography–mass spectrometry	kb	kilobase (1000 nucleotide bases, in a nucleic acid or polynucleotide fragment)
GFR	glomerular filtration rate		
GGT	γ-glutamyltransferase	kcal	kilocalorie
GH	growth hormone	kDa	kilodalton
GI	gastrointestinal	kg	kilogram
GIP	glucose-dependent insulinotrophic peptide	kPa	kilopascal
		L	litre (the SI unit of volume in medicine)
Gn-RH	gonadotrophin-releasing hormone		
		LCAT	lecithin cholesterol acyltransferase
GTT	glucose tolerance test		
h	hour	LD	lactate dehydrogenase
Hb	haemoglobin	LDL	low-density lipoprotein
HCC	hydroxycholecalciferol	LH	luteinizing hormone
hCG	human chorionic gonadotrophin	LH-RH	luteinizing hormone-releasing hormone
HDL	high-density lipoprotein	β-LPH	β-lipotrophin

MCT	medullary carcinoma of the thyroid	PKU	phenylketonuria
MCV	mean cell volume	Po_2	the partial pressure of O_2 in the gas phase in equilibrium with O_2 (units kPa)
MEN	multiple endocrine neoplasia		
min	minute	PP	pyridoxal phosphate
MIT	mono-iodotyrosine	PRA	plasma renin activity
MMA	methylmalonic acid	PRPP	5-phosphoribosyl-1-pyrophosphate
mol. mass	molecular mass (see also M_r)		
M_r	relative molecular mass	PSA	prostate-specific antigen
MR	magnetic resonance	PTH	parathyroid hormone
MRI	magnetic resonance imaging	PTHrP	parathyroid hormone-related protein
mRNA	messenger ribonucleic acid		
MSAFP	maternal serum [α_1-fetoprotein]	q.i.d.	quater in die, four times daily
		RDS	respiratory distress syndrome
NABQI	N-acetyl-p-benzoquinoneimine	RFLP	restriction fragment length polymorphism
NAD	nicotinamide adenine dinucleotide		
		RNA	ribonucleic acid
NADH	reduced nicotinamide adenine dinucleotide	rT3	reverse tri-iodothyronine
		SD	standard deviation
NADP	nicotinamide adenine dinucleotide phosphate	SG	specific gravity
		SHBG	sex hormone-binding globulin
NIDDM	non–insulin-dependent diabetes mellitus	SI	Système Internationale
		SIADH	inappropriate secretion of antidiuretic hormone
NSE	neurone-specific enolase		
NTI	nonthyroidal illness	T3	tri-iodothyronine
17-OHP	17-hydroxyprogesterone	T4	thyroxine
Pa	pascal (the SI unit of pressure)	Taq	Thermus aquaticus
PABA	p-aminobenzoic acid	TBG	thyroxine-binding globulin
PBG	porphobilinogen	TIBC	total iron-binding capacity
Pco_2	the partial pressure of CO_2 in the gas phase in equilibrium with CO_2 dissolved in blood (units kPa)	TPN	total parenteral nutrition
		TPP	thiamin pyrophosphate
		TRAb	thyrotrophin-receptor antibody
		TRH	thyrotrophin-releasing hormone (thyroliberin)
PCOS	polycystic ovary syndrome		
PCR	polymerase chain reaction	TSH	thyroid-stimulating hormone (thyrotrophin)
PEM	protein-energy malnutrition		
PHP	pseudohypoparathyroidism	UDP	uridine 5′-pyrophosphate (formerly called uridine diphosphate, hence UDP)
pK_a	the logarithm to the base 10 of the reciprocal of the ionization constant of an acid in a buffer solution. The pK_a of an acid is equal to the pH at which the [acid] and [buffer] are equal, and is the pH at which the buffering power is greatest		
		U&E	Urea and electrolytes
		VLDL	very low density lipoprotein
		YAC	yeast artificial chromosome
		WHO	World Health Organization

CHAPTER 1

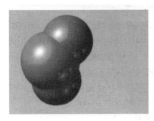

Requesting and Interpreting Tests

Introduction, 1
Requesting investigations, 1

Collection of specimens, 3
Near-patient testing, 3

Interpreting and using
   laboratory data, 3

Introduction

There can now be few patients admitted to hospital on whom no biochemical tests are performed. In general practice, there is also increasing use of such tests. Their selection, ordering and interpretation occupy a significant portion of the doctor's time, particularly that of the junior doctor.

In this first chapter, we set out some of the principles of requesting tests and of the interpretation of results. The effects of analytical errors and of physiological factors, as well as of disease, on test results are stressed. The role of biochemical testing in differential diagnosis and in screening is discussed.

Requesting investigations

There are two principal approaches to test requesting:

1 *Discretionary* or *selective* requesting, in which tests are requested on the basis of the patient's symptoms, signs and previous history (including results of investigations).

2 *Screening*, in which a predetermined set of tests is performed, even when there is not necessarily a clinical indication for them.

Discretionary requesting

The case for discretionary requesting has been put admirably (Asher, R. (1954) Straight and crooked thinking in medicine. *British Medical Journal,* **2,** 460–462.):

1 Why do I request this test?
2 What will I look for in the result?
3 If I find what I am looking for, will it affect my diagnosis?
4 How will this investigation affect my management of the patient?
5 Will this investigation ultimately benefit the patient?

In about 80% of patients presenting at surgeries or out-patient departments, a provisional diagnosis can be made after taking the history. The clinical examination, and possibly other tests such as 'side-room' tests on urine, may further clarify the diagnosis. Thereafter, tests may be requested on a logical basis:

• *To confirm a diagnosis*, e.g. plasma [free T4] and [TSH] in suspected hyperthyroidism.
• *To aid differential diagnosis*, e.g. to distinguish between different forms of jaundice.
• *To refine a diagnosis*, e.g. use of adreno-corticotrophic hormone (ACTH) to localize Cushing's syndrome (Chapter 16).
• *To assess the severity of disease*, e.g. plasma [urea] or [creatinine] in renal disease.
• *To monitor progress*, e.g. plasma [glucose] and [K+] to follow the treatment of patients with diabetic ketoacidosis.
• *To detect complications or side-effects*, e.g. aminotransferase measurements in patients being treated with hepatotoxic drugs.

• *To monitor therapy*, e.g. plasma drug concentrations in patients treated with anti-epileptic drugs.

Screening

Screening tests are generally investigations carried out without a clear clinical indication. Because of the low incidence of disease in the population being studied, false-positive results (see below) are common in relation to true-positive results.

Well-population screening

In this, tests are carried out on people from an apparently healthy population to try to detect presymptomatic or early disease. Programmes should only be initiated when:

• The disease is common or life-threatening.
• The tests used are sensitive and specific (p. 8), acceptable to the people to be screened, and able to be carried out in large numbers.
• Clinical, laboratory and other facilities are available for follow-up of abnormalities.
• Effective treatment is available.
• The financial aspects have been clarified and the implications accepted.

Only a few programmes of this nature have gained acceptance. *Case-finding programmes* are more selective and yield a higher proportion of useful results (Table 1.1).

Case-finding programmes

In these, appropriate tests are performed on a population sample known to be at high risk of a particular disease, e.g. blood [lead] in lead battery workers.

Screening of patients

Many laboratories analyse and report some tests as functional or organ-related groups. For example, a 'liver function test' group might consist of plasma bilirubin, alanine aminotransferase (ALT), alkaline phosphatase (ALP), γ-glutamyltransferase (GGT) and albumin measurements.

In other instances, to simplify requesting, a wide range of tests are routinely requested on all patients in a particular category, e.g. admission screening on all those admitted through the Accident and Emergency Department.

Medical advantages and disadvantages of screening

Advantages. Firstly, an uncommon or unexpected disease may be found and treated (Table 1.2). Secondly, the early requesting of a battery of tests might be expected to expedite man-

Table 1.1 Examples of tests used in case-finding programmes.

CASE-FINDING PROGRAMMES

Programmes to detect diseases in	Chemical investigations
Neonates	
Phenylketonuria	Serum [phenylalanine]
Hypothyroidism	Serum [TSH] and/or [thyroxine]
Adolescents and young adults	
Substance abuse	Drug screen
Pregnancy	
Diabetes mellitus in the mother	Plasma and urine [glucose]
Open neural tube defect in the fetus	Maternal serum [α-fetoprotein]
Industry	
Industrial exposure to lead	Blood [lead]
Industrial exposure to pesticides	Plasma cholinesterase activity
Elderly	
Malnutrition	Plasma [albumin] and/or [pre-albumin]
Thyroid dysfunction	Plasma [TSH] and/or [thyroxine]

SCREENING: UNEXPECTED TEST RESULTS	
Disease	Unexpected abnormal test result
Hyperparathyroidism	Raised plasma [calcium]
Hypothyroidism	Raised plasma [TSH] and/or a low [total T4] or [free T4]
Diabetes mellitus	High random plasma [glucose]
Renal tract disease	Raised plasma [creatinine] or [urea]
Liver disease	Increased plasma ALT, AST, GGT or ALP

Table 1.2 Advantages of screening in identifying unexpected test results.

agement of the patient. Most studies have not shown this to be so.

Disadvantages. It is easy to miss significant abnormalities in the 'flood' of data coming from the laboratory, even when the abnormalities are 'flagged' in some way. Most of the abnormalities detected will be of little or no significance, yet may need additional time-consuming and often expensive tests to clarify their importance (or lack of it).

Collection of specimens

Most quantitative chemical investigations are carried out on blood, less often on urine and other materials such as cerebrospinal fluid, intestinal secretions, faeces, calculi, sweat, amniotic fluid and fluids obtained by paracentesis, and occasionally saliva.

It is extremely important that the correct specimen is collected at the right time into an appropriate container. This is discussed in more detail in Appendix A.

Near-patient testing

An increasing number of chemical tests on blood can now be performed outside the main laboratory. Some use visual inspection of dipsticks, while others are performed on small analysers simple enough to be used by a wide range of staff in the ward or out-patient clinic.

Their use eliminates the need to send the specimen to the laboratory, and will usually allow a more rapid turnaround time. Thus, they are particularly suitable for use in intensive-care, high-dependency and accident and emergency units. Limited use of more specialized equipment may be of value in specialist clinics (e.g. glucose and HbA$_{1c}$ in a diabetic clinic). Simple analysers are used to a more limited extent in general practice surgeries. Near-patient testing is discussed in Appendix B.

Interpreting and using laboratory data

Most reports issued by clinical biochemistry laboratories contain numerical measures of concentration or activity, expressed in the appropriate units. The following questions should be considered when interpreting the results:

• Is each result normal or abnormal? Reference ranges (often incorrectly called normal ranges) are needed in order to answer questions about quantitative data.

• Does each result fit in with my previous assessment of this patient? If not, can I explain the discrepancy?

• Has a significant change occurred in any of the results from those previously reported?

• Do any of the results alter my diagnosis of this patient's illness or influence the way in which the illness should be managed?

• If I cannot explain a result, what do I propose to do about it?

This section discusses the interpretation of laboratory results and the factors that may cause them to vary, under the following main headings:

I *Analytical factors*. These cause errors in measurement.

2 *Biological and pathological factors*. Both these sets of factors affect the concentrations of analytes in blood, urine and other fluids sent for analysis.

Sources of variation in test results

Analytical sources of variation

Systematic and random variation
Analytical results are subject to error, no matter how good the laboratory and no matter how skilled the analyst. These errors may be due to lack of accuracy, i.e. always tend to be either high or low, or may be due to random effects and lack precision, i.e. may be unpredictably high or low.

Accuracy. An accurate method will, on average, yield results close to the true value of what is being measured. It has no systematic bias.

Precision. A precise method yields results that are close to one another (but not necessarily close to the true value) on repeated analysis. If multiple measurements are made on one specimen, the spread of results will be small for a precise method and large for an imprecise one.

The quantitative aspects of lack of precision, or imprecision, need to be considered in more detail. If a very large number of measurements of plasma [K^+] were to be made on a sample, by both an imprecise and a precise method, a histogram of the scatter of results would in each case show a normal (Gaussian) distribution, but with the results of the precise method being clustered more tightly about the mean, say, 3.6 mmol/L.

The standard deviation (SD) is the usual measure of scatter around a mean value. If the spread of results is wide, the SD is large, whereas if the spread is narrow, the SD is small. For data that have a Gaussian distribution, as is nearly always the case for analytical errors, the shape of the curve (Fig. 1.1) is completely defined by the mean and the SD, and these characteristics are such that:
- About 67% of results lie in the range mean ± 1 SD.
- About 95% of results lie in the range mean ± 2 SD.
- Over 99% of results lie in the range mean ± 3 SD.

Most clinical biochemistry laboratories

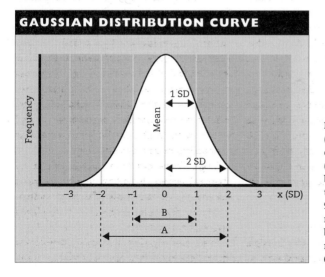

GAUSSIAN DISTRIBUTION CURVE

Fig. 1.1 Diagram of a Gaussian (normal or symmetrical) distribution curve. The span (A) of the curve, the distance between the mean −2 SD and the mean +2 SD, includes about 95% of the 'population'. The narrower span (B), the distance between the mean −1 SD and mean +1 SD, includes about 67% of the 'population'.

publish SD data for their analytical imprecision figures, thus allowing more ready interpretation of results. This allows clinicians to interpret the results as far as potential analytical errors are concerned.

Blunders

These are grossly inaccurate results that bear no constant or predictable relation to the true value. They arise, for instance, from mislabelling of specimens at the time of collection, or transcription errors when preparing or issuing reports.

If a very unexpected result is obtained from the laboratory, the doctor looking after the patient should always discuss the result with the laboratory immediately, so that laboratory staff can check whether a blunder has been made in the laboratory. Blunders, when they occur, may be due to the hitherto undetected interchange of two specimens, in which case the results for another patient may also be grossly in error.

Serial results in the same patient

Doctors often have to interpret two or more sets of results for the same analysis or group of analyses performed on different occasions on the same patient. If the results differ, this raises the following question: is the difference between two measurements of the same analyte significant? In other words, are such differences due to deterioration or improvement of a patient's condition, or could they be due mainly to laboratory imprecision? Without elaborating on the statistical aspects of this, the following rule may be applied: if the results for analyses performed on specimens collected on different occasions, but under otherwise identical conditions, differ by more than 2.8 times the analytical SD, it is very likely (i.e. there is a chance of over 95%) that a genuine change in concentration of the substance has occurred.

Biological causes of variation

We can only begin to consider the possible biological significance of results after their analytical significance has been assessed. The key questions now are:
- How do results vary in health?
- How do results vary in different diseases?

How do results vary in health?

The concentrations of all analytes in blood vary with time due to diverse physiological factors *within* the individual. There are also differences *between* individuals.

Within-individual variation

The following may be important causes of within-individual variation:
- *Diet*. Variations in diet can affect the results of many tests, including plasma [triglyceride], the response to glucose tolerance tests, urinary calcium excretion.
- *Time of day*. Several plasma constituents show diurnal variation (variation with the time of day), or a sleep/wake cycle. Examples include plasma iron, ACTH and cortisol concentrations.
- *Posture*. Proteins and all protein-bound constituents of plasma show significant differences in concentration between blood collected from upright individuals and blood from recumbent individuals. Examples include plasma calcium, cholesterol, cortisol and total thyroxine concentrations.
- *Muscular exercise*. Recent exercise, especially if vigorous or unaccustomed, may increase plasma creatine kinase activity and blood [lactate], and lower blood [pyruvate].
- *Menstrual cycle*. Several substances show variation with the phase of the cycle. Examples include plasma [iron], and the plasma concentrations of the pituitary gonadotrophins, ovarian steroids and their metabolites, as well as the amounts of these hormones and their metabolites excreted in the urine.
- *Drugs*. These can have marked effects on chemical results. Attention should be drawn particularly to the many effects of oestrogen containing oral contraceptives on plasma constituents (p. 239).

Even after allowing for known physiological factors that may affect plasma constituents and for analytical imprecision, there is still considerable residual individual variation (Table 1.3). The magnitude of this variation depends on the analyte, but it may be large and must be taken into account when interpreting successive values from a patient.

Between-individual variation

Differences between individuals can affect the concentrations of analytes in the blood. The following are the main examples:

- *Age.* Examples include plasma [phosphate] and alkaline phosphatase activity, and plasma and urinary concentrations of the gonadotrophins and sex hormones.
- *Sex.* Examples include plasma creatinine, iron, urate and urea concentrations and GGT activity, and plasma and urinary concentrations of the sex hormones.
- *Race.* Racial differences have been described for plasma [cholesterol] and [protein]. It may be difficult to distinguish racial from environmental factors, such as diet.

Reference ranges

When looking at results, we need to compare each result with a set of results from a particular defined (or reference) population. This reference range is determined, in practice, by measuring a set of reference values from a sample of that population, usually of healthy individuals. However, reference ranges can relate to any definable population (e.g. patients with myocardial infarction, or a previous set of results from the same individual – see below).

The nature of the reference population should be given whenever reference ranges are quoted, although a healthy population is usually assumed.

To interpret results in a particular patient, the most suitable reference ranges would be results for analyses obtained for that individual before becoming ill. For example, in a patient undergoing elective surgery, a preoperative set of values can be obtained, to compare with results obtained postoperatively. However, for most patients, baseline data obtained when they were healthy will not be available. Even age-matched and sex-matched reference ranges are often difficult to obtain, since fairly large numbers of individuals are needed. In practice, blood donors are very often selected as the most readily available reference population.

Distribution of results in reference population

When results of analyses for a reference population are analysed, they are invariably found to cluster round a central value, with a distribution that may be symmetrical (often Gaussian, Fig. 1.2a) or asymmetrical (often log-Gaussian, Fig. 1.2b). However, reference ranges can be calculated from these data without making any assumptions about the distribution of the data, using non-parametric methods.

Because of geographical, racial and other biological sources of variation between individuals, as well as differences in analytical methods, each laboratory should define and

WITHIN-INDIVIDUAL VARIATION OF PLASMA CONSTITUENTS

Plasma constituent	CV (%)	Plasma constituent	CV (%)
[Sodium]	1	ALT activity	25
[Calcium]	1–2	AST activity	25
[Potassium]	5	[Iron]	25
[Urea]	10		

CV: coefficient of variation.

Table 1.3 Residual individual variation of some plasma constituents (expressed as the approximated day-to-day, within-individual coefficient of variation).

PLASMA [Na⁺] AND GGT ACTIVITIES

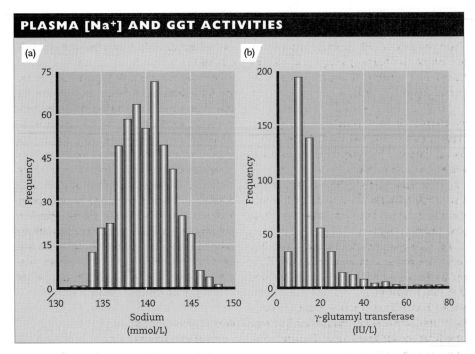

Fig. 1.2 Histograms showing the relative frequency with which results with the values indicated were obtained when plasma [Na+] and γ-glutamyltransferase (GGT) activities were measured in a reference population of healthy adult women. The sodium data are symmetrically distributed about the mean (a), whereas the GGT data show a log-Gaussian distribution (b).

publish its own reference ranges. Conventionally, these include the central 95% of the results obtained for each analysis from the reference population. This 95% figure is arbitrary, selected in order to minimize the overlap between results from diseased populations and from healthy individuals.

Analytical factors can affect the reference ranges for individual laboratories. If an *inaccurate* method is used, the reference range will reflect the method bias. If an *imprecise* method is used, the reference range will be widened, i.e. the observed span of results (reflected in the SD) will be greater. In statistical terms – the observed variance (i.e. the square of the SD) of the population results will equal the sum of the true or biological variance of the population plus the analytical variance of the method.

'Normal ranges'

The expression 'normal range' is commonly equated with the reference range. However, 'reference range' is more appropriate, since:

• As defined above, about 5% of results from healthy people will be outside the reference range – so the term 'normal range' is clearly inappropriate, since it implies that 5% of healthy people are not normal.

• The practice of relating the reference range to a defined reference population, without necessarily implying either health or disease, is a useful one.

Effect of disease on chemical results

Biochemical test results do not exist in isolation, since, by the time tests are requested, the doctor will often have made a provisional diagnosis and a list of differential diagnoses based on each patient's symptoms and signs.

For example, in a patient with severe abdominal pain, tenderness and rigidity, there may be several differential diagnoses to consider – including, for example, acute pancreatitis, perforated peptic ulcer and acute cholecystitis. In all three conditions, the plasma amylase activity may be raised, i.e. above the upper reference value for healthy adults. So healthy adult reference ranges (in this instance) are irrelevant, since healthy adults do not have abdominal pain, tenderness and rigidity! Instead, we need to know how the plasma amylase activity might vary in the clinically likely differential diagnoses. It would be useful to know, for instance, whether very high plasma amylase activities are associated with one of these diagnostic possibilities, but not with the other two.

To summarize, to interpret results on patients adequately, we need to know:

1 The reference range for healthy individuals of the appropriate age range and of the same sex.

2 The values to be expected (reference range) for patients with the disease, or diseases, under consideration.

3 The prevalence of the disease, or diseases, in the population to which the patient belongs.

The assessment of diagnostic tests

In evaluating and interpreting a test, it is necessary to know how it behaves in health and disease. We shall use the following terms:

1 *Sensitivity (true-positive rate)*. This is the incidence (percentage) of positive results for a test in patients with the particular disease. A test which is always abnormal (or positive) in patients with the disease has 100% sensitivity.

2 *False-positive rate*. This is the incidence (percentage) of positive results in people known or subsequently proved to be free from the particular disease. If a test is always normal in individuals who do not have the disease, that test has a false-positive rate of 0%. The term *specificity* (100% minus the percentage false-

positive rate) is often used in the same context as false-positive rate.

3 The *predictive value of a positive test result*. This is the percentage of positive results that are true positives (i.e. the patient has the condition) when a test is performed on a defined population containing both healthy and diseased individuals. It must be stressed that this measure is critically dependent on the incidence of the disease in this defined population (see below).

The ideal test is 100% sensitive and has a 0% false-positive rate (100% specificity), shown diagrammatically in Fig. 1.3a. This ideal is rarely achieved; there is usually overlap between the healthy and diseased populations (Fig. 1.3b). In practice, we have to decide where to draw dividing lines that most effectively separate 'healthy' from 'diseased' groups, or disease A from disease B. We can illustrate this by means of the following hypothetical example.

Suppose that we wish to distinguish patients with acute myocardial infarction from those with other causes of acute chest pain. In blood taken 24 h after the onset of pain, we know that plasma creatine kinase (CK) activity is *usually* raised in patients who have had a myocardial infarction, and that it is *sometimes* raised in patients with other causes of chest pain. The overlap is illustrated in Fig. 1.4, which we assume portrays results obtained from a study of very large numbers of patients in both categories.

To identify *every* patient with myocardial infarction, we must take a *low* cut-off figure for plasma CK activity (say, 200 IU/L). The test is then 100% sensitive, but the false-positive rate is unacceptably high, since only about 70% of patients without infarction are correctly classified by the test. If, on the other hand, we wish to identify *only* patients who have had a myocardial infarct and exclude all those without an infarct, then a *high* cut-off must be selected, at a plasma CK activity of about 450 IU/L. The false-positive rate is now 0%, but the sensitivity has suffered, since only about 75% of patients with myocardial infarction have been identified with this higher cut-off figure.

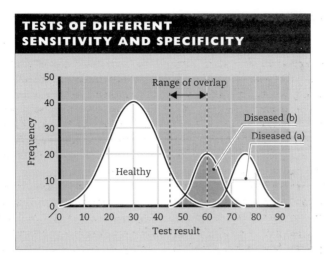

Fig. 1.3 Diagrammatic representations of the distributions of results obtained with a test (a) that completely separates healthy people from people with a disease without any overlap between the distribution curves (i.e. an ideal test with 100% sensitivity and 100% specificity), and a test (b) that is less sensitive and less specific, in which there is an area of overlap between the distribution curves for healthy people and people with disease.

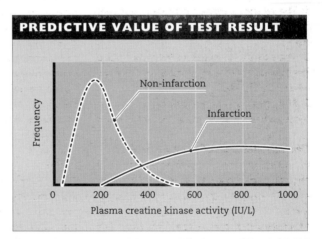

Fig. 1.4 The predictive value of a positive (abnormal) result for a diagnostic test. The text describes the implications for the sensitivity, specificity and predictive value of an abnormal result of setting the cut-off value for abnormality at 200 IU/L and at 450 IU/L.

These two extremes show that it is usually possible to increase the sensitivity of a test, but only at the expense of a high false-positive rate. Conversely, the false-positive rate can be decreased, but only at the expense of a loss of sensitivity.

In practice, the bias towards sensitivity, or a low rate of false positives, will depend on clinical objectives. For example, if all patients with myocardial infarction are to be admitted to a coronary care unit, a low cut-off figure is desirable to maximize sensitivity. The 'price' of this decision will be that more patients without myocardial infarction will also be admitted to the unit, thereby incurring additional expense and, very possibly, straining the specialist facilities unnecessarily and unacceptably.

Disease prevalence

Before discussing the effect of disease prevalence on diagnostic decision-making, predictive values need to be considered further. These are defined as follows:

$$\frac{\text{Predictive value of}}{\text{a positive test result}} = \frac{\text{True positives}}{\text{All positives}} \times 100$$

$$\frac{\text{Predictive value of}}{\text{a negative test result}} = \frac{\text{True negatives}}{\text{All negatives}} \times 100$$

Predictive values are arrived at most easily if a table is constructed (Table 1.4). In practice, predictive values are very important diagnostically, since they give the *probability* that an abnormal result being interpreted by a doctor comes from someone with disease.

Knowledge of the sensitivity and of the false-positive rate, combined with clinical considerations, can affect the cut-off values for any test. Decisions about cut-off values are also crucially dependent on the prevalence of the disease in question, since this will affect the predictive value of the test. To illustrate this point, we shall again use the example of plasma CK activity measurements in the diagnosis of myocardial infarction in two diagnostic circumstances:

Coronary care unit, where the incidence of myocardial infarction is high, i.e. about half the patients admitted to the unit. We shall also assume that 2000 patients have been admitted and that a cut-off plasma CK activity value of 350 IU/L has been selected, giving (for illustrative purposes) a sensitivity of 95 % and a false-positive rate of approximately 10 %. As expected (Table 1.5), most of the abnormal results come from patients with myocardial infarction, and most of the negative results from patients without myocardial infarction – the test seems to perform adequately.

General medical ward, where we can assume only that about 5 % of admissions with chest pain are due to myocardial infarction. The same sensitivity, false-positive rate and cut-off value (350 IU/L) are assumed. Table 1.6 shows that an abnormal test result, *after changing only the prevalence of the disease*, is now twice as likely to be associated with the absence as with the presence of myocardial infarction. Thus, in this instance, the predictive value of a positive result for the test is less in the general medical unit than in the coronary care unit.

In other words, in the general medical ward, plasma CK measurements by themselves are of relatively little diagnostic value for identifying

Table 1.4 The predictive value of the results of analyses.

PREDICTIVE VALUES: CALCULATION

Diagnostic category	Positive results	Negative results	Totals
Disease present	True positives (TP)	False negatives (FN)	Numbers with disease (TP + FN)
Disease absent	False positives (FP)	True negatives (TN)	Numbers without disease (TN + FP)
Totals	Total positives (TP + FP)	Total negatives (TN + FN)	Total numbers studied (TP + FP + TN + FN)
Predictive value of a positive result	TP/(TP + FP) (times 100 for %)		
Predictive value of a negative result		TN/(TN + FN) (times 100 for %)	

PLASMA CREATINE KINASE ACTIVITY IN CORONARY CARE UNIT

Diagnostic category	Positive results (>350 IU/L)	Negative results (<350 IU/L)	Totals
Infarct confirmed	950	50	1000
No infarct	100	900	1000
Totals	1050	950	2000
Predictive value of a positive result	950/1050 × 100 = 90.5 %		
Predictive value of a negative result		900/950 × 100 = 94.7 %	

Assumptions: sensitivity 95 %, false positive rate 10 % (specificity 90 %), prevalence of myocardial infarction 50 %. The data relate to 2000 patients.

Table 1.5 A hypothetical set of results for plasma creatine kinase activity measurements in patients admitted to a coronary care unit with chest pain.

PLASMA CREATINE KINASE ACTIVITY IN GENERAL MEDICAL UNIT

Diagnostic category	Positive results (>350 IU/L)	Negative results (<350 IU/L)	Totals
Infarct confirmed	95	5	100
No infarct	190	1710	1900
Totals	285	1715	2000
Predictive value of a positive result	95/285 × 100 = 33.3 %		
Predictive value of a negative result		1710/1715 × 100 = 99.7 %	

Assumptions: sensitivity 95 %, false positive rate 10 % (specificity 90 %), prevalence of myocardial infarction 5 %. The data relate to 2000 patients.

Table 1.6 A hypothetical set of results for plasma creatine kinase activity measurements in patients admitted to a general medical unit with chest pain.

patients who have had a myocardial infarction. If the test is to be used for this purpose, the cut-off value should probably be increased so that the test is less sensitive but gives rise to fewer false positives.

Screening for rare diseases

The interpretation to be placed on a positive result for a test depends heavily on the prevalence of the disease for which that test is being used. For diseases that are rare, tests of extremely high sensitivity and specificity are required. To illustrate this, consider an inherited metabolic disorder with an incidence of 1 : 5000; this is similar to that of some of the commoner, treatable, inherited metabolic diseases such as phenylketonuria or congenital hypothyroidism (Table 19.2, p. 248). Assume that we

SCREENING TEST IN NEONATES

Diagnostic category	Positive results	Negative results	Totals
Disease present	199	1	200
Disease absent	4999	994 801	999 800
Totals	5198	994 802	1 000 000
Predictive value	3.8 %	100 %	

Assumptions: Sensitivity of the test 99.5 %, false positive rate 0.5 % (specificity 99.5 %), prevalence of the disorder, 1 : 5000; 1 000 000 neonates screened.

Note that the prevalence of phenylketonuria and of hypothyroidism in the UK are about 1 : 5000 live births (Table 19.2, p. 248), and that about 800 000 neonates in the UK are screened annually.

Table 1.7 A hypothetical set of results of a screening test for a relatively common inherited metabolic disorder in neonates.

have a test with a good performance, i.e. a sensitivity of 99.5 % and a false-positive rate of 0.5 % (Table 1.7).

Table 1.7 shows that, for every neonate affected by the disorder who has a positive test result, there will be about 25 (4999/199) neonates who also have a positive test but who do not have the disease. Two important points emerge:
• Tests with very high sensitivity and with very low false-positive rates are required when screening for rare disorders.
• A heavy investigative load will result from the screening programme, since all the false positives will have to be followed up to determine whether or not they indicate the presence of disease.

The traditional 95 % reference range (see above) is not relevant to screening for rare conditions, since the rate of false positives would be far too high. The cut-off value has to be altered to decrease the false-positive rate, at the probable expense of missing some patients who have the condition for which screening is being carried out.

Audit

Audit is the process whereby the procedures involved in patient care are monitored in order to give high priority to the delivery of an efficient and cost-effective service. The measure of health outcome is benefit to the patient.

The value of audit can most readily be seen in those specialties concerned directly with patient care, but the principles are applicable to all clinical and investigational specialties (e.g. radiology), as well as laboratory-based specialties such as clinical biochemistry.

The audit process

There is an essential sequence to auditing activities (Fig. 1.5):
• Identify an area of concern or interest, particularly if it is felt that there is room for improvement in the service, or if the same quality of service can be provided more economically.
• Review and analyse the present procedures.
• Identify specific aspects that might be capable of improvement.
• Identify alternative procedures or standards that might lead to improvement.
• Take the practical steps necessary to implement any changes proposed.
• Compare the performance after the changes with those before them.
• It must be emphasized that the final stage of analysis of the effects of any change is an integral part of the audit process; it is essential to know whether the measures taken have improved the service or made it more cost-

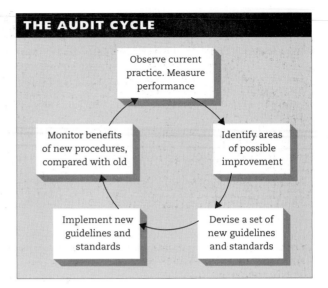

THE AUDIT CYCLE

Observe current practice. Measure performance

Identify areas of possible improvement

Devise a set of new guidelines and standards

Implement new guidelines and standards

Monitor benefits of new procedures, compared with old

Fig. 1.5 The audit cycle.

effective. Sometimes, changes have no effect, or even adverse effects.

Audit in clinical biochemistry

Laboratories monitor their performance:
- Internally, by day-to-day within-laboratory checks on the accuracy and precision of all assays.
- Externally, by participation in national and international quality assurance schemes.

Factors other than accuracy and precision are also monitored:

Test requesting, specimen collection and transport. Is advice about the selection of suitable tests available? Are request forms easy to use? Are appropriate containers for specimens readily available? Is the specimen transport system convenient, rapid and efficient? Is there a phlebotomy service, and if so, how effective is it?

Analytical aspects of the service. Are there too many grossly inaccurate results (blunders) due, for example, to transcription errors? Is the test repertoire appropriate? Are tests being offered that are now out of date and due to be replaced?

Reporting and interpretation. Are reports getting to the right place at the right time (or

should near-patient testing be considered)? Are handbooks, details of protocols and reference ranges readily available to service users? Are comments on reports adequate and helpful? Is expert advice on the selection and interpretation of results always readily available?

Emergency service. Is this being provided in the most cost-effective manner?

Clinical guidelines. Is there a case for introducing standardized clinical guidelines for the investigation and treatment of well-defined clinical conditions? Such guidelines would define the appropriate investigations, and their timing, in relation to patients with, for example, myocardial infarction, liver disease, thyroid disease, the acute abdomen, etc.

Education and research. Are users of the diagnostic service being educated in the proper use of laboratory facilities? Is the laboratory playing its part in fulfilling a more general educative role in the hospital and the community? Is there appropriate investment in research and development?

To an increasing extent, laboratories are required to satisfy certain standards in meeting the above requirements, and achievement of the standards is recognized through accreditation by an external body.

KEY POINTS

1 As a rule, only those tests that may contribute to diagnosis and management of patients should be requested.

2 Population screening is indicated where reliable tests are able to detect important and treatable disease; case-finding screening is valuable in groups at high risk of a specific disorder.

3 There is an overlap between test results obtained in health and those obtained in disease or (where the test is being used for screening) results from affected individuals.

4 Effective tests reduce this overlap to a minimum, but there will always be a trade-off between maximizing the sensitivity of a test, i.e. detecting as many affected individuals as possible, and maximizing its specificity, i.e. minimizing the number of non-affected individuals classified as abnormal by the test.

5 Strategies to maximize a test's value depend both on the test itself and on the prevalence of the disease in the population being studied.

Case 1.1

The resident on a surgical ward was called by the nursing staff to examine a patient whose condition was thought to have deteriorated two days after a hemicolectomy. The doctor obtained a specimen of venous blood and requested plasma urea and electrolyte measurements as an emergency. The results (column B), together with those for the same analyses on a specimen collected the previous day (column A), were as follows:

Analysis	A (mmol/L)	B (mmol/L)	Reference range (mmol/L)
[Urea]	8.5	1.8	2.5–6.6
[Na+]	131	144	132–144
[K+]	3.2	1.4	3.3–4.7
[Total CO$_2$]	24	10	24–30

What is the likely explanation for these changes? What should the resident do next?

Comments on Case 1.1

The results in column B are typical of those reported when a blood specimen has been obtained from a site close to where an intravenous infusion of 0.9 % NaCl (150 mmol/L) is being given. The analysis should be repeated on a fresh blood specimen. When the plasma analyses were repeated in this patient, the results were as follows (data in mmol/L): [urea] 9.0; [Na+] 130; [K+] 3.4; [total CO$_2$], 22.

CHAPTER 2

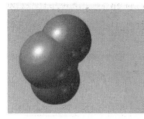

Disturbances of Water, Sodium and Potassium Balance

Water and sodium balance, 15
Disorders of water and sodium
  homeostasis, 19
Other chemical investigations
  in fluid balance disorders, 24

Potassium balance, 26
Abnormalities of plasma
  potassium concentration, 26
Other investigations in
  disordered K+ metabolism, 30

Fluid and electrolyte balance
  in surgical patients, 30
Metabolic response to
  trauma, 30

Fluid loss, retention or redistribution are common clinical problems in many areas of clinical practice. The management of these conditions is often urgent, and requires a rapid assessment of the history and examination, and of biochemical and other investigations.

In this chapter we consider:

- The distribution of water, Na+ and K+ in the different fluid compartments of the body, and its control by hormonal and other factors.
- Clinical effects and management of different types of loss, retention or redistribution of fluid.
- Causes and investigation of hypernatraemia and hyponatraemia.
- Causes and investigation of hyperkalaemia and hypokalaemia.
- Fluid and electrolyte problems in surgical patients, and the metabolic response to trauma.

Water and sodium balance

In considering the balance of any substance, both the internal and external balance of the substance must be borne in mind. The internal balance relates to the distribution between different body compartments, while the external balance matches input with output.

The movements of Na+ and water that occur all the time between plasma and glomerular filtrate, or between plasma and gastrointestinal (GI) secretions, provide the potential for large losses, with serious and rapid alterations in internal balance. For example, about 25 000 mmol Na+ are filtered at the glomerulus over 24 hours, normally with subsequent reabsorption of more than 99%. Likewise, 1000 mmol Na+ enter the GI tract in various secretions each day, but less than 0.5% (5 mmol) is normally lost in the faeces.

Internal distribution of water and sodium

In a 70 kg adult, the total body water is about 42 L – about 28 L of intracellular fluid (ICF) and 14 L of extracellular fluid (ECF) water. The ECF water is distributed as 3 L plasma water and 11 L interstitial water. The total body Na+ is about 4200 mmol – about 50% in the ECF, 40% in bone, and 10% in the ICF. Thus, Na+ is mainly extracellular.

Two important factors influence the distribution of fluid between the ICF and the intravascular and extravascular compartments of the ECF:

Osmolality. This affects the movement of water across cell membranes.

Colloid osmotic pressure. Together with hydrodynamic factors, this affects the movement of water and low molecular mass solutes (predominantly NaCl) between the intravascular and extravascular compartments.

Osmolality, osmolarity and tonicity

The *osmolality* is the number of solute particles per unit weight of water, irrespective of the size or nature of the particles. Therefore, on a weight basis, low molecular weight solutes contribute much more to the osmolality than high molecular weight solutes. The units are mmol/kg of water. This determines the osmotic pressure exerted by a solution across a membrane. Most laboratories can measure plasma osmolality directly, but it is also possible to calculate the approximate osmolality of plasma using the following formula (all concentrations must be in mmol/L):

Calculated osmolality :

$$= 2[Na^+] + 2[K^+] + [glucose] + [urea]$$

This formula includes all the low molecular weight solutes contributing to plasma osmolality. Values for Na^+ and K^+ are doubled so as to allow for their associated anions. The formula is approximate and is not a complete substitute for direct measurement. Calculated osmolality is usually close to measured osmolality, but the two may differ considerably when there are gross increases in plasma protein or lipid concentrations, both of which decrease the plasma water per unit volume. They also differ considerably when large amounts of unmeasured low molecular mass solutes (e.g. ethanol) are present in plasma.

The osmolality of urine is usually measured directly, but is also linearly related to its specific gravity (SG), unless there are significant amounts of glucose, protein or X-ray contrast media present.

Osmolarity is the number of particles of solute per litre of solution. Its units are mmol/L. Its measurement or calculation has been largely replaced by osmolality.

Tonicity is a term often used interchangeably with osmolality. However, it should only be used in relation to the osmotic pressure due to those solutes (e.g. Na^+) that exert their effects across cell membranes, thereby causing movement of water into or out of the cells. Substances that can readily diffuse into cells down their concentration gradients (e.g. urea, alcohol) contribute to plasma osmolality but not to plasma tonicity, since after equilibration their concentration will be equal on both sides of the cell membrane. Tonicity is not readily measurable.

The tonicity of ICF and ECF equilibrate with one another by movement of water across cell membranes. An increase in ECF tonicity causes a reduction in ICF volume as water moves from the ICF to the ECF to equalize the tonicity of the two compartments, whereas a decrease in ECF tonicity causes an increase in ICF volume as water moves from the ECF to the ICF.

Colloid osmotic pressure (oncotic pressure)

The osmotic pressure exerted by plasma proteins across cell membranes is negligible compared with the osmotic pressure of a solution containing NaCl and other small molecules, since they are present in much lower molar concentrations. However, although small molecules diffuse freely across the capillary wall, and so are not osmotically active at this site, plasma proteins do not readily do so. This means that plasma [protein] and hydrodynamic factors together determine the distribution of water and solutes across the capillary wall, and hence between the intravascular and interstitial compartments (Fig. 2.1).

Regulation of external water balance

Typical intakes and outputs of water are given in Table 2.1.

Water intake is normally controlled by the sensation of thirst, and its output by the action of vasopressin, also known as antidiuretic hormone (ADH). In states of pure water deficiency, plasma tonicity increases, causing a sensation of thirst and stimulating vasopressin secretion, both mediated by hypothalamic osmoreceptors. Vasopressin then promotes water reabsorption in the distal nephron, with consequent production of small volumes of concentrated urine. Conversely, a large intake of water causes a fall in tonicity, suppresses

WATER AND SOLUTE MOVEMENT

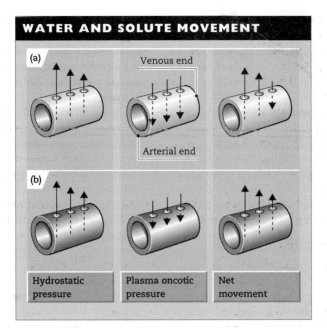

Fig. 2.1 Movements of water and low molecular mass solutes across the capillary wall when the plasma [protein] concentration is (a) normal and (b) low. The effects shown are: hydrostatic pressure, which drives water and low molecular mass solutes *outwards* and decreases along the length of the capillary; and plasma oncotic pressure, which attracts water and low molecular mass solutes *inwards* and is constant along the length of the capillary. The net movement of water and low molecular mass solutes across the capillary wall is governed by the net effect of hydrostatic and plasma oncotic pressures.

WATER INTAKE AND OUTPUT

Intake of water	mL	Output of water	mL
Water drunk	1500	Urine volume	1500
Water in food	750	Water content of faeces	50
Water from metabolism of food	250	Losses in expired air and insensible perspiration	950
Total	2500	Total	2500

Table 2.1 Average daily water intake and output of a normal adult in the United Kingdom.

thirst and reduces vasopressin secretion, leading to a diuresis, producing large volumes of dilute urine.

Secretion of vasopressin is normally controlled by small changes in ECF tonicity, but it is also under tonic inhibitory control from baroreceptors in the left atrium and great vessels on the left side of the heart. Where haemodynamic factors (e.g. excessive blood loss, heart failure) reduce the stretch on these receptors, often without an accompanying change in ECF tonicity, a reduction in tonic inhibitory control stimulates vasopressin secretion. The resulting water retention causes hyponatraemia and is relatively ineffective in expanding the intravascular compartment, since water diffuses freely throughout all compartments (Fig. 2.2).

Regulation of external sodium balance

Dietary intakes of Na^+ (and Cl^-) are very variable world-wide, but are usually closely matched by their corresponding urinary losses. There is normally little loss of these ions through the skin or in the faeces. A typical 'Western' diet provides 100–200 mmol of both Na^+ and Cl^- daily.

The amount of Na^+ excreted in the urine controls the ECF volume since, when osmoregulation is normal, the amount of extracellular water is maintained in a constant quantitative ratio to the amount of extracellular Na^+. At least four mechanisms are probably important regulators of Na^+ excretion:

The renin–angiotensin–aldosterone system. Renin is secreted in response to a fall in renal afferent arteriolar pressure or to a reduction in supply of Na^+ to the distal tubule. It converts angiotensinogen in plasma to angiotensin I (AI), which in turn is converted to angiotensin II (AII) by angiotensin-converting enzyme (ACE). Both AII and its metabolic product angiotensin III (AIII) are pharmacologically active, and stimulate the release of aldosterone from the adrenal cortex. Aldosterone acts on the distal tubule

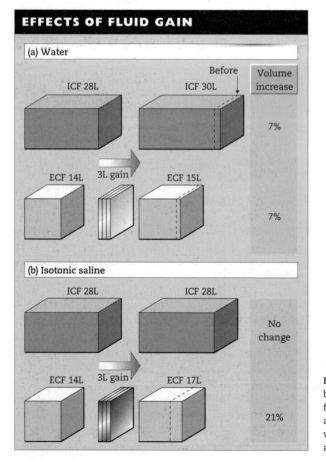

EFFECTS OF FLUID GAIN

(a) Water

Before | Volume increase

ICF 28L   ICF 30L

7%

ECF 14L   3L gain   ECF 15L

7%

(b) Isotonic saline

ICF 28L   ICF 28L

No change

ECF 14L   3L gain   ECF 17L

21%

Fig. 2.2 Different effects on the body's fluid compartments of fluid gains of 3 L of (a) water and (b) isotonic saline. The volumes shown relate to a 70 kg adult.

to promote Na+ reabsorption in exchange for urinary loss of H+ or K+. Since Na+ cannot enter cells freely, its retention (with iso-osmotically associated water) contributes solely to ECF volume expansion, unlike pure water retention (Figs 2.2 and 2.3). Although the renin–angiotensin–aldosterone system causes relatively slow responses to Na+ deprivation or Na+ loading, evidence suggests that this is the main regulatory mechanism for Na+ excretion.

The glomerular filtration rate (GFR). The rate of Na+ excretion is often related to the GFR. When the GFR falls acutely, less Na+ is excreted, and vice versa.

Atrial natriuretic peptide (ANP). Several similar peptides in the atrium of the heart promote Na+ excretion by the kidney, apparently by causing a marked increase in GFR. The importance of the ANP regulatory mechanism is not yet clear.

Dopamine. An increase in filtered Na+ load causes increased dopamine synthesis by proximal tubule cells. The dopamine then acts on the distal tubule to stimulate Na+ excretion.

Disorders of water and sodium homeostasis

Whereas losses or gains of pure water are distributed across all fluid compartments, losses or gains of Na+ and water, as isotonic fluid, are borne by the much smaller ECF compartment (Figs 2.2 and 2.3). Thus, it is usually more urgent to replace losses of isotonic fluid than losses of

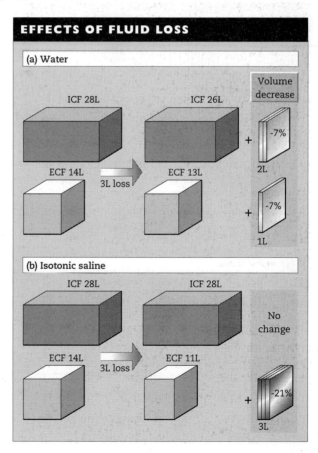

EFFECTS OF FLUID LOSS

(a) Water

ICF 28L   ICF 26L   Volume decrease

ECF 14L   ECF 13L   3L loss   +   -7%   2L

+   -7%   1L

(b) Isotonic saline

ICF 28L   ICF 28L

ECF 14L   ECF 11L   3L loss   No change

+   -21%   3L

Fig. 2.3 Different effects on the body's fluid compartments of fluid losses of 3 L of (a) water and (b) isotonic saline. The volumes shown relate to a 70 kg adult.

water. For the same reason, circulatory overload is more likely with excessive administration of isotonic Na+-containing solutions than with isotonic dextrose (the dextrose is metabolized, leaving water behind).

Plasma [Na+] cannot be used as a simple measure of body Na+ status (Fig. 2.2), since it is very often abnormal as a result of losses or gains of water rather than of Na+. The plasma [Na+] must be interpreted in relation to the patient's history and the findings on clinical examination, and if necessary backed up by other investigations.

The main causes of depletion and excess of water are summarized in Table 2.2, and of Na+

Table 2.2 Causes of depletion and of excess of water.

DEPLETION AND EXCESS OF WATER	
Categories	Examples
Depletion of water	
Inadequate intake	Infants, patients in coma or who are very sick, or have symptoms such as nausea or dysphagia
Abnormal losses via	
Lungs	Inadequate humidification in mechanical ventilation
Skin	Fevers and in hot climates
Renal tract	Diabetes insipidus, lithium therapy
Excess of water	
Excessive intake	
Oral	Psychogenic polydipsia
Parenteral	Hypotonic infusions after operations
Renal retention	Excess of vasopressin (SIADH, Table 2.5), hypoadrenalism, hypothyroidism

DEPLETION AND EXCESS OF SODIUM	
Categories	Examples
Depletion of sodium	
Inadequate oral intake	Rare, by itself
Abnormal losses via	
Skin	Excessive sweating, dermatitis, burns
GI tract	Vomiting, aspiration, diarrhoea, fistula, paralytic ileus, blood loss
Renal tract	Osmotic diuresis, diuretic therapy, renal tubular disease, mineralocorticoid deficiency
Excess of sodium	
Excessive intake	
Oral	Sea water (drowning), salt tablets, hypertonic NaCl administration (this is rare)
Parenteral	Post-operatively, infusion of hypertonic NaCl
Renal retention	Acute and chronic renal failure, primary and secondary hyperaldosteronism, Cushing's syndrome

Table 2.3 Causes of depletion and of excess of sodium.

in Table 2.3. Although some of these conditions may be associated with abnormal plasma [Na⁺], it must be emphasized that this is not necessarily the case. For example, patients with acute losses of isotonic fluid (e.g. plasma, ECF, blood) may be severely and dangerously hypovolaemic and Na⁺-depleted, and very possibly in shock, but their plasma [Na⁺] may nevertheless be normal or even raised.

Hyponatraemia

Most patients with hyponatraemia also have a low plasma osmolality (reference range 280–290 mmol/kg). Unless an unusual cause of hyponatraemia is suspected (see 'Other causes of hyponatraemia', p. 23), measurement of plasma osmolality contributes little or no extra information.

Patients with hyponatraemia can be divided into three categories, on the basis of the ECF volume being low, normal or increased. These categories in turn reflect a total body Na⁺ that is low, normal or increased, respectively. The value of this classification is twofold. Firstly, the clinical history and examination often indicate the ECF volume and therefore the total body Na⁺ status. Secondly, treatment often depends on the total body Na⁺ status rather than the [Na⁺].

Hyponatraemia with low ECF volume (Table 2.4)

The patient has lost Na⁺ and water in one or more body fluids (e.g. GI tract secretions, urine, inflammatory exudate). This leads to tachycardia, orthostatic hypotension, reduced skin turgor and oliguria. The hypovolaemia causes secondary aldosteronism with a low urinary [Na⁺] (usually less than 20 mmol/L) and a 'volume stimulus' to vasopressin secretion, resulting in oliguria and a concentrated urine.

Table 2.4 Causes of hyponatraemia.

HYPONATRAEMIA

ECF volume	Categories	Examples
Decreased total body Na⁺ (loss of Na⁺ > H₂O)		
Extrarenal losses of Na⁺ (urine [Na⁺] < 20 mmol/L)	GI tract	Vomiting, diarrhoea
	Skin	Burns, severe dermatitis
	'Internal'	Paralytic ileus, peritoneal fluid
Renal losses of Na⁺ (urine [Na⁺] > 20 mmol/L)	Diuretics	
	Kidneys	Renal tubular acidosis
	Adrenals	Mineralocorticoid deficiency
Normal or near-normal total body Na⁺	Acute conditions	Parenteral administration of water, after surgery or trauma, or during or after delivery
	Chronic conditions	
	Antidiuretic drugs	Opiates, chlorpropamide
	Kidneys	Chronic renal failure
	Adrenals	Glucocorticoid deficiency
	Vasopressin excess	SIADH (Table 2.5)
	Osmoregulator	Low setting in carcinomatosis
Increased total body Na⁺	Acute conditions	Acute renal failure
	Chronic conditions	Oedematous states (p. 23)

The consequent water retention contributes to the hyponatraemia.

Treatment requires administration of isotonic saline and volume expanders (e.g. albumin, dextran) if there is hypotension.

Hyponatraemia with normal ECF volume (Table 2.4)

The hyponatraemia results from excessive water retention, due to inability to excrete a water load. This may develop acutely, or it may be chronic.

Acute water retention. Plasma [vasopressin] is acutely increased after trauma or major surgery, as part of the metabolic response to trauma, and during delivery and postpartum. Administration of excessive amounts of water (e.g. as 5% dextrose) in these circumstances may exacerbate the hyponatraemia and cause acute water intoxication (p. 30).

Chronic water retention. Perhaps the most widely known chronic 'cause' of this form of hyponatraemia is the syndrome of inappropriate secretion of ADH (SIADH) (Table 2.5). Whether this concept is of value in understanding its aetiology, or valid in terms of altered physiology, is uncertain. As the name implies, ADH (or rather vasopressin) is being secreted in the absence of an 'appropriate' physiological stimulus, of either hypernatraemia or fluid depletion. As water

Table 2.5 The syndrome of inappropriate secretion of ADH (SIADH).

is retained, the potential for expansion of the ECF volume is limited by a reduction in renin and an increase in sodium excretion. A new steady state is achieved, with essentially normal, or only mildly increased, ECF volume. If the causative disorder (Table 2.5) is transient, plasma [Na^+] returns to normal when the primary disorder (e.g. pneumonia) is treated. However, in patients with cancer, the hyponatraemia is presumably due to production of vasopressin or a related substance by the tumour, and is usually persistent. If symptoms are mild, they may be treated by severe fluid restriction (i.e. 500 mL/day or less), but if this is ineffective, treatment with a drug that antagonizes the renal effects of vasopressin (e.g. lithium carbonate, demeclocycline) may be tried.

Other causes of chronic retention of water include:

Chronic renal disease. Damaged kidneys may be unable to concentrate or to dilute urine normally, tending to produce a urine of osmolality 300 mmol/kg (i.e. about that of plasma). Thus, the ability to excrete a water load is severely impaired, and excess water intake (oral or intravenous) readily produces a dilutional hyponatraemia. These patients may also be overloaded with Na^+ (p. 23).

Glucocorticoid deficiency. Whether due to anterior pituitary disease or abrupt withdrawal of long-term glucocorticoid therapy, this may lead to inability to excrete a water load, and to hyponatraemia.

SIADH	
Characteristics of the syndrome	Causes (and examples)
Low plasma [Na^+] and osmolality	Malignant disease of the bronchus, prostate, pancreas, etc.
Inappropriately high urine osmolality	Chest diseases, e.g. pneumonia, bronchitis, tuberculosis
Excessive renal excretion of Na^+	CNS diseases, including brain trauma, tumours,
No evidence of volume depletion	meningitis
No evidence of oedema	Drug treatment, e.g. carbamazepine, chlorpropamide,
Normal renal and adrenal function	opiates
	Miscellaneous conditions, including porphyria, psychosis, postoperative states

Resetting of the osmostat. Some patients with malnutrition, carcinomatosis and tuberculosis seem to have their osmostat reset at a low level, with plasma [Na^+] of 125–130 mmol/L. The cause is uncertain.

Hyponatraemia with increased ECF volume (Table 2.4)

Significant increases in total body Na^+ give rise to clinically detectable oedema. Generalized oedema is usually associated with secondary aldosteronism, caused by a reduction in renal blood flow, which stimulates renin production. Patients fall into at least three categories:

Renal failure. Excess water intake in a poorly controlled patient with acute or chronic renal disease can lead to hyponatraemia with oedema.

Congestive cardiac failure. The failing heart, with reduced renal perfusion and 'apparent' volume deficit, and the increased venous pressure, with altered fluid distribution between the intravascular and interstitial compartments (Fig. 2.1), lead to secondary aldosteronism and increased vasopressin secretion. This produces Na^+ overload and hyponatraemia.

Hypoproteinaemic states. Low plasma [protein], especially low [albumin], leads to excessive losses of water and low molecular mass solutes from the intravascular to the interstitial compartments (Fig. 2.1). Hence interstitial oedema is accompanied by reduced intravascular volume, with consequent secondary aldosteronism and stimulation of vasopressin release.

'Sick cell syndrome'

Patients with oedema and hyponatraemia may be very ill, and are often very resistant to treatment. Although the total ECF volume is increased, the effective arterial plasma volume is often contracted. Secondary hyperaldosteronism (which causes Na^+ retention) and vasopressin secretion (which causes water retention) may not be the whole explanation, since plasma [aldosterone] and [vasopressin] are not always raised. The hyponatraemia may

be due, at least in part, to the 'sick cell syndrome', in which there is an inability to maintain an Na^+ gradient across the cell membrane.

Other causes of hyponatraemia

Artefact. 'Hyponatraemia' is often caused by collection of a blood specimen from a vein close to a site at which fluid (typically 5% dextrose) is being administered intravenously.

In all the examples of hyponatraemia discussed above, the low plasma [Na^+] occurs in association with reduced plasma osmolality. Where this is not the case, the following possibilities should be considered:

Pseudohyponatraemia. This is due to a reduction in plasma water caused by marked hyperlipidaemia or hyperproteinaemia (e.g. multiple myeloma). The diagnosis can be confirmed by measuring plasma [Na^+] in undiluted plasma, using a direct ion-selective electrode, or by measuring plasma osmolality. In the absence of another cause of true hyponatraemia, the results of these measurements will be normal.

Hyperosmolar hyponatraemia. This may be due to hyperglycaemia, administration of mannitol, or occasionally other causes. The hyponatraemia mainly reflects the shift of water out of the cells into the ECF in response to osmotic effects, other than those due to Na^+, across cell membranes. Treatment should be directed to the cause of the hyperosmolality rather than to the hyponatraemia.

Hypernatraemia

This is the commonest cause of increased tonicity of body fluids. It is nearly always due to water deficit rather than Na^+ excess. The ICF volume is decreased due to movement of water out of the cells.

Hypernatraemia with decreased body sodium (Table 2.6)

This is the commonest group. It is usually due to extrarenal loss of hypotonic fluid. The nature and effects of the disturbance of fluid

HYPERNATRAEMIA

Body sodium	Categories	Examples
Decreased body Na+ *(loss of $H_2O > Na^+$)*	Extrarenal	Sweating, diarrhoea
	Renal	Osmotic diuresis (e.g. diabetes mellitus)
Normal body Na+ *(loss of H_2O only)*	Extrarenal	Fever, high-temperature climates
	Via kidneys	Diabetes insipidus, prolonged unconsciousness
Increased body Na+ *(retention of $Na^+ > H_2O$)*	Steroid excess	Steroid treatment, Cushing's syndrome, Conn's syndrome
	Intake of Na+	Self-induced or iatrogenic, oral or parenteral

Table 2.6 Causes of hypernatraemia.

balance can be thought of as comprising two components:

1 Loss of water, which causes volume reduction of both ICF and ECF and consequent hypernatraemia.

2 Loss of isotonic fluid, which causes reduction in ECF volume, with hypotension, shock and oliguria. Urine osmolality is high, and urine [Na+] is less than 20 mmol/L.

Urinary loss of hypotonic fluid sometimes occurs, due to renal disease or to osmotic diuresis; in these patients, urine [Na+] is likely to be greater than 20 mmol/L. The commonest cause of hypernatraemia associated with an osmotic diuresis is hyperglycaemia.

Treatment should initially aim to replace the deficit of isotonic fluid by infusing isotonic saline or, if the deficit is large, hypotonic saline.

Hypernatraemia with normal body sodium (Table 2.6)

These patients have a pure water deficit, as may occur when insensible water losses are very high (e.g. in hot climates, in unconscious patients, or in patients with a high fever) and insufficient water is drunk as replacement. The urine has a high osmolality, and its Na+ content depends on Na+ intake.

Hypernatraemia with normal body Na+ also occurs in diabetes insipidus (p. 57) due to excessive renal water loss. This loss is normally replaced by drinking. However, dehydration may develop if the patient is unable to drink, as may occur in very young children or in unconscious patients. The urine has a low osmolality and its Na+ content depends on Na+ intake.

Treatment should aim to rehydrate these patients fairly slowly, to avoid causing acute shifts of water into cells, especially those of the brain, which may have accommodated to the hyperosmolality by increasing its intracellular solute concentration. Water, administered orally, is the simplest treatment. Intravenous therapy may be necessary, with 5% glucose or glucose–saline.

Hypernatraemia with increased body sodium (Table 2.6)

This is relatively uncommon. Mild hypernatraemia may be caused by an excess of mineralocorticoids or glucocorticoids. More often, it occurs if excess Na+ is administered therapeutically (e.g. $NaHCO_3$ during resuscitation). Treatment may be with diuretics or, rarely, by renal dialysis.

Other chemical investigations in fluid balance disorders

Several other chemical investigations, in addition to plasma [Na+], may help when the history or clinical examination suggests that there is a disorder of fluid balance.

Blood specimens

Plasma albumin. This may help to assess acute changes in intravascular volume. It is also often useful in following changes in patients with fluid balance disorders over time. Plasma [albumin] should be measured in patients with oedema, to find out whether hypoalbuminaemia is present as a contributory cause, and to determine its severity.

Plasma urea and plasma creatinine. Hypovolaemia is usually associated with a reduced GFR, and so with raised plasma [urea] and [creatinine]. Plasma [urea] may increase before plasma [creatinine] in the early stages of water and Na^+ depletion (p. 21).

Plasma chloride. Alterations in plasma [Cl^-] parallel those in plasma [Na^+], except in the presence of some acid–base disturbances (p. 45). Chloride measurements are rarely of value in assessing disturbances of fluid balance.

Plasma osmolality. Plasma osmolality usually parallels plasma [Na^+] and can be estimated by calculation (p. 16), but may be of value when a defect in vasopressin action is suspected to be responsible for a fluid–electrolyte disorder. Plasma osmolality measurements are also of interest when it seems likely that the calculated osmolarity and measured osmolality might differ significantly. This occurs when:

1 There is marked hyperproteinaemia or hypertriglyceridaemia, causing a low plasma water concentration.

2 Significant amounts of foreign low molecular mass materials (e.g. ethanol, ethylene glycol) which will not contribute to calculated osmolarity are present in plasma.

In both these examples, the finding of a marked discrepancy between the measured osmolality and the calculated osmolarity may be of diagnostic value.

Urine specimens

Urine osmolality

Measurements of urine osmolality are of value in the investigation of:

Polyuria. A relatively concentrated urine suggests that polyuria is due to an osmotic diuretic (e.g. glucose), whereas a dilute urine suggests that there is primary polydipsia or diabetes insipidus (p. 57). Patients with chronic renal failure may also have polyuria, with a urine osmolality that is usually within 50 mmol/kg of the plasma value.

Oliguria. Where acute renal failure is suspected (p. 60).

SIADH. In patients with SIADH (p. 22), the urine osmolality is not maximally dilute, despite a dilutional hyponatraemia.

Urine sodium

This normally varies with Na^+ intake. Measurements of 24-hour output, taken with the clinical findings, may be useful in the diagnosis of disturbances in Na^+ and water handling, and in planning fluid replacement.

Patients with low urine [Na^+]. This is an appropriate response in patients who are volume-depleted, with oliguria and normally functioning kidneys; urine [Na^+] is usually less than 10 mmol/L, and urine flow increases after volume repletion. Na^+ retention and low urine [Na^+] occur in the secondary hyperaldosteronism associated with congestive cardiac failure, liver disease and hypoproteinaemic states, and in Cushing's syndrome and Conn's syndrome.

Patients with natriuresis. In hyponatraemic patients with evidence of ECF volume depletion, continuing natriuresis (i.e. urine [Na^+] greater than 20 mmol/L) suggests either:

1 Volume depletion that is so severe as to have led to acute renal failure. The patient will be oliguric, with rising plasma [urea] and [creatinine]; diuresis fails to occur after volume repletion.

2 In the absence of acute renal failure, this occurs with over-zealous diuretic use, with salt-losing nephritis, and with defects in the hypothalamic–pituitary–adrenal axis, including Addison's disease.

Natriuresis may also occur in hyponatraemic states associated with SIADH or acute water intoxication and where ECF volume is normal or even increased.

Potassium balance

Potassium is the main intracellular cation. About 98% of total body K^+ is in cells; only 2% (about 50 mmol) in the ECF. There is a large concentration gradient across cell membranes, the ICF $[K^+]$ being about 150 mmol/L compared with about 4 mmol/L in ECF.

Internal distribution

This is determined by movements across the cell membrane. Factors causing K^+ to move out of cells include hypertonicity, acidosis, insulin lack, and severe cell damage or cell death. Potassium moves into cells if there is alkalosis, or when insulin is given.

External balance

This is mainly determined, in the absence of GI disease, by intake of K^+ and by its renal excretion. A typical 'Western' diet contains 20–100 mmol K^+ daily; this intake is normally closely matched by the urinary excretion. The control of renal K^+ excretion is not fully understood, but the following points have been established:

• Nearly all the K^+ filtered at the glomerulus is reabsorbed in the proximal tubule. Less than 10% reaches the distal tubule, where the main regulation of K^+ excretion occurs. Secretion of K^+ in response to alterations in dietary intake occurs in the distal tubule, the cortical collecting tubule and the collecting duct.

• The distal tubule is an important site of Na^+ reabsorption. When Na^+ is reabsorbed, the tubular lumen becomes electronegative in relation to the adjacent cell, and cations in the cell (e.g. K^+, H^+) move into the lumen to balance the charge. The rate of movement of K^+ into the lumen depends on there being sufficient delivery of Na^+ to the distal tubule, as well as on the rate of urine flow and on the concentration of K^+ in the tubular cell.

• The concentration of K^+ in the tubular cell depends largely on adenosine triphosphatase-dependent (ATPase-dependent) Na^+/K^+ exchange with peritubular fluid (i.e. the ECF). This is affected by mineralocorticoids, by acid–base changes and by ECF $[K^+]$. The tubular cell $[K^+]$ tends to be increased by hyperkalaemia, by mineralocorticoid excess and by alkalosis, all of which tend to cause an increase in K^+ excretion.

Abnormalities of plasma potassium concentration

The reference range for plasma $[K^+]$ is 3.3–4.7 mmol/L. The important, and often life-threatening, clinical manifestations of abnormalities of plasma $[K^+]$ are those relating to disturbances of neuromuscular excitability and of cardiac conduction. Any patient with an abnormal plasma $[K^+]$ who also shows signs of muscle weakness or of a cardiac arrhythmia should have cardiac monitoring with electrocardiography (ECG). The abnormal plasma $[K^+]$ should be corrected, with appropriate monitoring during treatment.

Hypokalaemia must not be equated with K^+ depletion, and hyperkalaemia must not be equated with K^+ excess. Although most patients with K^+ depletion have hypokalaemia, and most patients with K^+ excess may have hyperkalaemia, acute changes in the distribution of K^+ in the body can offset any effects of depletion or excess. To generalize, acute changes in plasma $[K^+]$ are usually caused by redistribution of K^+ across cell membranes, whereas chronic changes in plasma $[K^+]$ are usually due to abnormal external K^+ balance.

Hypokalaemia (Table 2.7)

Altered internal distribution: shift of K^+ into cells

Acute shifts of K^+ into the cell may occur in *alkalosis*, but the hypokalaemia may be more closely related to the increased renal excretion of K^+. Patients with respiratory alkalosis caused by voluntary hyperventilation rarely show hypokalaemia, but patients on pro-

HYPOKALAEMIA

Cause	Categories	Examples
Artefact		Specimen collected from an infusion site or near to one
Redistribution of K+ between ECF and ICF		Alkalosis, familial periodic paralysis (hypokalaemic form), treatment of hyperglycaemia
Abnormal external balance	Inadequate intake	Anorexia nervosa, alcoholism (both rare)
	Abnormal losses from the GI tract	Vomiting, nasogastric aspiration, diarrhoea, fistula, laxative abuse, villous adenoma of the colon
	Abnormal losses from the renal tract	Diuretics, osmotic diuresis, renal tubular acidosis, aldosteronism, Cushing's syndrome, Bartter's syndrome

Table 2.7 Causes of hypokalaemia.

longed assisted ventilation may have low plasma [K+] if the alveolar P_{CO_2} is low for a relatively long period.

Insulin in high dosage, given intravenously, promotes the uptake of K+ by liver and muscle. Acute shifts of K+ into the cells may occur in diabetic ketoacidosis shortly after starting treatment.

Adrenaline and other β-adrenergic agonists stimulate the uptake of K+ into cells. This may contribute to the hypokalaemia appearing in patients after myocardial infarction, since catecholamine levels are likely to be increased in these patients. Hypokalaemic effects of salbutamol (a synthetic β-adrenergic agonist) have also been described.

Cellular incorporation of K+ may cause hypokalaemia in states where cell mass rapidly increases. Examples include the treatment of severe megaloblastic anaemia with vitamin B_{12} or folate, and the parenteral re-feeding of wasted patients (especially if insulin is also administered). It also occurs when there are rapidly proliferating leukaemic cells.

Altered external balance: deficient intake of K+

Prolonged deficient intake of K+ can lead to a decrease in total body K+, eventually mani-

fested as hypokalaemia. This may occur in chronic and severe malnutrition in the Third World, in the elderly on deficient diets, in anorexia nervosa, and in patients receiving prolonged postoperative parenteral nutrition but with inadequate K+ replacement.

Altered external balance: excessive losses of K+

Hyperaldosteronism, both primary and secondary, and Cushing's syndrome (including that due to steroid administration) cause excessive renal K+ loss due to increased K+ transfer into the distal tubule in response to increased reabsorption of Na+ from the tubular lumen. Mineralocorticoid excess also favours transfer of K+ into the tubular cell in exchange for Na+ at the peritubular border of the cell. Urinary K+ loss in hyperaldosteronism returns to normal if there is dietary Na+ restriction, which limits distal tubular delivery of Na+.

Diuretic therapy increases renal K+ excretion by causing increased delivery of Na+ to the distal tubule and increased urine flow rate. Diuretics may also cause hypovolaemia, with consequent secondary hyperaldosteronism.

Acidosis and alkalosis both affect renal K+ excretion in ways that are not fully understood. Acute acidosis causes K+ retention, and acute alkalosis causes increased K+

excretion. However, chronic acidosis and chronic alkalosis both cause increased K^+ excretion.

Gastrointestinal fluid losses often cause K^+ depletion. However, if gastric fluid is lost in large quantity, renal K^+ loss due to the resultant metabolic alkalosis is the main cause of the K^+ depletion, rather than the direct loss of K^+ in gastric juice. In diarrhoea or laxative abuse, the increased losses of K^+ in faeces may cause K^+ depletion.

Renal disease does not usually cause excessive K^+ loss. However, a few tubular abnormalities are associated with K^+ depletion, in the absence of diuretic therapy:

Renal tubular acidosis. The K^+ loss is caused both by the chronic acidosis and, in patients with proximal renal tubular acidosis (p. 58), by increased delivery of Na^+ to the distal tubule. In distal renal tubular acidosis, the inability to excrete H^+ may cause a compensatory transfer of K^+ to the tubular fluid.

Table 2.8 Causes of hyperkalaemia.

Bartter's syndrome. The syndrome consists of persistent hypokalaemia with secondary hyperaldosteronism in association with a metabolic alkalosis; patients are normotensive. There is increased delivery of Na^+ to the distal tubule, caused by an abnormality of chloride reabsorption in the loop of Henle.

Other causes of hypokalaemia

Artefact. Collection of a blood sample from a vein near to a site of an intravenous infusion, where the fluid has a low $[K^+]$.

Excessive sweating. Sweat $[K^+]$ is normally between 5 and 20 mmol/L.

Hyperkalaemia (Table 2.8)

Plasma $[K^+]$ over 6.5 mmol/L requires urgent treatment. Intravenous calcium gluconate has a rapid but short-lived effect in countering the neuromuscular effects of hyperkalaemia. Treatment with glucose and insulin causes K^+ to pass into the ICF. However, treatment with ion-exchange resins or renal dialysis may be needed.

HYPERKALAEMIA		
Cause	Categories	Examples
Artefact		Trauma during blood collection, delay in separating plasma/serum, freezing blood
Redistribution of K^+ between ECF and ICF		Acidosis, hypertonicity, tissue and tumour necrosis (e.g. burns, leukaemia), haemolytic disorders, hyperkalaemic familial periodic paralysis, insulin deficiency
Abnormal external balance	Increased intake	Excessive oral intake of K^+ (rare by itself)
	Decreased renal output* Renal causes	1 Renal failure, oliguric (acute and chronic); inappropriate oral intake in chronic failure 2 Failure of renal tubular response, due to systemic lupus erythematosus, K^+-sparing diuretics, chronic interstitial nephritis
	Adrenal causes	Addison's disease, selective hypoaldosteronism

*With or without inappropriate intake.

Altered internal distribution of K^+

Acidosis. The effects of acidosis on internal K^+ balance are complicated. As a general rule, acidotic states are often accompanied by hyperkalaemia, as K^+ moves from the ICF into the ECF. Although this is the case for acute respiratory acidosis, and for both acute and chronic metabolic acidosis, it is more unusual to find hyperkalaemia in chronic respiratory acidosis. It is important to note that a high plasma $[K^+]$ may be accompanied by a reduced total body K^+ as a result of excessive urinary K^+ losses in both chronic respiratory acidosis and in metabolic acidosis.

Hypertonic states. In these, K^+ moves out of cells, possibly because of the increased intracellular $[K^+]$ caused by the reduction in ICF volume.

Uncontrolled diabetes mellitus. The lack of insulin prevents K^+ from entering cells. This results in hyperkalaemia, despite the K^+ loss caused by the osmotic diuresis.

Cellular necrosis may lead to excessive release of K^+ and may result in hyperkalaemia. Extensive cell damage may be a feature of rhabdomyolysis (e.g. crush injury), haemolysis, burns, or tumour necrosis (e.g. in the treatment of leukaemias).

Digoxin poisoning prevents K^+ from entering into cells, but therapeutic doses do not have this effect.

Altered external balance: increased intake of K^+

Increased K^+ intake only rarely causes accumulation of K^+ in the body, since the normal kidney can excrete a large K^+ load. However, if there is renal impairment, K^+ may accumulate if salt substitutes are administered, or excessive amounts of some fruit drinks are drunk, or if excessive potassium replacement therapy accompanies diuretic administration.

Altered external balance: decreased excretion of K^+

Intrinsic renal disease is an important cause of hyperkalaemia. It may occur in acute renal failure and in the later stages of chronic renal failure. In patients with renal disease that largely affects the renal medulla, hyperkalaemia may occur earlier. This may be because increased K^+ secretion from the collecting duct, an important adaptive response in the damaged kidney, is lost earlier in patients with medullary disease.

Mineralocorticoid deficiency may occur in Addison's disease and in secondary adrenocortical hypofunction. In both, K^+ retention may sometimes occur. This is not an invariable feature, presumably because other mechanisms can facilitate K^+ excretion. Selective hypoaldosteronism, accompanied by normal glucocorticoid production, may occur in patients with diabetes mellitus in whom juxtaglomerular sclerosis probably interferes with renin production. ACE inhibitors, by reducing AII (and therefore aldosterone) levels, may lead to increased plasma $[K^+]$, but severe problems are only likely to occur in the presence of renal failure.

Patients treated with K^+-sparing diuretics (e.g. spironolactone, amiloride) may fail to respond to aldosterone. If the K^+ intake is high in these patients, or if they have renal insufficiency or selective hypoaldosteronism, these can all lead to dangerous hyperkalaemia.

Other causes of hyperkalaemia

Artefact. This is the commonest cause of hyperkalaemia. When red cells or, occasionally, white cells and platelets are left in contact with plasma or serum for too long, K^+ leaks from the cells. In any blood specimen that does not have its plasma or serum separated from the cells within about three hours, $[K^+]$ is likely to be spuriously high. Blood specimens collected into potassium EDTA, an anticoagulant widely used for haematological specimens, have greatly increased plasma $[K^+]$. Sometimes, doctors decant part of a blood specimen initially collected by mistake into potassium EDTA into another container, and send this for biochemical analysis. A clue to the source of this artefact, which may increase plasma $[K^+]$ to 'lethal' levels (e.g. over 8 mmol/L), is an accompanying very low plasma [calcium], due to chelation of Ca^{2+} with EDTA.

Pseudohyperkalaemia. Pseudohyperkalaemia can occur in acute and chronic myeloproliferative disorders, chronic lymphocytic leukaemia, and severe thrombocytosis as a result of cell lysis during venepuncture, or if there is any delay in the separation of plasma following specimen collection.

Other investigations in disordered K+ metabolism

Urine K+ measurements may be of help in determining the source of K^+ depletion in patients with unexplained hypokalaemia, but are otherwise of little value. A 24-hour urine collection should be made.

Plasma total [CO_2] (p. 44) may prove helpful in the investigation of disorders of K^+ balance, since metabolic acidosis and metabolic alkalosis are commonly associated with abnormalities of K^+ homeostasis. It is rarely necessary to assess acid–base status fully when investigating disturbances of K^+ metabolism; plasma [total CO_2] often suffices.

Other investigations may be indicated by the history of the patient's illness and the findings on clinical examination.

Fluid and electrolyte balance in surgical patients

Patients admitted for major elective surgery, who may be liable to develop disturbances of water and electrolyte balance postoperatively, require preoperative determination of baseline values for plasma urea, creatinine, Na^+ and K^+.

Patients who present for emergency surgery, with disturbances of water and electrolyte metabolism already developed, require to have the severity of the disturbances assessed and corrective measures instituted preoperatively. This usually involves the measurement of plasma urea, creatinine, Na^+ and K^+ as an emergency. Ideally, fluid and electrolyte disturbances should be corrected before surgery.

Metabolic response to trauma

Accidental and operative trauma produce several metabolic effects. These include breakdown of protein, release of K^+ from cells and a consequent K^+ deficit due to urinary loss, temporary retention of water, use of glycogen reserves, gluconeogenesis, mobilization of fat reserves and a tendency to ketosis that sometimes progresses to a metabolic acidosis. Hormonal responses include increased secretion of adrenal corticosteroids, with temporary abolition of negative feedback control, and increased secretion of aldosterone and vasopressin.

The metabolic responses to trauma are physiological and appropriate. They are the reason why postoperative states are such frequent causes of temporary disturbances in electrolyte metabolism. Most patients after major surgery have a temporarily impaired ability to excrete a water load or a Na^+ load; they also have a plasma [urea] that is often raised due to tissue catabolism. Injudicious fluid therapy, especially in the first 48 h after operation, may 'correct' the chemical abnormalities, e.g. by lowering the plasma [urea], but only by causing retention of fluid and the possibility of acute water intoxication.

Postoperatively, any tendency for patients to develop disturbances of water and electrolyte balance can be minimized by regular clinical assessment. In addition to plasma 'electrolytes', fluid balance charts and measurement of 24-hour urinary losses of Na^+ and K^+, or losses from a fistula, can provide information of value in calculating the approximate volume and composition of fluid needed to replace continuing losses.

Acute water intoxication is a severe and dangerous disorder associated with acute neurological symptoms (drowsiness, fits) and later with coma and often death. The symptoms are due to acute swelling of the brain cells caused by the entry of water from the ECF, which has become hypotonic relatively rapidly with respect to the ICF. There is controversy about the appropriate treatment. However, in most centres this would be instituted as a matter of urgency with the infusion of hypertonic saline; a diuretic may also be given to avoid causing fluid overload.

KEY POINTS

1 Compared to the extracellular fluid (ECF) compartment (volume about 14 L), the intracellular fluid (ICF) is much larger (about 28 L) and has a relatively low [Na+] and high [K+].
2 Gains or losses of water are distributed through both ECF and ICF. Intake and output are controlled by thirst and vasopressin, respectively.
3 In general, the ECF volume parallels total body sodium, and is normally mainly controlled by aldosterone. Sodium retention will expand ECF volume, and vice versa.
4 Acute losses of isotonic fluid cause hypovolaemia, with clinical symptoms of hypotension, etc., but not hyponatraemia, at least in the short term.

5 Losses of hypotonic fluid, e.g. in sweat, or of water often result in hypernatraemia.
6 Increased vasopressin secretion is part of the metabolic response to trauma or surgery. Care should be taken to avoid giving excess hypotonic fluids during or after surgery, since there is a danger of acute water intoxication.
7 Changes in plasma [K+] usually result from acute movements across the cell membrane or, in the longer term, whole-body gains or losses.
8 Hyperkalaemia, especially of acute onset, can cause potentially lethal neuromuscular abnormalities, and should be treated urgently with appropriate biochemical and electrocardiography (ECG) monitoring.

Case 2.1

A 45-year-old man was brought into the accident and emergency department late at night in a comatose state. It was impossible to obtain a history from him, and clinical examination was difficult, but it was noted that he smelt strongly of alcohol. The following analyses were requested urgently.

	Plasma analyses	Reference range
[Urea] (mmol/L)	4.7	2.5–6.6
[Na+] (mmol/L)	137	132–144
[K+] (mmol/L)	4.3	3.3–4.7
[Total CO$_2$] (mmol/L)	20	24–30
[Glucose] (mmol/L)	4.2	3.6–5.8 (fasting)
Osmolality (mmol/kg)	465	280–290

Why is his measured osmolality so high?

Comments on Case 2.1

The osmolality can be calculated as 291.5, using the formula on p. 16. The difference between this figure and the value for the directly measured osmolality (465 mmol/L) could be explained by the presence of another low molecular mass solute in plasma. From the patient's history, it seemed that ethanol might be contributing significantly to the plasma osmolality, and plasma [ethanol] was measured the following day, on the residue of the specimen collected at the time of emergency admission. The result was 170 mmol/L, very close to the difference between the measured and calculated osmolalities.

Case 2.2

A 76-year-old man was making reasonable postoperative progress following major abdominal surgery for a carcinoma of the colon.

Two days after the operation he appeared well, and there were no signs of dehydration or oedema. The following results were obtained:

	Plasma analyses (mmol/L)	Reference range (mmol/L)
[Urea]	4.3	2.5–6.6
[Na+]	128	132–144
[K+]	4.3	3.3–4.7
[Total CO₂]	25	24–30

What is the most likely cause of this man's low plasma [Na+]?

Comments on Case 2.2

Hyponatraemia is often seen in postoperative patients receiving intravenous fluids. At this time the ability to excrete water is reduced as part of the metabolic response to trauma. If excessive amounts of hypotonic fluids (usually 5 % dextrose) are given, hyponatraemia will result. It may also be at least partly due to the 'sick cell syndrome'. There are usually no clinical features of water intoxication, and all that is required is review of the patient's fluid balance, and adjustment of the prescription for intravenous fluids. This man had received a total of 4.5 L of fluid since his operation, and his fluid balance chart showed that he had a positive balance of 2 L.

Case 2.3

A 63-year-old coal miner had had a persistent chest infection, with cough and sputum, for the previous two months. He was a smoker. Clinical examination revealed finger clubbing, crackles and wheezes throughout the chest, and a small pleural effusion. There were no signs of dehydration or oedema. Examination of blood and of a random urine specimen yielded the following results:

	Plasma analyses	Reference range
[Urea] (mmol/L)	2.3	2.5–6.6
[Na+] (mmol/L)	118	132–144
[K+] (mmol/L)	4.3	3.3–4.7
[Total CO₂] (mmol/L)	26	24–30
Osmolality (mmol/kg)	260	280–290
Urine analyses		
[Na+]	74	
Osmolality	625	

What is the most likely cause of this man's low plasma [Na+] and osmolality?

Comments on Case 2.3

This patient is not diluting his urine in response to low plasma osmolality and hyponatraemia: this suggests inappropriate ADH secretion. There tends to be a continuing natriuresis despite the hyponatraemia in these patients, as the retention of water leads to mild expansion of the ECF, and hence reduced aldosterone secretion. The presence of a dilutional hyponatraemia is also supported by the low plasma [urea].

Before diagnosing the syndrome of inappropriate ADH secretion (SIADH, p. 22), it is important to exclude adrenal, pituitary and renal disease. In this patient, possible explanations relate to the recurrent chest infections, or an underlying bronchogenic carcinoma, with ectopic secretion of ADH.

Case 2.4

A 71-year-old woman was found by a neighbour drowsy and unwell. She had had an upper respiratory tract infection several weeks previously, and had been very slow to recover from this. She had been increasingly thirsty over this period. The only past history was of diabetes mellitus, diagnosed about five years previously and controlled by diet. On examination, she was very dehydrated, but her breath did not smell of ketones. The following results were obtained:

	Plasma analyses (mmol/L)	Reference range (mmol/L)
[Urea]	28.2	2.5–6.6
[Na+]	156	132–144
[K+]	4.4	3.3–4.7
[Total CO$_2$]	26	24–30
[Glucose]	38.2	3.6–5.8 (fasting)

Why is her sodium so high?

Comments on Case 2.4

She has hyperglycaemic, hyperosmolar, nonketotic metabolic decompensation of her diabetes. The onset of this is usually slower than that of ketoacidosis, and, possibly because vomiting is less likely, patients do not become acutely ill so rapidly. The prolonged osmotic diuresis due to the severe hyperglycaemia results in large losses of water, often in excess of the sodium loss, resulting in hypernatraemia. GFR is reduced, causing raised plasma [urea].

Treatment requires the replacement of the fluid and electrolyte losses, and the use of insulin to restore the glucose concentration to normal and prevent the continuing osmotic diuresis. (See also Chapter 11.)

Case 2.5

A young man was trapped underneath a car in a road traffic accident, and suffered multiple fractures. Despite adequate fluid intake over the next 36 h, at that time he was noted to be oliguric. The following results were obtained:

	Plasma analyses	Reference range
[Urea] (mmol/L)	22.1	2.5–6.6
[Na+] (mmol/L)	133	132–144
[K+] (mmol/L)	6.1	3.3–4.7
[Creatinine] (μmol/L)	214	55–120

Why is the potassium high?

Comments on Case 2.5

The crush injuries, with associated rhabdomyolysis, may have caused hyperkalaemia for at least two reasons: release of K+ from the damaged muscle; acute renal failure caused by release of myoglobin, which is filtered at the glomerulus but precipitates in the distal nephron. This impairs the ability of the kidney to excrete K+.

Case 2.6

A 64-year-old man was admitted on a Sunday for an elective operation on his nasal sinuses; his previous hospital notes were not available. He appeared to be fit for operation on clinical examination, and his preoperative ECG was normal, but the following results were obtained on a blood specimen analysed as part of the routine preoperative assessment:

	Plasma analyses (mmol/L)	Reference range (mmol/L)
[Urea]	7.0	2.5–6.6
[Na⁺]	135	132–144
[K⁺]	8.8	3.3–4.7
[Total CO₂]	30	24–30

How would you interpret the hyperkalaemia in relation to the findings on clinical examination and the normal ECG recording? Would your comments be influenced by the information that became available later that day, when the patient's medical records were received, that he had chronic lymphocytic leukaemia?

Comments on Case 2.6

The ECG changes that are associated with hyperkalaemia are not correlated closely with the level of plasma [K⁺], but it would be most unlikely for the ECG to be normal in a patient whose plasma [K⁺] was 8.8 mmol/L. It is much more likely that the hyperkalaemia was an artefact caused by release of K⁺ from blood cells (in this case from lymphocytes).

CHAPTER 3

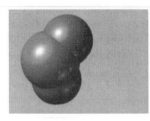

Acid–Base Balance and Oxygen Transport

Transport of carbon dioxide, 35
Renal mechanisms for HCO₃⁻ reabsorption and H⁺ excretion, 36
Buffering of hydrogen ions, 37
Investigating acid–base balance, 38

Disturbances of acid–base status, 39
Interpretation of results of acid–base assessment, 42
Other investigations in acid–base assessment, 44
Oxygen transport, 45

Indications for full blood acid–base and oxygen measurements, 46
Respiratory insufficiency, 46
Treatment of acid–base disturbances, 46

The hydrogen ion concentration of extracellular fluid (ECF) is normally maintained within very close limits. To achieve this, each day the body must dispose of:

1 About 20 000 mmol of CO_2 generated by tissue metabolism. CO_2 itself is not an acid, but combines with water to form the weak acid, carbonic acid.

2 About 40–80 mmol of non-volatile acids, mainly sulphur-containing organic acids, which are excreted by the kidneys.

This chapter deals with the clinical disturbances that may arise in respiratory disorders, when gaseous exchange of O_2 or CO_2 or both in the lung is impaired, and in metabolic disorders when there is either an excessive production, or loss, of nonvolatile acid or an abnormality of excretion.

Transport of carbon dioxide

The CO_2 produced in tissue cells diffuses freely down a concentration gradient across the cell membrane into the ECF and red cells. This gradient is maintained because red blood cell metabolism is anaerobic, so that no CO_2 is produced there, and the concentration remains low. The following reactions then occur:

$$CO_2 + H_2O \leftrightarrow H_2CO_3 \qquad (1)$$

$$H_2CO_3 \leftrightarrow H^+ + HCO_3^- \qquad (2)$$

Reaction 1, the hydration of CO_2 to form carbonic acid (H_2CO_3), is slow, except in the presence of carbonate dehydratase as a catalyst. This limits its site in the blood mainly to erythrocytes, where carbonate dehydratase is located. The second reaction, the ionization of carbonic acid, then occurs rapidly and spontaneously. As a result, erythrocytes are the principal site of H^+ and HCO_3^- formation in the blood. The H^+ ions are mainly buffered inside the red cell by haemoglobin. Haemoglobin is a more effective buffer when deoxygenated, so its buffering capacity increases as it passes through the capillary beds and gives up oxygen to the tissues. Bicarbonate ions, meanwhile, pass from the erythrocytes down their concentration gradient into plasma, in exchange for chloride ions, to maintain electrical neutrality.

In the lungs, the $P\text{CO}_2$ in the alveoli is maintained at a low level by ventilation. The $P\text{CO}_2$ in the blood of the pulmonary capillaries is therefore higher than the $P\text{CO}_2$ in the alveoli, so the gradient is reversed. The above reaction sequence shifts to the left, carbonate dehydratase again catalysing reaction 1. CO_2 then diffuses into the alveoli down its concentration gradient, and is excreted by the lungs.

Renal mechanisms for HCO_3^- reabsorption and H^+ excretion

Glomerular filtrate contains the same concentration of HCO_3^- as plasma. At normal $[HCO_3^-]$, renal tubular mechanisms are responsible for reabsorbing virtually all this HCO_3^-. If this did not occur, large amounts of HCO_3^- would be lost in the urine, reducing the body's buffering capacity and resulting in an acidosis. In addition, the renal tubules are responsible for excreting 40–80 mmol of acid per day under normal circumstances. This will increase when there is an acidosis.

The mechanism of reabsorption of HCO_3^- is shown in Figure 3.1. HCO_3^- is not able to cross the luminal membrane of the renal tubular cells. H^+ is pumped from the tubular cell into the lumen, in exchange for Na^+. The H^+ combines with HCO_3^- to form H_2CO_3 in the lumen. This dissociates to give water and CO_2, which readily diffuses into the cell. In the cell, CO_2 recombines with water under the influence of carbonate dehydratase, to give H_2CO_3. This dissociates to H^+ and HCO_3^-. The HCO_3^- then passes across the basal membrane of the cell into the interstitial fluid. This mechanism results in the reabsorption of filtered HCO_3^-, but no net excretion of H^+.

The net excretion of H^+ relies on the same renal tubular cell reactions as HCO_3^- reabsorption, but occurs after luminal HCO_3^- has been reabsorbed, and depends on the presence of other suitable buffers in the urine (Fig. 3.2). The main urinary buffer is phosphate, most of which is present as HPO_4^{2-}, which can

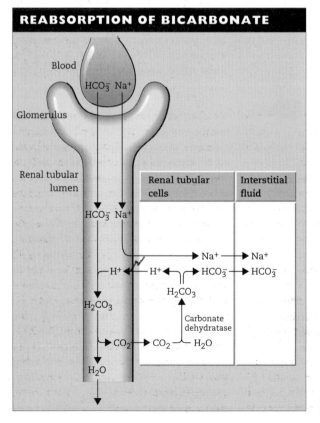

REABSORPTION OF BICARBONATE

Fig. 3.1 Reabsorption of bicarbonate in the renal tubule.

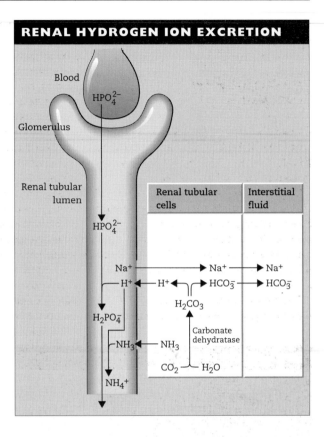

RENAL HYDROGEN ION EXCRETION

Fig. 3.2 Renal hydrogen ion excretion.

combine with H^+ to form $H_2PO_4^-$. Ammonia can also act as a urinary buffer, and is formed by the deamination of glutamine in renal tubular cells under the influence of the enzyme glutaminase. Ammonia readily diffuses across the cell membrane into the tubular lumen, where it combines with H^+ to form NH_4^+. This does not pass across cell membranes, so passive reabsorption is prevented. Glutaminase is induced in chronic acidoses, stimulating increased ammonia production and therefore increased H^+ excretion in the form of NH_4^+ ions.

Buffering of hydrogen ions

The lungs and the kidneys together maintain overall acid–base balance. However, the ECF needs to be protected against rapid changes in $[H^+]$. This is achieved by various buffer systems.

A buffer system consists of a weak (incompletely dissociated) acid in equilibrium with its conjugate base and H^+. The capacity of a buffer for H^+ is related to its concentration and the position of its equilibrium, being most effective at the $[H^+]$ at which the acid and conjugate base are present in equal concentration. Thus, haemoglobin and plasma proteins act as efficient buffers in blood, since they are abundant and at a physiological $[H^+]$ of approximately 40 nmol/L have side groups that exist in an appropriate equilibrium. At this $[H^+]$, the bicarbonate buffer system has an equilibrium that is far removed from the ideal, with $[HCO_3^-]$ being about twenty times greater than $[H_2CO_3]$. However, the effectiveness of the bicarbonate system is greatly enhanced *in vivo* by the fact that H_2CO_3 is readily produced or disposed of by interconversion with CO_2. Furthermore, physiological control mechanisms act to maintain both P_{CO_2} and $[HCO_3^-]$ within limits, and hence to control $[H^+]$.

Any physiological buffer system can be used to investigate and define acid–base status, but the H_2CO_3/HCO_3^- buffer system has proved to be the most appropriate for this purpose, because of its physiological importance.

The Henderson equation simply applies the law of mass action to this buffer system, to give:

$$\left[H^+\right] = K \times \left[H_2CO_3\right]/\left[HCO_3^-\right] \qquad (3)$$

The $[H_2CO_3]$ term can be replaced by $S.P_{CO_2}$, where S is the solubility coefficient of CO_2, since H_2CO_3 is in equilibrium with dissolved CO_2. Substituting numerical values, at $37\,^{\circ}C$ this equation becomes:

$$\left[H^+\right] = 180 \times P_{CO_2}/\left[HCO_3^-\right] \qquad (4)$$

(when $[H^+]$ is measured in nmol/L, P_{CO_2} in kPa, and $[HCO_3^-]$ in mmol/L).

The changes discussed in the above paragraphs are caused by changes in the equilibria of chemical reactions, and must be distinguished from the acid–base changes that occur as a result of respiratory or renal physiological mechanisms operating to return plasma $[H^+]$ towards normal. For example, if there is a rise in P_{CO_2}, this will be immediately reflected by a rise in both plasma $[H^+]$ and $[HCO_3^-]$ due to a shift to the right in reactions 1 and 2 above. Only after several hours, however, would the effect of physiological renal compensatory changes become evident.

Investigating acid–base balance

The acid–base status of a patient can be fully characterized by measuring $[H^+]$ and P_{CO_2} in arterial or arterialized capillary blood specimens; $[HCO_3^-]$ is then obtained by calculation (eqn 4). Plasma $[HCO_3^-]$ has largely replaced terms such as standard bicarbonate, base excess and base deficit, although these derived values are still sometimes reported. They are not necessary for the understanding of acid–base disturbances.

Collection and transport of specimens

Arterial blood specimens are the most appropriate for assessment of acid–base status. However, unless an arterial cannula is *in situ*, these specimens may be difficult to obtain for repeated assessment of patients whose clinical condition is rapidly changing. Arterialized capillary blood specimens are also widely used, especially in infants and children. It is essential for the capillary blood to flow freely, and collection of satisfactory samples may be impossible if there is peripheral vasoconstriction or the blood flow is sluggish.

Patients must be relaxed, and their breathing pattern should have settled after any temporary disturbance (e.g. due to insertion of an arterial cannula), before specimens are collected. Some patients may hyperventilate temporarily because they feel apprehensive.

Blood is collected into syringes or capillary tubes that contain sufficient heparin to act as anticoagulant; excess heparin, which is acidic, must be avoided. Specimens must be free from air bubbles, since these will equilibrate with the sample, causing a rise in P_{O_2} and a fall in P_{CO_2}.

Acid–base measurements should be performed immediately the sample has been obtained, or the specimen should be chilled until analysis can be performed. Otherwise, glycolysis (with production of lactic acid) occurs, and the acid–base composition of the blood alters rapidly. Specimens chilled in iced water can have their analysis delayed as long as four hours. However, the clinical reasons that gave rise to the need for full acid–base studies usually demand much more rapid answers.

Temperature effects

Acid–base measurements are nearly always made at $37\,^{\circ}C$, but some patients may have body temperatures that are higher or lower than $37\,^{\circ}C$. Equations are available to relate $[H^+]$, P_{CO_2} and P_{O_2}, determined at $37\,^{\circ}C$, to 'equivalent' values that correspond to the patient's body temperature. However, reference ranges for acid–base data have only been established by most laboratories for measurements made at $37\,^{\circ}C$. Adjustment of analytical results to values that would have been obtained at the patient's temperature, according to these equations, may therefore be misleading. If treatment aimed at reducing an acid–base disturbance (e.g. $NaHCO_3$ infusion) is given to a severely hypothermic patient, the effects of the treatment should be monitored frequently by repeating the acid–base measurements (at $37\,^{\circ}C$).

Disturbances of acid–base status

Acid–base disorders fall into two main categories, respiratory and metabolic:

1 *Respiratory disorders*. A primary defect in ventilation affects the P_{CO_2}.

2 *Metabolic disorders*. The primary defect may be production of nonvolatile acids, or ingestion of substances that give rise to them, in excess of the kidney's ability to excrete these substances. Alternatively, the primary defect may be the loss of H^+ from the body, or it may be loss or retention of HCO_3^-.

Acid–base status can be understood and described on the basis of the relationships represented by reactions 1 and 2, and consideration of the Henderson equation. The following discussion is restricted mainly to consideration of simple acid–base disturbances, in which there is a single primary disturbance, normally

Table 3.1 Illustrative data for patients with simple disturbances of acid–base balance.

accompanied by compensatory physiological changes that usually tend to correct plasma $[H^+]$ towards normal. We shall not consider mixed disturbances, where two or more primary simple disturbances are present, in any detail. Sets of illustrative acid–base results for patients with the four categories of simple disorders of acid–base status are given in Table 3.1.

Respiratory acidosis (Table 3.2)

This is caused by CO_2 retention due to hypoventilation. It may accompany defects in the control of ventilation, or diseases affecting the nerve supply or muscles of the chest wall or diaphragm, or disorders affecting the respiratory cage or intrinsic lung disease.

In acute respiratory acidosis, a rise in P_{CO_2} causes the equilibria in reactions 1 and 2 to shift to the right, as a result of which plasma $[H^+]$ and $[HCO_3^-]$ both increase. Equilibration of H^+ with body buffer systems limits the potential rise in $[H^+]$, and a new steady state is achieved within a few minutes.

Unless the cause of the acute episode of acidosis resolves, or is treated quickly and successfully, renal compensation causes HCO_3^- retention and H^+ excretion, thereby returning plasma $[H^+]$ towards normal while $[HCO_3^-]$ increases even further. These compensatory changes occur over a period of hours to days, by which time a new steady state is achieved and the daily renal H^+ excretion and HCO_3^- retention return to normal. The patient then has the pattern of acid–base abnormalities of chronic respiratory acidosis.

ACID–BASE DISORDERS

	[H+] (nmol/L)	Pco₂ (kPa)	Plasma [HCO₃] (mmol/L)	Plasma [total CO₂] (mmol/L)
Reference ranges	36–44	4.4–6.1	21.0–27.5	24–30
Respiratory acidosis	58 ↑	9.3 ↑	29 ↑ renal comp	32 ↑
Respiratory alkalosis	29 –	3.2 ↓	20 ↓	22 –
Metabolic acidosis	72 ↑	3.2 ↓	8 ↓ buffers	11 ↓
Metabolic alkalosis	28 ↓	6.0 ~	39 ↑	43 ↑

RESPIRATORY ACIDOSIS

Mechanism	Examples of causes
Alveolar P_{CO_2} increased due to defect in respiratory control mechanisms	CNS disease—stroke, trauma CNS depression—anaesthetics, opiates, severe hypoxia Neurological disease—motor neurone disease, spinal cord lesions, poliomyelitis
Alveolar P_{CO_2} increased due to defect in respiratory function	Pulmonary disease—chronic bronchitis, severe asthma, pulmonary oedema, fibrosis Mechanical disorders—thoracic trauma, pneumothorax, myopathies

Table 3.2 Respiratory acidosis.

RESPIRATORY ALKALOSIS

Mechanism	Examples of causes
Alveolar P_{CO_2} lowered due to hyperventilation	Voluntary hyperventilation, mechanical ventilation Reflex hyperventilation—chest wall disease, decreased pulmonary compliance Stimulation of respiratory centre—pain, fever, salicylate overdose, hepatic encephalopathy, hypoxia

Table 3.3 Respiratory alkalosis.

Respiratory alkalosis (Table 3.3)

This is due to hyperventilation. The reduced P_{CO_2} that results causes the equilibrium positions of reactions 1 and 2 to move to the left. As a result, plasma [H+] and [HCO$_3^-$] both fall, although the relative change in [HCO$_3^-$] is small.

If conditions giving rise to a low P_{CO_2} persist for more than a few hours, the kidneys increase HCO$_3^-$ excretion and reduce H+ excretion. Plasma [H+] returns towards normal, whereas plasma [HCO$_3^-$] falls even further. A new steady state will be achieved in hours to days, if the respiratory disorder persists. It is unusual for chronic respiratory alkalosis to be severe, and plasma [HCO$_3^-$] rarely falls below 12 mmol/L.

Metabolic acidosis (Table 3.4)

Increased production or decreased excretion of H+ leads to accumulation of H+ within the ECF. This disturbs the equilibrium in reaction 2, with a shift to the left as the extra H+ ions combine with HCO$_3^-$ to form H$_2$CO$_3$. However, since there is no ventilatory abnormality, any increase in plasma [H$_2$CO$_3$] is only transient, as the related slight increase in dissolved CO$_2$ is immediately excreted by the lungs. The net effect is that a new equilibrium rapidly establishes itself in which the product, [H+]×[HCO$_3^-$], remains unchanged, since [H$_2$CO$_3$] is unchanged. In consequence, the rise in plasma [H+] is limited, but at the expense of a fall in [HCO$_3^-$].

The rise in ECF [H+] stimulates the respiratory centre, causing compensatory hyperventilation. As a result, due to the fall in P_{CO_2}, plasma [H+] returns back towards normal, while plasma [HCO$_3^-$] falls even further.

Plasma [H+] will not, however, become completely normal, since it is the low [H+] that is the drive to the compensatory hyperventilation – as the [H+] falls, that drive becomes correspondingly reduced. In addition, if renal function is normal, H+ will be excreted by the kidney. It is quite common for patients with metabolic acidosis to have very low plasma [HCO$_3^-$], often below 10 mmol/L.

Metabolic alkalosis (Table 3.5)

This is most often due to prolonged vomiting, but may be due to other causes. The loss of H+ upsets the equilibrium in reaction 2, causing it to shift to the right as H_2CO_3 dissociates to form H+ and HCO$_3^-$. However, because there is no disturbance of ventilation, plasma PCO$_2$ remains constant, with the net effect that plasma [H+] falls and [HCO$_3^-$] rises. Respiratory compensation (i.e. hypoventilation) for the alkalosis is usually minimal, since any rise in PCO$_2$ will be a potent stimulator of ventilation. HCO$_3^-$ is freely filtered at the glomerulus, and is therefore available for excretion in the urine, which would tend to restore the acid–base status towards normal. The continuing presence of an alkalosis means that there is inappropriate reabsorption of filtered HCO$_3^-$ from the distal nephron. This can be due to extracellular fluid volume depletion, potassium deficiency, or mineralocorticoid excess.

Table 3.4 Metabolic acidosis.

METABOLIC ACIDOSIS

Mechanism	Examples of causes
Increased H+ production in excess of body's excretory capacity	Ketoacidosis—diabetic, alcoholic Lactic acidosis—hypoxic, shock, drugs, inherited metabolic disease Poisoning—methanol, salicylate
Failure to excrete H+ at the normal rate	Acute and chronic renal failure Distal renal tubular acidoses
Loss of HCO$_3$	Loss from the GI tract—severe diarrhoea, pancreatic fistula Loss in the urine—uretero-enterostomy, proximal renal tubular acidosis, carbonate dehydratase inhibitors (acetazolamide)

METABOLIC ALKALOSIS

Mechanism	Examples of causes
Saline-responsive	H+ loss from GI tract—vomiting, nasogastric drainage H+ loss in urine—thiazide diuretics (especially in cardiac failure), nephrotic syndrome Alkali administration—sodium bicarbonate
Saline-unresponsive	Associated with hypertension—primary and secondary aldosteronism, Cushing's syndrome Not associated with hypertension—severe K+ depletion, Bartter's syndrome

Table 3.5 Metabolic alkalosis.

Interpretation of results of acid–base assessment

Results of acid–base measurements must be considered in the light of clinical findings, and the results of other chemical tests (e.g. plasma creatinine, urea, Na^+ and K^+); other types of investigation (e.g. radiological) may also be important.

Interpretation of acid–base results is based on the equilibria represented by reactions 1 and 2 and the related Henderson equation. After reviewing the clinical findings, acid–base results can be considered in the following order:

1 Plasma [H+]. Reference range 36–44 nmol/L.
2 Plasma P_{CO_2}. Reference range 4.5–6.1 kPa.
3 Plasma [HCO_3^-]. Reference range 21.0–27.5 mmol/L.

This procedure immediately identifies those patients in whom there is an uncompensated acidosis or an alkalosis, and is the starting point for their further classification, as considered below.

Alternatively, the results can be plotted on a diagram of [H+] against P_{CO_2} (Fig. 3.3). On this diagram, simple acid–base disturbances represent bands of results, as shown. Careful consideration needs to be given to results falling between the bands due to metabolic acidosis and respiratory alkalosis, or between those due to respiratory acidosis and metabolic alkalosis. These may represent either a combination of two acid–base disorders, or compensation for a simple disorder.

Plasma [H+] is increased

The patient has an acidosis. The P_{CO_2} result is considered next, as follows:

1 P_{CO_2} is decreased. The patient has a *metabolic acidosis*. The reduced P_{CO_2} is due to hyperventilation, the physiological compensatory response (e.g. the overbreathing in patients with diabetic ketoacidosis). Plasma [HCO_3^-] is

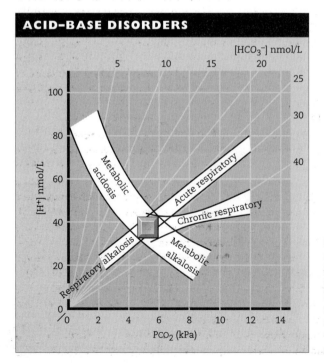

ACID–BASE DISORDERS

Fig. 3.3 On this plot of [H+] against P_{CO_2}, lines of equal [HCO_3^-] radiate from the origin, increasing in value towards the bottom right corner. The bands of values marked show the expected results in patients with simple acid–base disorders.

reduced in these patients, often to below 10 mmol/L.

2 P_{CO_2} is normal. The patient has an *uncompensated metabolic acidosis*. Plasma $[HCO_3^-]$ will be decreased. However, the normal compensatory response should lower the P_{CO_2} in patients with a simple metabolic acidosis (see above), so there is a coexisting respiratory pathology causing CO_2 retention – in other words, there is a simultaneous respiratory acidosis. This combination of results is seen, for example, in patients with combined respiratory and circulatory failure, such as occurs during a cardiac arrest.

3 P_{CO_2} is increased. The patient has a *respiratory acidosis*. If this is a simple disturbance, plasma $[HCO_3^-]$ will be increased. The pattern of results will tend to differ, however, depending on whether the respiratory acidosis is acute or chronic:

Acute. The patient will have a high plasma $[H^+]$ and high P_{CO_2}, with a slightly raised plasma $[HCO_3^-]$, since the renal response has not yet had time to develop.

Chronic. The patient will have a normal or slightly raised plasma $[H^+]$, a high P_{CO_2}, and a markedly raised plasma $[HCO_3^-]$ that is usually over 32 mmol/L, due to renal retention of HCO_3^-.

Plasma [H+] is decreased

The patient has an alkalosis. The P_{CO_2} result should be assessed next:

1 P_{CO_2} is decreased. The patient has a *respiratory alkalosis*. If this is a simple disturbance, plasma $[HCO_3^-]$ will be decreased (not below about 12 mmol/L).

2 P_{CO_2} is normal. The patient has an *uncompensated metabolic alkalosis*, and the plasma $[HCO_3^-]$ will be increased.

3 P_{CO_2} is increased. It is unlikely that this patient has a simple acid–base disturbance. The patient may have a metabolic alkalosis with some respiratory compensation. However, significant hypoventilation is not often a feature of the compensatory response to a metabolic alkalosis, so it is unlikely. A commoner explanation for a low plasma $[H^+]$ and an increased

P_{CO_2} is that the patient has a mixed acid–base disturbance, consisting of a metabolic alkalosis and a respiratory acidosis. Plasma $[HCO_3^-]$ will also be increased.

Plasma [H+] is normal

The patient either has no acid–base disturbance, or no net acid base disturbance, as a result of one of the mechanisms described below. Considering the P_{CO_2} result next:

1 P_{CO_2} is decreased. The patient most probably has a mixed acid–base disturbance consisting of a respiratory alkalosis and a metabolic acidosis. Both these types of acid–base disturbance cause a decreased plasma $[HCO_3^-]$, and the distinction can usually be made on clinical grounds. A fully compensated respiratory alkalosis is another possibility.

2 P_{CO_2} is normal. There is no significant acid–base disturbance. Since both plasma $[H^+]$ and P_{CO_2} are normal, plasma $[HCO_3^-]$ must be normal; see eqn 4.

3 P_{CO_2} is increased. The patient either has a fully compensated respiratory acidosis, or there is a mixed acid–base disturbance consisting of a respiratory acidosis and a metabolic alkalosis. Both these possibilities give rise to increased plasma $[HCO_3^-]$, to over 30 mmol/L. They can usually be distinguished on clinical grounds, which must include consideration of any treatment that the patient may have received (e.g. $NaHCO_3$).

Mixed acid–base disturbances

It may not always be possible to differentiate some mixed acid–base disturbances from simple ones by the scheme described above. For instance, some patients with chronic renal failure (which causes a primary metabolic acidosis) may also have chronic obstructive airways disease (which causes a primary respiratory acidosis). Plasma $[H^+]$ will be increased in these patients, but the results for plasma P_{CO_2} and $[HCO_3^-]$ cannot be predicted. The history and clinical findings must be taken into account.

Plotting the results on a diagram of $[H^+]$ against P_{CO_2} (Fig. 3.3) may help. Results falling between the bands of respiratory and metabolic acidoses are due to a combination of these two conditions. Likewise, results between the bands due to respiratory and metabolic alkaloses are due to a combination of these two disorders.

Other investigations in acid–base assessment

The full characterization of acid–base status requires arterial or arterialized capillary blood samples, since venous blood P_{CO_2} (even if 'arterialized') bears no constant relationship to alveolar P_{CO_2}. However, other investigations can provide some useful information.

Total CO_2 (reference range 24–30 mmol/L)

This test, performed on venous plasma or serum, includes contributions from HCO_3^-, H_2CO_3, dissolved CO_2 and carbamino compounds. However, about 95% of 'total CO_2' is contributed by HCO_3^-. Total CO_2 measurements have the advantages of ease of sample collection and suitability for measurement in large numbers, but they cannot define a patient's acid–base status, since plasma $[H^+]$ and P_{CO_2} are both unknown. For example, an increased plasma [total CO_2] may be due to

either a respiratory acidosis or a metabolic alkalosis. However, when interpreted in the light of the clinical findings, plasma [total CO_2] can often give an adequate assessment of whether an acid–base disturbance is present and, if one is present, provide an indication of its severity. This is particularly true when there is a metabolic disturbance. However, patients with respiratory disturbances are much more likely to require full assessment of acid–base status, both for their definition and for monitoring and controlling their treatment.

Anion gap (AG) (reference range 10–20 mmol/L)

The anion gap (or *ion difference*) derives from plasma electrolyte results, as follows:

$$AG = \left(\left[Na^+\right]+\left[K^+\right]\right)-\left(\left[Cl^-\right]+\left[total\ CO_2\right]\right)$$

The difference between the cations and the anions represents the unmeasured anions or anion gap and includes proteins, phosphate, sulphate and lactate ions. It serves as a pointer to the presence of certain types of acid–base disturbance, especially a metabolic acidosis. The anion gap may be increased because of an increase in unmeasured anions or, less often, a decrease in unmeasured cations (Table 3.6). A reduction in the anion gap occurs much less frequently, and can usually be traced to laboratory error.

One value of the anion gap is that it draws attention to the possibility that there is present

Table 3.6 Causes of an increased anion gap.

ANION GAP	
Mechanism	Examples of causes
Plasma [unmeasured anions] increased with or without changes in [Na+] and [Cl-]	Metabolic acidosis—uraemic acidosis, lactic acidosis, diabetic ketoacidosis, salicylate overdose, methanol ingestion
Increase in plasma [Na+]	Treatment with sodium salts, e.g. salts of some high-dose antibiotics such as carbenicillin; this increases plasma [unmeasured anions]
Artefact	Improper handling of specimens after collection, causing loss of CO_2

in plasma a significant amount of an analyte that is much less frequently measured, such as lactate or a drug metabolite. In addition, in the presence of a metabolic acidosis, a raised anion gap points to the cause being excessive production of hydrogen ions or failure to excrete them. A normal anion gap indicates that the cause is a loss of bicarbonate with its counterbalancing cations (Table 3.4, and see below).

Plasma chloride (reference range 95–107 mmol/L)

The causes of metabolic acidosis are sometimes divided into those with an increased anion gap (Table 3.6) and those with a normal anion gap. In the latter group, the fall in plasma [total CO_2], which accompanies the metabolic acidosis, is associated with an approximately equal rise in plasma [Cl^-]. Patients with a metabolic acidosis and a normal anion gap are sometimes described as having a hyperchloraemic acidosis. Chronic renal failure is the commonest cause of hyperchloraemic acidosis.

Increased plasma [Cl^-], out of proportion to any accompanying increase in plasma [Na^+], may occur in patients with chronic renal failure, ureteric transplants into the colon or renal tubular acidosis, or in patients treated with carbonate dehydratase inhibitors. Increased plasma [Cl^-] may also occur in patients who develop respiratory alkalosis as a result of prolonged assisted ventilation. An iatrogenic cause of increased plasma [Cl^-] is the intravenous administration of excessive amounts of isotonic or 'physiological' saline, which contains 155 mmol/L NaCl.

Patients who lose large volumes of gastric secretion (e.g. due to pyloric stenosis) often show a disproportionately marked fall in plasma [Cl^-] compared with any hyponatraemia that may develop. They develop a metabolic alkalosis, and are often dehydrated.

Oxygen transport

The full characterization of the oxygen composition of a blood sample requires measurement of Po_2, haemoglobin (Hb) concentration and percentage oxygen saturation.

Measurements of Po_2 in arterial blood (reference range 12–15 kPa) are important, and are often valuable in assessing the efficiency of oxygen therapy, when high Po_2 values may be found. Above a Po_2 of 10.5 kPa, however, Hb is almost fully saturated with O_2 (Fig. 3.4). Results of Po_2 measurements may be misleading in conditions where the oxygen-carrying capacity of blood is grossly impaired, as in severe anaemia, carbon monoxide poisoning and when abnormal Hb derivatives (e.g. methaemoglobin) are present. Measurement of both the blood [Hb] and the percentage oxygen saturation are required in addition to Po_2 under these circumstances.

Haemoglobin measurements are widely available, and Po_2 is one of the measurements automatically performed by most blood gas analysers as part of the full acid–base assessment of patients.

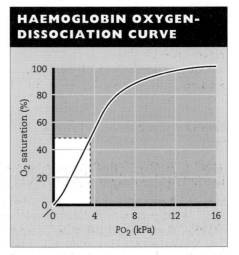

HAEMOGLOBIN OXYGEN-DISSOCIATION CURVE

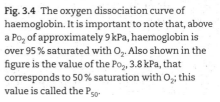

Fig. 3.4 The oxygen dissociation curve of haemoglobin. It is important to note that, above a Po_2 of approximately 9 kPa, haemoglobin is over 95 % saturated with O_2. Also shown in the figure is the value of the Po_2, 3.8 kPa, that corresponds to 50 % saturation with O_2; this value is called the P_{50}.

Indications for full blood acid–base and oxygen measurements

The main indications for full acid–base assessment, coupled with Po_2 or oxygen saturation measurements, are in the investigation and management of patients with pulmonary disorders, severely ill patients in intensive care units, and patients in the operative and perioperative periods of major surgery who may often be on assisted ventilation. Other important applications include the investigation and management of patients with vascular abnormalities involving the shunting of blood.

Full acid–base assessment is less essential in patients with metabolic acidosis or alkalosis, for whom measurements of plasma [total CO_2] on venous blood may give sufficient information.

Respiratory insufficiency

This term is applied to two types of disorder in which lung function is impaired sufficiently to cause the Po_2 to become abnormally low, usually less than 8.0 kPa.

Type I: Low Po_2 with normal or low Pco_2

Hypoxia without hypercapnia occurs in patients in whom there is a preponderance of alveoli that are adequately perfused with blood, but inadequately ventilated. It occurs, for example, in emphysema, pulmonary oedema and asthma. Type II respiratory insufficiency can also occur in some of these conditions, if they are sufficiently severe.

In type I respiratory insufficiency there is, in effect, a partial right-to-left shunt, bringing unoxygenated blood to the left side of the heart. Increased ventilation of the adequately perfused and ventilated alveoli is able to compensate for the tendency for the Pco_2 to rise. It cannot, however, restore the Po_2 to normal, since the blood perfusing the normal alveoli conveys haemoglobin that is already nearly saturated with O_2.

Type II: Low Po_2 with high Pco_2

This combination means that there is hypoventilation. The cause may be central in origin, or due to airways obstruction, or it may be neuromuscular. There may be altered ventilation/perfusion relationships, with an excessive number of alveoli being inadequately perfused; this causes 'wasted' ventilation and an increase in 'dead space'.

Chronic obstructive airways disease is an important cause of type II respiratory insufficiency. It also occurs with mechanical defects in ventilation (e.g. chest injuries, myasthenia gravis). In severe asthma, if serial measurements show a rising Pco_2 and falling Po_2, more intensive treatment is urgently needed.

Treatment of acid–base disturbances

A thorough clinical assessment is the basis on which the results of acid–base analyses are interpreted, and treatment initiated. Having defined the nature of an acid–base disturbance, treatment should aim to correct the primary disorder and to assist the physiological compensatory mechanisms. In some cases, more active intervention may be necessary (e.g. treatment with $NaHCO_3$). It is often possible to correct an acid–base disturbance by treatment aimed only at the causative condition (e.g. diabetic ketoacidosis is usually corrected without the administration of $NaHCO_3$). Where active treatment of the acid–base disturbance is necessary, this is usually needed for metabolic disturbances.

In metabolic acidosis, treatment with HCO_3^- is usually not indicated unless $[H^+]$ is very high (i.e. over 90 nmol/L), except for patients with proximal renal tubular acidosis, who lose HCO_3^- because of the primary defect.

In metabolic alkalosis many patients inappropriately retain HCO_3^- because of volume depletion, potassium depletion, or mineralocorticoid excess, perpetuating the alkalosis. These patients respond to the administration of isotonic saline. Nonresponders include patients with mineralocorticoid excess, either due to primary adrenal hyperfunction or to those causes of secondary adrenal hyperfunction that are not due to hypovolaemia and ECF depletion. These include renal artery stenosis, magnesium deficiency and Bartter's syndrome. Treatment of these is directed at the primary disorder.

KEY POINTS

1 Meaningful acid–base studies on blood usually require arterial specimens, and need to be analysed soon after collection.
2 Respiratory acidosis is common in chronic obstructive airways disease. There is a raised P_{CO_2}, [H+] and [HCO_3^-]. Compensatory renal HCO_3^- retention tends to return [H+] towards normal.
3 Respiratory alkalosis is usually transient and due to overbreathing, or occasionally artificial ventilation. P_{CO_2}, [HCO_3^-] and [H+] are reduced.
4 Metabolic acidosis is due to acid overproduction, e.g. diabetic ketoacidosis, to failure to excrete acid, e.g. renal disease, or loss of base. [H+] is increased and [HCO_3^-] is decreased, and there is often compensatory reduction in P_{CO_2} due to overbreathing.
5 Metabolic alkalosis is most often due to loss of gastric acid, e.g. pyloric stenosis. [H+] is low and [HCO_3^-] is raised.
6 Respiratory insufficiency is said to be present when the P_{O_2} is below 8.0 kPa. In Type I, the P_{CO_2} is normal or low, in Type II it is raised.

Case 3.1

A 70-year-old man was admitted to hospital as an emergency. He gave a history of dyspepsia and epigastric pain extending over many years. He had never sought medical attention for this. One week prior to admission, he had started to vomit, and had since vomited frequently, being unable to keep down any food. He was clinically dehydrated, and had marked epigastric tenderness, but no sign of abdominal rigidity. Analysis of an arterial blood specimen gave the following results:

	Plasma analyses (mmol/L)	Reference range (mmol/L)
[Urea]	17.3	2.5–6.6
[Na+]	117	132–144
[K+]	2.2	3.3–4.7
[Creatinine]	250	55–120

	Blood gas analyses	Reference range
[H+] (nmol/L)	26	36–44
P_{CO_2} (kPa)	6.2	4.4–6.1
[Bicarbonate] (mmol/L)	44	21.0–27.5
P_{O_2} (kPa)	9.5	12–15

Continued on p. 48

Case 3.1 *continued*

How would you describe this patient's acid–base status? What might have caused the various abnormalities revealed by these results? Why is the plasma [K+] so low?

Comments on Case 3.1

The patient had a metabolic alkalosis. This was caused by his persistent vomiting, the vomit being likely to consist almost entirely of gastric contents. In this age group, the cause could be carcinoma of the stomach or chronic peptic ulceration with associated fibrosis, leading to obstruction of gastric outflow.

Gastric juice [K+] is about 10 mmol/L. Also, in the presence of an alkalosis, K+ shifts from the ECF into cells. Furthermore, dehydration causes secondary hyperaldosteronism, in order to maintain ECF volume, and Na+ is avidly retained by the kidneys in exchange for H+ and K+. Patients such as this man, despite having an alkalosis and despite being hypokalaemic, often excrete an acid urine containing large amounts of K+.

Case 3.2

The junior doctor first on call for the accident and emergency (A&E) department examined a 22-year-old man who was having an acute attack of asthma. The patient was very distressed, so the doctor treated him with a nebulized bronchodilator immediately and returned 10 min later to examine him, when he was more settled and was breathing air. He decided to check the patient's arterial blood gases, the results of which were:

	Blood gas analyses	Reference range
[H+] (nmol/L)	44	36–44
P_{CO_2} (kPa)	6.0	4.4–6.1
[Bicarbonate] (mmol/L)	27.0	21.0–27.5
P_{O_2} (kPa)	10.2	12–15

The doctor asked the A&E consultant whether he could send the patient home. Would you consider that these results suggested that it would be safe to do so?

Comments on Case 3.2

It would not be safe to send this patient home. In a moderately severe asthmatic attack, the ventilatory drive from hypoxia and from mechanical receptors in the chest normally results in a P_{CO_2} at or below the lower end of the reference range. A P_{CO_2} greater than this is a serious prognostic sign, indicative either of extensive 'shunting' of blood through areas of the lung that are underventilated because of bronchoconstriction or plugging with mucus, or of the patient becoming increasingly tired. A rising P_{CO_2} in an asthmatic attack is an indication for ventilating these patients.

Case 3.3

A 75-year-old widow, a known heavy smoker and chronic bronchitic, and a patient in a long-stay hospital, became very breathless and wheezy. The senior nurse called the doctor who was on duty, but he was unable to come at once because he was treating another emergency. He asked the nurse to start the patient on 24% oxygen. One hour later, when the doctor arrived, he examined the patient and took an arterial specimen to determine her blood gases. The results were as follows:

Continued on p. 49

Case 3.3 continued

	Blood gas analyses	Reference range
[H+] (nmol/L)	97	36–44
P_{CO_2} (kPa)	21.8	4.4–6.1
[Bicarbonate] (mmol/L)	42	21.0–27.5
P_{O_2} (kPa)	22.5	12–15

How would you describe the patient's acid–base status? Do you think that she was breathing 24 % oxygen?

Comments on Case 3.3

This patient had a respiratory acidosis. Although she gave a long history of chest complaints, the history of the recent illness was short, and it was most unlikely that renal compensation could have accounted in that short time for the very high arterial plasma [HCO_3^-].

From the arterial P_{O_2} result, it was apparent that the patient was breathing a much higher concentration of O_2 than 24 %. Atmospheric pressure is approximately 100 kPa, and the P_{O_2} of inspired air (in kPa) is numerically equal, approximately, to the percentage of O_2 inspired. Further, it is approximately true that:

$$\text{Inspired } P_{O_2} = \text{alveolar } P_{O_2} + \text{alveolar } P_{CO_2}$$

Since alveolar P_{CO_2} equals arterial P_{CO_2}, this equation can be rewritten as:

$$\text{Inspired } P_{O_2} = \text{alveolar } P_{O_2} - \text{arterial } P_{CO_2}$$

Alveolar P_{O_2} must be greater than arterial P_{O_2}, so it was possible to conclude that the patient must have been breathing O_2 at a concentration of at least 40 %. On checking, it was found that the wrong mask had been fitted, and that O_2 was being delivered at 60 %.

It was concluded that the patient had an underlying chronic (compensated) respiratory acidosis with CO_2 retention (type II respiratory failure), and that the administration of oxygen at high concentration had removed the hypoxic drive to ventilation, thereby superimposing an acute respiratory acidosis on the underlying chronic acid–base disturbance.

Case 3.4

A young woman was admitted in a confused and restless condition. History taking was not easy, but it seemed that she had been becoming progressively unwell over the preceding week or two. Acid–base analysis was performed, and results were as follows:

	Blood gas analyses	Reference range
[H+] (nmol/L)	78	36–44
P_{CO_2} (kPa)	3.2	4.4–6.1
[Bicarbonate] (mmol/L)	6	21.0–27.5
P_{O_2} (kPa)	11.8	12–15

What is her acid–base disorder? What are the most likely causes, and what investigations could narrow this down?

Comments on Case 3.4

She has a metabolic acidosis. Despite the long list of possible causes of metabolic acidoses, the commonest causes are diabetic ketoacidosis, renal failure, salicylate overdose and lactic acidosis. These can usually be differentiated on the basis of the history; by measuring U&Es, glucose, and salicylate if indicated; and performing urinalysis (using a dipstick, and looking especially for ketones). Lactate can also be measured if required, but is not often necessary. This woman was a newly presenting Type I diabetic.

Case 3.5

An elderly man was brought into the accident and emergency department after collapsing in the street. He was deeply comatose and cyanosed, with unrecordable blood pressure. The results of acid base analysis were as follows:

	Blood gas analyses	Reference range
[H+] (nmol/L)	124	36–44
Pco$_2$ (kPa)	10.4	4.4–6.1
[Bicarbonate] (mmol/L)	15.4	21.0–27.5
Po$_2$ (kPa)	4.8	12–15

What is his acid–base status? What are possible causes?

Comments on Case 3.5

He has a combined metabolic and respiratory acidosis. The combination of the elevated H+ and Pco$_2$ may initially suggest that he has a respiratory acidosis, but the bicarbonate would not be reduced in a simple respiratory acidosis. This means that there is an additional component of a metabolic acidosis present. Results of this sort are seen in patients with markedly impaired circulatory and respiratory function, such as occurs after a cardiac arrest. This man had a large abdominal aortic aneurysm that had ruptured.

Case 3.6

A 60-year-old man with insulin-treated Type II diabetes experienced severe central chest pain, associated with nausea. He refused to let his wife call the doctor, but went to bed, and since he felt too ill to eat he stopped taking his insulin. Two days later, he had another episode of chest pain and became breathless. His wife called an ambulance, and he was admitted. He was shocked, with central cyanosis, pulse 120/min, blood pressure 65/35, respiratory rate 30/min. An electrocardiogram (ECG) demonstrated a large anterior myocardial infarct. The results of acid–base analyses were as follows:

	Blood gas analyses	Reference range
[H+] (nmol/L)	39	36–44
Pco$_2$ (kPa)	2	4.4–6.1
[HCO$_3^-$] (mmol/L)	9.4	21.0–27.5
Po$_2$ (kPa)	7	12–15

What is his acid–base status, and what may have caused it?

Comments on Case 3.6

He has a combination of a metabolic acidosis (causing elevated H+, and low Pco$_2$), and a respiratory alkalosis (causing low H+ and low Pco$_2$). The combination explains the normal H+ with the very low Pco$_2$. The metabolic acidosis could be due to diabetic ketoacidosis (caused by inappropriately stopping his insulin in the face of his severe illness) and/or to lactic acidosis (caused by impaired tissue perfusion because of his circulatory failure). The respiratory alkalosis is due to hyperventilation, caused by pulmonary oedema and/or hypoxia and/or anxiety.

CHAPTER 4

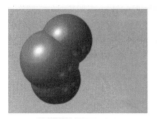

Renal Disease

Tests of glomerular function, 51   Renal handling of sodium and   Renal failure, 59
Tests of tubular function, 55   potassium, 58   Proteinuria, 61
                                                                                                  Renal stones, 63

Many diseases affect renal function. In some, several functions are affected; in others, there is selective impairment of glomerular function or of one or more tubular functions.

In this chapter, we discuss the use of chemical tests to investigate glomerular and tubular function. In general, chemical tests are mainly of value in detecting the presence of renal disease by its effects on renal function, and in assessing its progress. They are of less value in determining the causes of disease.

Tests of glomerular function

The glomerular filtration rate (GFR) depends on the net pressure across the glomerular membrane, the physical nature of the membrane and its surface area, which in turn reflects the number of functioning glomeruli. All three factors may be modified by disease, but in the absence of large changes in filtration pressure or in the structure of the glomerular membrane, the GFR provides a useful index of the numbers of functioning glomeruli. It gives an estimate of the degree of renal impairment by disease.

Accurate measurement of the GFR by clearance tests requires determination of the concentrations, in plasma and urine, of a substance that is filtered at the glomerulus, but which is neither reabsorbed nor secreted by the tubules; its concentration in plasma needs to remain constant throughout the period of

urine collection. It is convenient if the substance is present endogenously, and important for it to be readily measured. Its clearance is given by:

$$\text{Clearance} = U.V/P$$

where U is the concentration in urine, V is the volume of urine produced per minute, and P is the concentration in plasma.

Inulin meets these criteria, apart from the fact that it is not an endogenous compound, but needs to be administered by intravenous infusion. This makes it impractical for routine clinical use.

Creatinine clearance or plasma [creatinine]?

Creatinine meets some of the criteria above. It is freely filtered, but its concentration may not remain constant over the period of urine collection, it is secreted by the tubules and its measurement in plasma is subject to analytical overestimation. In practice, the effects of tubular secretion and analytical overestimation tend to cancel each other out at normal levels of GFR, and the creatinine clearance is a fair approximation to the GFR. As the GFR falls progressively, however, creatinine clearance deviates further and further from the true GFR.

Creatinine clearance is usually about 110 mL/min in the 20–40 year-old age-group. Thereafter, it falls slowly but progressively to about 70 mL/min in people over eighty. In children, the GFR should be related to surface area; when this is done, results are similar to those found in young adults.

Measurement of plasma [creatinine] is more precise than creatinine clearance, as there are two extra sources of imprecision in clearance measurements, i.e. timed measurement of urine volume and urine [creatinine]. Accuracy of urine collections is very dependent on patients' co-operation and the care with which the procedure has been explained or supervised; inaccuracies of 20–30% are not uncommon in the timed collection of urine specimens. The combination of these errors causes an imprecision (1 standard deviation, SD) of about 10% under ideal conditions with 'good' collectors; this increases to 20–30% under less ideal conditions.

It will be apparent that creatinine clearance measurements are potentially unreliable. Although creatinine clearance measurements are commonly made, accurate measurement of GFR is not often required. Indications for its measurement include determining the dose of a number of potentially toxic drugs that are cleared from the body by renal excretion, investigation of patients with minor abnormali-

ties of renal function, and assessment of possible kidney donors.

If endogenous production of creatinine remains constant, the amount of it excreted in the urine each day becomes constant and the plasma [creatinine] will then be inversely proportional to creatinine clearance. The consequence of the form of this relationship is that a raised plasma [creatinine] is a good indicator of impaired renal function, but a normal [creatinine] does not necessarily indicate normal renal function (Fig. 4.1). In most circumstances, however, assessment of glomerular function can be made and changes in GFR over time can be monitored, biochemically, by measurement of plasma [creatinine] rather than by measurement of creatinine clearance, because:

• Plasma [creatinine] normally remains fairly constant throughout adult life, whereas creatinine clearance declines with advancing age.

• Plasma [creatinine] correlates as well with GFR, as does creatinine clearance in patients with renal disease.

• Measurements of plasma [creatinine] are as effective in detecting early renal disease as creatinine clearance.

• Plasma [creatinine] measurements enable

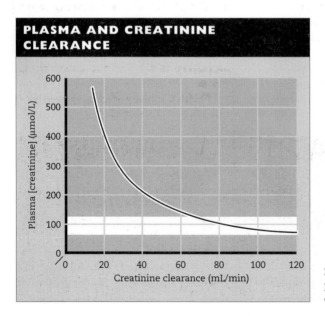

PLASMA AND CREATININE CLEARANCE

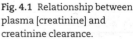

Fig. 4.1 Relationship between plasma [creatinine] and creatinine clearance.

the progress of renal disease to be followed with better precision than creatinine clearance.

Plasma creatinine

Creatine is synthesized in the liver, kidneys and pancreas, and is transported to its sites of usage, principally muscle and brain. About 1–2% of the total muscle creatine pool is converted daily to creatinine through the spontaneous, non-enzymatic loss of water. Creatinine is an end-product of nitrogen metabolism, and as such undergoes no further metabolism, but is excreted in the urine. Creatinine production reflects the body's total muscle mass.

Creatinine in the plasma is filtered freely at the glomerulus. A small amount of this undergoes tubular reabsorption. A larger amount, up to 10% of urinary creatinine, is secreted into the urine by the tubules.

The reference range of serum [creatinine] in adults is 55–120 μmol/L. However, individual subjects maintain their [creatinine] within much tighter limits than this. This means that a progressive rise in serial creatinine measurements, even within the reference range, can indicate impaired renal function.

Low plasma [creatinine] (Table 4.1)

A low [creatinine] is found in subjects with a small total muscle mass. A low plasma [creati-nine] may therefore be found in children, and values are, on average, normally lower in women than in men. Abnormally low values may be found in wasting diseases and starvation, and in patients treated with corticosteroids, due to their protein catabolic effect. Creatinine synthesis is increased in pregnancy, but this is more than offset by the combined effects of the retention of fluid and the physiological rise in GFR that occur in pregnancy, so plasma [creatinine] is usually low.

High plasma [creatinine] (Table 4.1)

Plasma [creatinine] tends to be higher in subjects with a large muscle mass. Other nonrenal causes of increased plasma [creatinine] include:
• A high meat intake can cause a temporary increase.
• Transient, small increases may occur after vigorous exercise.
• Some analytical methods are not specific for creatinine. For example, plasma [creatinine] will be overestimated using some methods in the presence of high concentrations of acetoacetate or cephalosporin antibiotics.
• Some drugs (e.g. salicylates, cimetidine) compete with creatinine for the tubular transport mechanism, thereby reducing tubular secretion of creatinine and elevating plasma [creatinine].

If non-renal causes can be excluded, the finding of an increased plasma [creatinine] indicates a fall in GFR. The renal causes of this include:
• Any disease in which there is impaired renal

Table 4.1 Causes of an abnormal plasma [creatinine].

ABNORMAL PLASMA [CREATININE]

Reduced plasma [creatinine]	
Physiological	Pregnancy
Pathological	Reduced muscle bulk (e.g. starvation, wasting diseases, steroid therapy)
Increased plasma [creatinine]	
No pathological significance	High meat intake, strenuous exercise
	Drug effects (e.g. salicylates)
	Analytical interference (e.g. due to cephalosporin antibiotics)
Pathological	Renal causes, i.e. any cause (acute or chronic) of a reduced GFR

perfusion (e.g. reduced blood pressure, fluid depletion, renal artery stenosis).

• Most diseases in which there is loss of functioning nephrons (e.g. acute and chronic glomerulonephritis).

• Diseases where pressure is increased on the tubular side of the nephron (e.g. urinary tract obstruction due to prostatic enlargement).

Plasma urea

Urea is formed in the liver from ammonia released by deamination of amino acids. Over 75% of non-protein nitrogen is excreted as urea, mainly by the kidneys; small amounts are lost through the skin and the gastrointestinal (GI) tract. Urea measurements are widely available, and have come to be accepted as giving a measure of renal function. However, as a test of renal function, plasma [urea] is inferior to plasma [creatinine], since 50% or more of urea filtered at the glomerulus is passively reabsorbed through the tubules, and this fraction increases if urine flow rate decreases, such as in dehydration.

High plasma [urea] (Table 4.2)

It is convenient to subdivide the causes of a high plasma [urea] into prerenal, renal and postrenal.

Prerenal uraemia may develop whenever there is impaired renal perfusion, and is essentially the result of a physiological response to

hypovolaemia or a drop in blood pressure. This causes renal vasoconstriction and a redistribution of blood such that there is a decrease in GFR, but preservation of tubular function. Stimulation of vasopressin secretion and of the renin–angiotensin–aldosterone system causes the excretion of small volumes of concentrated urine with a low Na content. This reduced urine flow in turn causes increased passive tubular reabsorption of urea. Thus shock, due to burns, haemorrhage or loss of water and electrolytes (e.g. severe diarrhoea), may lead to increased plasma [urea]. Renal blood flow also falls in congestive cardiac failure, and may be further reduced if such patients are treated with potent diuretics. If prerenal uraemia is not treated adequately and promptly by restoring renal perfusion, it can progress to intrinsic renal failure.

Increased production of urea in the liver occurs on high protein diets, or as a result of increased protein catabolism (e.g. due to trauma, major surgery, extreme starvation). It may also occur after haemorrhage into the upper GI tract, which gives rise to a 'protein meal' of blood.

Plasma [urea] increases relatively more than plasma [creatinine] in pre-renal uraemia. This is because tubular reabsorption of urea is increased significantly in these patients, whereas relatively little reabsorption of creatinine occurs.

Renal uraemia may be due to acute or chronic renal failure, with reduction in

Table 4.2 Causes of an abnormal plasma [urea].

ABNORMAL PLASMA [UREA]	
Reduced plasma [urea]	Low protein diet, severe liver disease, water retention
Increased plasma [urea]	
Prerenal causes	High protein diet, GI haemorrhage ('meal' of blood)
	Any cause of increased protein catabolism (e.g. trauma, surgery, extreme starvation)
	Any cause of impaired renal perfusion (e.g. ECF losses, cardiac failure, hypoproteinaemia)
Renal causes	Any cause (acute or chronic) of a reduced GFR
Postrenal causes	Any cause of obstruction to urine outflow (e.g. benign prostatic hypertrophy, malignant stricture or obstruction, stone)

glomerular filtration. Plasma [urea] increases until a new steady state is reached at which urea production equals the amount excreted in the urine, or continues to rise in the face of near-total renal failure. Although frequently measured as a test of renal function, it is always important to remember that plasma [urea] may be increased for reasons other than intrinsic renal disease (prerenal and postrenal uraemia).

Postrenal uraemia occurs due to outflow obstruction, which may occur at different levels (i.e. in the ureter, bladder or urethra), due to various causes (e.g. renal stones, prostatism, genitourinary cancer). Back-pressure on the renal tubules enhances back-diffusion of urea, so that plasma [urea] rises disproportionately more than plasma [creatinine].

Impaired renal perfusion and urinary tract obstruction, each in themselves possible causes of uraemia, may in turn cause damage to the kidney and thus cause renal uraemia.

Low plasma [urea] (Table 4.2)

Less urea is synthesized in the liver if there is reduced availability of amino acids for deamination, as may occur in starvation or malabsorption. However, in extreme starvation plasma [urea] may rise as increased muscle protein breakdown then provides the major source of fuel. In patients with severe liver disease (usually chronic), urea synthesis may be impaired leading to a fall in plasma [urea].

Plasma [urea] may fall as a result of water retention associated with inappropriate vasopressin secretion or dilution of plasma with intravenous fluids.

Tests of tubular function

Specific disorders affecting the renal tubules may affect the ability to concentrate urine or to excrete an appropriately acidic urine, or may cause impaired reabsorption of amino acids, or glucose, or phosphate, etc. In some conditions these defects occur singly; in others, multiple defects are present. Renal tubular disorders may be congenital or acquired, the congenital disorders all being very rare. Chemical investigations are needed for specific identification of these abnormalities and may include amino acid chromatography, or investigation of calcium and phosphate metabolism (Chapter 5), or an oral glucose tolerance test (p. 152). The functions tested most often are renal concentrating power and the ability to produce an acid urine.

The healthy kidney has a considerable reserve capacity for reabsorbing water, and for excreting H^+ and other ions, only exceeded under exceptional physiological loads. Moderate impairment of renal function may reduce this reserve, and this is revealed when loading tests are used to stress the kidney. Tubular function tests are only used when there is reason to suspect that a specific abnormality is present.

Urine osmolality and renal concentration tests

Urine osmolality varies widely in health, between 50 and 1250 mmol/kg, depending upon the body's requirement to produce a maximally dilute or a maximally concentrated urine.

The failing kidney loses its capacity to concentrate urine at a relatively late stage. A patient with polyuria due to chronic renal failure is unable to produce either a dilute or a concentrated urine. Instead, urine osmolality is generally within 50 mmol/kg of the plasma osmolality (i.e. between about 240 and 350 mmol/kg). This has important implications. To excrete the obligatory daily solute load of about 600 mmol requires approximately two litres of water at a maximum urine osmolality of 350 mmol/kg, compared to 500 mL of the most concentrated urine achieved by the normal kidney. Hence, patients with chronic renal disease require a daily water intake of at least two litres to maintain their water balance. On the other hand, a large intake of water can lead to dangerous hyponatraemia, since water excretion is limited by the inability to produce a sufficiently dilute urine.

Urine osmolality is directly proportional to the osmotic work done by the kidney, and is the correct measure of concentrating power. Urine specific gravity, which can be estimated using urinalysis dipsticks, is usually directly proportional to osmolality, but gives spuriously high results if there is significant glycosuria or proteinuria.

Renal concentration tests are not normally required in patients with established chronic renal failure, and indeed may be positively dangerous. However, the tests may be indicated in patients with polyuria in whom common causes (e.g. diabetes mellitus) have first been excluded. In a number of conditions, the kidney loses its ability to maintain medullary hyperosmolality, and hence to excrete a concentrated urine, but these should have been excluded before renal concentration tests are performed. Causes of failure to concentrate urine are shown in Table 4.3.

In cases of polyuria, measurement of the osmolality of early morning urine specimens, or of several specimens passed during the day, should be made before proceeding to formal concentration tests. If urinary osmolality greater than 800 mmol/kg (or specific gravity more than 1.020) is observed in any specimen, as should be the case in most patients who can concentrate urine normally, there is no point in

Table 4.3 Causes of failure to concentrate urine.

performing further tests of concentrating ability.

Formal tests of renal concentrating power measure the concentration of urine produced in response either to fluid deprivation or to intramuscular injection of 1-deamino,8-D-arginine vasopressin (DDAVP), a synthetic analogue of the vasopressin. If the patient is receiving drugs that affect the renal concentrating ability (e.g. carbamazepine, chlorpropamide, DDAVP), these should be stopped for at least 48 h before testing. A fluid deprivation test is performed first. Then, if the patient is unable to concentrate the urine adequately following fluid deprivation, a DDAVP test follows on immediately.

Fluid deprivation test

This test is effectively a bioassay of vasopressin, which is difficult to measure itself. The test can be hazardous in a patient excreting large volumes of dilute urine, and requires close supervision. There are a number of ways of performing a fluid deprivation test, differing in detail but all involving fluid deprivation over several hours, with the patient under observation to ensure that no fluid is taken, and that excessive fluid losses do not occur. Local directions for test performance should be followed. For instance, beginning at 10 p.m., the patient is told not to drink overnight, and urine specimens are collected whilst the patient continues not to drink between 8 a.m. and 3 p.m. the next

FAILURE TO CONCENTRATE URINE

Causal mechanism	Examples of causes
Insufficient secretion of vasopressin	Lesions of the supra-optic–hypothalamic–hypophyseal tract (e.g. trauma, neoplasm)
Inhibition of vasopressin release	Psychogenic polydipsia, lesions of the thirst centre causing polydipsia
Inability to maintain renal medullary hyperosmolality	Chronic renal failure, hydronephrosis, lithium toxicity, hypokalaemia, hypercalcaemia, renal papillary necrosis (e.g. analgesic nephropathy)
Inability to respond to vasopressin	Renal tubular defects (e.g. nephrogenic diabetes insipidus, Fanconi's syndrome)
Increased solute load per nephron	Chronic renal failure, diabetes mellitus

day. During the test, the patient should be weighed every two hours, and the test should be stopped if weight loss of 3–5% occurs. Blood and urine specimens are collected for measurement of osmolality.

Normally, there is no increase in plasma osmolality (reference range 285–295 mmol/kg) over the period of water deprivation, whereas urine osmolality rises to 800 mmol/kg or more. A rising plasma osmolality and a failure to concentrate urine are consistent with either a failure to secrete vasopressin or a failure to respond to vasopressin at the level of the distal nephron. When this pattern of results is obtained, it is usual to proceed immediately to perform the DDAVP test.

DDAVP test

The patient is allowed a moderate amount of water to drink at the end of the fluid deprivation test, to alleviate thirst. An intramuscular injection of DDAVP is then given, and urine specimens are collected at hourly intervals for a further three hours and their osmolality measured.

Interpretation of tests of renal concentrating ability

These tests are of most value in distinguishing between hypothalamic–pituitary, psychogenic and renal causes of polyuria (Table 4.3).

Patients with diabetes insipidus of hypothalamic–pituitary origin produce insufficient vasopressin; they should therefore respond to the DDAVP test, but not to fluid deprivation. As a rule, these patients show an increase in plasma osmolality during the fluid deprivation test, to more than 300 mmol/kg, and a low urine osmolality (200–400 mmol/kg). There is a marked increase in urine osmolality, to 600 mmol/kg or more, in the DDAVP test.

Patients with psychogenic diabetes insipidus should respond to both fluid deprivation and to DDAVP. In practice, however, renal medullary hypo-osmolality often prevents the urine osmolality from reaching 800 mmol/kg after fluid deprivation or DDAVP injection in these tests, as normally performed. Also, the chronic suppression of the physiological mechanism that controls vasopressin release may impair the normal hypothalamic response to dehydration. These patients have a plasma osmolality that is initially low, but which rises during the tests. However, fluid deprivation may have to be continued for more than 24 hours in these patients before medullary hyperosmolality is restored; only then do they show normal responses to fluid deprivation or to DDAVP injection.

Polyuria of renal origin may be due to inability of the renal tubule to respond to vasopressin, as in nephrogenic diabetes insipidus. In this condition, there is failure to produce a concentrated urine in response either to fluid deprivation or to DDAVP injection, the urinary osmolality usually remaining below 400 mmol/kg; in these patients, plasma osmolality increases as a result of fluid deprivation.

Urinary acidification tests

Urine is normally acidic, compared to plasma, in healthy subjects on a meat-containing diet. An alkaline urine may be found in vegans, in patients ingesting alkali, or in patients with urinary tract infections. Urinalysis using dipsticks can be used to give a rough estimate of urine pH over the range 5–9. It is important to measure urine pH on freshly voided urine specimens.

Urine acidification is a function of the distal nephron, which can secrete H^+ until the limiting intraluminal pH of approximately 5.0 or less is reached. Acidification occurs as a result of the kidney reabsorbing the large amounts of the HCO_3^- that were filtered at the glomerulus, and excreting H^+ produced as nonvolatile acids during tissue metabolism. The amount of H^+ that can be secreted into the tubules before the limiting intraluminal pH is reached depends on the presence of urine buffers. The H^+ in urine is only partly eliminated as such, and it is mostly excreted as H^+ combined with buffer ions, principally inorganic phosphate (Figs 3.1, 3.2) or with ammonia as NH_4^+.

It is possible to assess the capacity of the kidney to produce an acid urine after a metabolic acidosis has been induced by administering ammonium chloride (NH_4Cl). In response to the NH_4Cl load, urine pH normally falls to below 5.3 in at least one specimen. It is essential to check that a satisfactory acidosis was induced, and this is assumed to have occurred if plasma [total CO_2] falls by about 4 mmol/L after NH_4Cl ingestion. More elaborate tests of urinary acidification (e.g. determining the renal threshold for HCO_3^-) are needed to differentiate between proximal and distal renal tubular acidosis.

Renal tubular acidosis

At least two distinct tubular abnormalities may give rise to conditions in which there is acidosis of renal origin but little or no change in plasma [creatinine], or other measure of the GFR.

Distal renal tubular acidosis (type I) is the more common type. It is due to an inability to maintain a gradient of [H^+] across the distal tubule and collecting ducts. It is usually caused by an inherited abnormality, but may occur in certain forms of acquired renal disease. Bone disease, commonly osteomalacia, results from the buffering of H^+ by bone, and there is often hypercalciuria and nephrocalcinosis. Loss of Na^+ and K^+ in the urine and hypokalaemia are common. Urinary pH rarely falls below 6.0 and never below 5.3 in the ammonium chloride test of urinary acidification.

Proximal renal tubular acidosis (Type II) is much less common. It is due to proximal tubular loss of HCO_3^- caused by a low renal threshold for HCO_3^-. Occasionally, this is an isolated abnormality. More often, it occurs as one of the features in some patients with Fanconi's syndrome (see below). If these patients are given enough NH_4Cl to reduce plasma [total CO_2] below the renal threshold for HCO_3^-, urinary pH may fall below 5.3. Diagnosis requires assessment of the renal threshold for HCO_3^-.

The amino acidurias

There are four groups of acids – the neutral, acidic and basic amino acids, and the imino acids proline and hydroxyproline. Each has its own specific mechanism for transport across the proximal tubular cell. Normally, the renal tubules reabsorb all the filtered amino acids except for small amounts of glycine, serine, alanine and glutamine. Amino aciduria may be due to disease of the renal tubule (renal or low threshold type), or to raised plasma [amino acids] (generalized or overflow type).

Renal amino aciduria may be due to impairment of one of the specific transport mechanisms. For example, in cystinuria there is a hereditary defect in the epithelial transport of cystine and the basic amino acids lysine, ornithine and arginine; it is a rare cause of renal (cystine) stones. Renal amino aciduria may also occur as a nonspecific abnormality due to generalized tubular damage, together with reabsorption defects affecting glucose or phosphate, or both.

The overflow types of amino aciduria result when the renal threshold for amino acids is exceeded, due to overproduction or to accumulation of amino acids in the body (e.g. phenylketonuria, p. 250; acute hepatic necrosis).

Fanconi's syndrome is a syndrome that may be inherited or secondary to a number of other disorders (e.g. heavy metal poisoning, multiple myeloma). The syndrome comprises multiple defects of proximal tubular function. There are excessive urinary losses of amino acids (generalized amino aciduria), phosphate, glucose and sometimes HCO_3^-, which gives rise to a proximal renal tubular acidosis. Distal tubular functions may also be affected. Sometimes globulins of low molecular mass may be detectable in urine, in addition to the amino aciduria. One of the inherited causes of Fanconi's syndrome is cystinosis.

Renal handling of sodium and potassium

Sodium excretion

The kidneys are essential for maintaining sodium balance, normally filtering about 21 000 mmol Na+/day. On a diet of 100 mmol Na+, and in the absence of any pathological loss of Na+, the kidney matches this intake with an excretion of 100 mmol Na+, which represents about 0.5% of the filtered Na+ load.

As the GFR declines in chronic renal failure, the proportion of the filtered Na+ that is excreted needs to increase progressively to maintain Na+ balance. The limit cannot generally exceed 20–30% of the filtered Na+ load. Once this is reached, any further reduction in GFR, or an increase in dietary Na+, leads to Na+ retention. Most patients with chronic renal failure tolerate normal levels of dietary Na+ if the GFR is more than 10 mL/min. However, if the GFR falls below this level, Na+ retention occurs, leading to expansion of the extracellular fluid (ECF), weight gain and worsening hypertension. In the presence of other Na+-retaining states (e.g. congestive cardiac failure or cirrhosis), Na+ retention will be even more pronounced. Treatment depends upon Na+ restriction and careful use of diuretic therapy.

Excessive Na+ loss may also occur in chronic renal failure. The kidneys' capacity to adapt to changes in Na+ intake is limited, and a requirement to conserve Na+ (e.g. in response to excessive use of diuretics or if the patient has severe diarrhoea) may not be met by the damaged kidneys. This leads on to a further fall in GFR. In chronic pyelonephritis and other disorders primarily affecting the renal tubules, large amounts of Na+ may be lost in the urine, and severe Na+ and water depletion can occur.

Potassium excretion

About 90% of K+ in the glomerular filtrate is normally reabsorbed in the proximal tubules, the distal tubules regulating the amount of K+ excreted in the urine. The rate of secretion of K+ by the distal tubules is influenced by the transtubular potential and by the tubular cell [K+], and is usually maintained adequately, provided the daily urine flow rate is greater than one litre.

In the presence of a normal GFR, about 550 mmol K+ are filtered daily at the glomerulus.

An average dietary intake of K+ is about 80 mmol/day, and external K+ balance is normally achieved by excreting about 15% of the filtered K+. A reduction in GFR to about 10 mL/min requires an increase in the proportion of the filtered K+ that is excreted to 150%. Distal tubular secretion of K+ is needed to achieve this. Generally, the normal daily intake of K+ can be tolerated if the GFR is 10 mL/min. At a GFR of about 5 mL/min, however, the limit of adaptation is reached, leading to K+ retention and hyperkalaemia. The ability of the GI tract to increase excretion of K+ helps to delay the onset of hyperkalaemia.

Excessive renal losses of K+ rarely occur in chronic renal disease, but the Na+ depletion that sometimes develops in renal disease may be associated with secondary aldosteronism, which in turn causes excessive loss of K+.

Measurement of urinary K+ output can prove very helpful in patients suspected of losing abnormal amounts of K+. Persistence of a relatively high urinary K+ output in the presence of hypokalaemia strongly suggests that the kidney is unable to conserve K+ adequately.

Renal failure

Acute renal failure

By definition, there is renal disease of acute onset, severe enough to cause failure of renal homeostasis. Often oliguric, diuretic and recovery phases can be recognized, although a few patients maintain a normal urine volume throughout the course of the illness. Chemical investigations help to determine the severity of the disease and to follow its course, but do not help much in determining the cause. Proteinuria is present, and haem pigments from the blood may make the urine dark.

Oliguric phase

Less than 400 mL urine is produced each day; there may be anuria in renal failure due to outflow obstruction. The oliguria is mainly due to a fall in GFR. The urine that is formed usually has an osmolality similar to plasma and a relatively high [Na$^+$], since the composition of the small amount of glomerular filtrate produced is little altered by the damaged tubules.

Plasma [Na$^+$] is usually low due to a combination of factors, including intake of water in excess of the amount able to be excreted, increase in metabolic water from increased tissue catabolism, and a shift of Na$^+$ from ECF to intracellular fluid (ICF). Plasma [K$^+$], on the other hand, is usually increased due to the impaired renal output and increased tissue catabolism, aggravated by the shift of K$^+$ out of cells that accompanies the metabolic acidosis which develops due to failure to excrete H$^+$ and to the increased formation of H$^+$ from tissue catabolism.

Retention of urea, creatinine, phosphate, sulphate and other waste products occurs. The rate at which plasma [urea] rises is affected by the rate of tissue catabolism; this, in turn, depends on the cause of the acute renal failure. In renal failure due to trauma (including renal failure developing after surgical operations), plasma [urea] tends to rise more rapidly than in patients with renal failure due to medical causes such as acute glomerulonephritis.

To differentiate the low urinary output of suspected acute renal failure from that due to severe circulatory impairment with reduced blood volume, the tests summarized in Table 4.4 may be helpful. However, none of these tests can be completely relied upon to make the important and urgent distinction between renal failure and hypovolaemia. Careful assessment of the patient's fluid status, possibly including measurement of the central venous pressure, is also required.

For monitoring patients in the oliguric phase of acute renal failure, plasma [creatinine] or [urea] and plasma [K$^+$] are particularly important, and need to be determined at least once daily. Decisions to use haemodialysis are reached at least partly on the basis of the results of these tests. The volume of urine and its electrolyte composition (and the volume and composition of any other measurable sources of fluid loss) should also be assessed in order to determine fluid and electrolyte replacement requirements.

Diuretic phase

With the onset of this phase, urine volume increases, but the clearance of urea, creatinine and other waste products may not improve to the same extent. Plasma [urea] and [creatinine] may therefore continue to rise, at least at the start of the diuretic phase. Large losses of electrolytes may occur in the urine and require to be replaced orally or parenterally. Measurement of these losses is needed so that correct replacement therapy can be given; this requires urine collections, for urine [Na$^+$] and [K$^+$] measurement, and calculation of daily outputs.

Plasma [K$^+$] tends to fall as the diuretic phase continues, due to the shift of K$^+$ back into the cells and to marked losses in urine resulting from impaired conservation of K$^+$ by the still-damaged tubules. Usually, Na$^+$ deficiency occurs also, due to failure of renal conservation. Throughout the diuretic phase, therefore, it is important to measure plasma [creatinine] or [urea] and both plasma [Na$^+$] and [K$^+$] at least once daily, and to monitor the output of Na$^+$ and K$^+$ in the urine.

Table 4.4 Investigation of low urinary output.

LOW URINARY OUTPUT		
Investigation	Simple hypovolaemia	Acute renal failure
Urine osmolality	Usually > 500 mmol/kg	Usually < 400 mmol/kg
Urine [urea] : plasma [urea]	Usually > 10	Usually < 5
Urine [Na$^+$]	Usually < 20 mmol/L	Usually > 40 mmol/L

Chronic renal failure

Most of the functional changes seen in chronic renal failure can be explained in terms of a full solute load falling on a reduced number of normal nephrons. The GFR is invariably reduced, associated with retention of urea, creatinine, urate, various phenolic and indolic acids, and other organic substances. The progress and severity of the disease are usually monitored by measuring plasma [creatinine] or [urea], or both.

Sodium, potassium and water

The renal handling of Na^+, K^+ and water by normal kidneys and in chronic renal failure has already been considered above (p. 58).

Acid–base disturbances

The total excretion of H^+ is impaired, mainly due to a fall in the renal capacity to form NH_4^+. Metabolic acidosis is present in most patients, but its severity remains fairly stable in spite of the reduced urinary H^+ excretion. There may be an extrarenal mechanism for H^+ elimination, possibly involving buffering of H^+ by calcium salts in bone; this would contribute to the demineralization of bone that often occurs in chronic renal failure.

Calcium and phosphate

Plasma [calcium] tends to be low, often due at least partly to reduced plasma [albumin]. Plasma [phosphate] is high, mainly due to the reduction of GFR.

Virtually all patients with chronic renal failure have secondary or, much less often, tertiary hyperparathyroidism, and they may develop osteitis fibrosa. Plasma [calcium], which is decreased or close to the lower reference value in patients with secondary hyperparathyroidism, increases later if tertiary hyperparathyroidism develops. Many patients with a low plasma [calcium] have reduced activity of renal cholecalciferol 1α-hydroxylase and develop osteomalacia or rickets. A few patients show a third type of bone abnormality, with increased bone density (osteosclerosis). It is not clear why any particular one of these various types of renal osteodystrophy should develop in an individual patient (p. 81).

Other metabolic abnormalities

Other findings in chronic renal failure may include impaired glucose tolerance and raised plasma [magnesium]. These are of no particular diagnostic significance.

Proteinuria

Glomerular filtrate normally contains about 30 mg/L protein; this corresponds to a total filtered load of about 5 g/24 h. Since less than 200 mg protein is normally excreted in the urine each day (half of which is Tamm–Horsfall mucoprotein, secreted by tubular cells), tubular reabsorption and catabolism are very efficient in health.

Proteinuria is described as glomerular proteinuria if the glomerulus becomes abnormally leaky, or as tubular proteinuria when tubular reabsorption of protein becomes defective. Abnormally large amounts of some plasma proteins may lead to an overflow proteinuria. Protein may also enter the urinary tract distal to the kidneys (e.g. due to inflammation), leading to postrenal proteinuria; if postrenal proteinuria is suspected, urine microscopy (including cytology) and culture should be carried out. Electrophoresis of a concentrated urine specimen may help to distinguish these forms of proteinuria. In tubular proteinuria, the proteins are mainly of low molecular weight, having been filtered through the glomerulus but not reabsorbed. In glomerular proteinuria, larger proteins that have filtered through the defective glomeruli are also present.

Side-room testing of urine for protein should be part of the full clinical examination of every patient. Dipstick tests for urine protein detect albumin at concentrations greater than 200 mg/L, but are less sensitive to other proteins, and in particular fail to detect the Bence Jones proteins that may be excreted in multiple myeloma. If the presence of proteinuria is confirmed, it should be quantified in a timed (usually 24-hour) urine collection, and simple tests of renal function performed. If the renal function tests are normal and the protein excretion is less than about 500 mg/24 h, it is probably not necessary to subject the patient to further investigation, although follow-up should be arranged. If the protein excretion is greater than this, or renal function is impaired, further investigation is necessary, and may include imaging techniques and biopsy.

Overflow proteinuria

Several conditions may give rise to abnormal amounts of low molecular mass proteins (i.e. less than about 70 kDa) in plasma and in urine. These proteins are filtered at the glomerulus and may then be neither reabsorbed nor catabolized completely by the renal tubular cells. The principal examples are listed in Table 4.5.

Glomerular proteinuria

Table 4.6 classifies glomerular proteinuria separately from tubular proteinuria, but many patients show features of both glomerular and tubular protein loss. Where quantitative measurements of urine protein loss are required (e.g. when monitoring treatment for the nephrotic syndrome), side-room tests are insufficiently precise; 24-hour collections of urine should be examined in the laboratory.

Some patients, typically with protein excretion rates of less than 1 g/24 h, have benign or functional proteinuria. This probably results from blood flow changes through the glomeruli, and is found in association with exercise, fever and congestive cardiac failure. Amongst these conditions, it is particularly important to recognize orthostatic proteinuria.

Nephrotic syndrome

In the nephrotic syndrome, large amounts of protein are lost in the urine, and hypopro-

Table 4.5 Overflow proteinuria.

OVERFLOW PROTEINURIA		
Protein	Molecular mass (kDa)	Cause
Amylase	45	Acute pancreatitis
Bence Jones protein	44	Multiple myeloma
Haemoglobin	68	Intravascular haemolysis
Lysozyme	15	Myelomonocytic leukaemia
Myoglobin	17	Crush injuries

GLOMERULAR AND TUBULAR PROTEINURIA	
Classification	Examples of causes
Glomerular proteinuria	
May or may not be of pathological significance	Orthostatic proteinuria, effort proteinuria, febrile proteinuria
Pathological significance	Glomerulonephritis, all forms; pathological causes of altered haemodynamics (e.g. renal artery stenosis)
Tubular proteinuria	Chronic nephritis and pyelonephritis, acute tubular necrosis, renal tubule defects (e.g. renal tubular acidosis), heavy metal poisoning, renal transplantation

Table 4.6 Glomerular and tubular proteinuria.

teinaemia and oedema (due to the low [albumin] and secondary hyperaldosteronism) develop. Usually, the protein losses in the urine are over 5 g/24 h. More than this is filtered at the glomerulus, but most is catabolized in the tubules and is therefore lost from the circulation, but does not appear in the urine. The amount of proteinuria does not correlate well with the severity of the renal disease. Patients with nephrotic syndrome may also have a secondary hyperlipidaemia.

Causes of nephrotic syndrome include glomerulonephritis, systemic lupus erythematosus and diabetic nephropathy.

Glomerulonephritis

This is the commonest group of causes of persistent proteinuria. Plasma proteins escape in varying amounts, depending on their molecular mass, on the amount of glomerular damage, and on the capacity of the renal tubule cells to reabsorb or metabolize the proteins that have passed the glomerulus.

The degree of proteinuria does not provide an index of the severity of renal disease. However, it is convenient to distinguish mild or moderate proteinuria, in which the loss is not sufficient to cause protein depletion, from severe proteinuria, in which the protein loss exceeds the body's capacity to replace losses by synthesis (usually 5–10 g/24 h). Severe, persistent proteinuria is one feature of the nephrotic syndrome, in which urinary protein loss is sometimes more than 30 g/24 h.

Orthostatic proteinuria

This is usually a benign condition that affects children and young adults, who exhibit proteinuria only after they have been standing up. For orthostatic (or postural) proteinuria to be diagnosed, protein is not detectable in an early morning urine specimen when tested by normal side-room methods (i.e. urine contains less than 100 mg/L). The patient is instructed to empty the bladder just before going to bed, and the test for protein is performed on a specimen of urine passed the following morning, collected immediately after getting up.

Orthostatic proteinuria is usually observed in only some of the urine specimens passed when up and about. For these individuals the prognosis is good, but it is less good for those in whom proteinuria is always detected when they are up and about.

Tubular proteinuria

This may be due to tubular or interstitial damage resulting from a variety of causes. The proteinuria is due to failure of the tubules to reabsorb some of the plasma proteins filtered by the normal glomerulus, or possibly due to abnormal secretion of protein into the urinary tract. The proteins excreted in tubular proteinuria mostly have a low molecular mass, e.g. β_2-microglobulin (11.8 kDa) and lysozyme (15 kDa). The loss of protein is usually mild, rarely more than 2 g/24 h.

Urinary β_2-microglobulin excretion is normally very small (under 0.4 mg/24 h). Its measurement has been used as a sensitive test of renal tubular damage. The test is of limited value for this purpose, however, if there is evidence of impaired renal function, e.g. increased plasma [creatinine].

Renal stones

Physicochemical principles govern the formation of renal stones, and are relevant to the choice of treatment aimed at preventing progression or recurrence. Stones may cause renal damage, often progressive.

The solubility of a salt depends on the product of the activities of its constituent ions. Frequently, the solubility product in urine is exceeded without the formation of a stone, provided there is no 'seeding' by particles present in urine, such as debris or bacteria, which promote crystal formation. Formation of stones can also be prevented by inhibitory substances that are normally present in the urine, such as citrate, which can chelate calcium, keeping it in solution.

People living or working in hot conditions are liable to become dehydrated, and show a greater tendency to form renal stones, as the urine becomes more concentrated. There are also several metabolic factors that can cause stones to form in the renal tract. However, in many patients, no cause can be found to explain why stones have formed. The main types of renal stone are listed in Table 4.7.

Hypercalciuria

Stones in the upper renal tract occur in 5–10% of adults in western Europe and the United States. These are mostly either pure calcium oxalate or a mixture of calcium oxalate and phosphate. Not every patient with renal stones, however, has hypercalciuria, since there is considerable overlap between the 24-hour urinary calcium excretion of healthy individuals on their normal diet (up to 12 mmol/24h) and the urinary calcium excretion of stone-formers.

Increased urinary calcium excretion may be associated with hypercalcaemia, for instance in primary hyperparathyroidism (p. 76), vitamin D overdosage and hypersensitivity to vitamin D (p. 78), or with normocalcaemia, as in idiopathic hypercalciuria, prolonged immobilization, and renal tubular acidosis. In many patients with what was previously considered to be 'idiopathic' hypercalciuria, the underlying disorder is an increase in intestinal calcium absorption.

Up to 10% of renal calculi, depending on the series, have been attributed to primary hyper-

parathyroidism (p. 76). It is important to investigate patients with renal calculi for primary hyperparathyroidism, as this condition can be cured.

Oxalate, cystine and xanthine excretion

The majority of urinary calculi contain oxalate, but excessive excretion of oxalate is primarily responsible for the formation of stones in only a small percentage of cases. Other occasional causes of stone formation include cystinuria (p. 58) and xanthinuria.

Primary hyperoxaluria is a rare condition in which there is increased excretion of oxalate and of glyoxylate, the latter due to deficiency of the enzyme responsible for converting glyoxylate to glycine. Patients with disease of the terminal ileum may have an increased tendency to form oxalate stones, due to the hyperoxaluria caused by increased absorption of dietary oxalate.

Chemical investigations on patients with renal stones

Stones should be analysed for some or all of the constituents listed in Table 4.7, as this can be helpful. The following tests may also be helpful in reaching a diagnosis:

• Plasma calcium, albumin, phosphate, total CO_2 and urate concentrations, and alkaline phosphatase activity. Full acid–base assessment is rarely needed.

• Urine dipstick testing (pH and protein), and 24-hour excretion of calcium, phosphate and

Table 4.7 Renal stones.

RENAL STONES		
Type of stone	Frequency in UK (%)	Metabolic cause or relevant factors
Calcium oxalate stones and mixed (calcium oxalate and phosphate stones)	80–55	Hypercalciuria (see text), excessive absorption of dietary oxalate, primary hyperoxaluria
Triple phosphate stones	5–10	Urinary tract infection (fall in [H+])
Urate stones	5–10	Gout, myeloproliferative disorders, high-protein diet, uricosuric drugs
Cystine stones	Approx. 1	Cystinuria
Xanthine stones	<1	Xanthinuria

urate. Occasionally, urinary excretion of oxalate, cystine or xanthine may be required, or urinary acidification tests.
• Renal function tests – plasma [creatinine] and/or plasma [urea].

In addition to chemical tests, microbiological examination of urine is usually performed. Radiological investigations of the urinary tract will be required to localize the stone.

KEY POINTS

1 The glomerular filtration rate (GFR) is the best single measure of the number of functioning nephrons, and is usually estimated routinely by measuring endogenous creatinine clearance.
2 When GFR is reduced, it tends to be overestimated by creatinine clearance.
3 Plasma [creatinine] is a more precise measurement than creatinine clearance, and is usually sufficient for following the progress of patients with renal disease.
4 Plasma [urea] is a less valuable test of renal function than [creatinine], since it is reabsorbed

by the tubule at low urine flow rates, as in prerenal uraemia.
5 Fluid deprivation or urinary acidification tests of tubular function are less often used.
6 Chemical tests are of value in following the progress of both acute and chronic renal failure, but not in determining the aetiology.
7 Side-room testing for urinary protein should form a part of all full clinical examinations.
8 Renal stones have a variety of causes, but it is important to investigate for hyperparathyroidism.

Case 4.1

An elderly man was struck by a car while crossing the road, and received multiple injuries. He was admitted to hospital, where he underwent emergency surgery. After 24 hours, he was observed to be clinically dehydrated, hypotensive and only to have passed 400 mL of urine. Results of biochemical investigations were as follows:

	Plasma	Reference range
[Urea] (mmol/L)	23.2	2.5–6.6
[Na+] (mmol/L)	143	132–144
[K+] (mmol/L)	4.8	3.3–4.7
[Creatinine] (μmol/L)	225	44–120

	Urine
[Urea] (mmol/L)	492
[Na+] (mmol/L)	6
Osmolality (mmol/kg)	826

Comments on Case 4.1

The patient has prerenal uraemia due to inadequate fluid replacement. He has passed a small volume of concentrated urine that is low in sodium. This is a normal physiological response by the kidney to impaired perfusion, due in this case to hypovolaemia. The [urea] has increased relatively more than the [creatinine] due to passive tubular reabsorption, and possibly also due to increased tissue catabolism as part of the response to trauma.

The biochemical features that distinguish pre-renal uraemia from established renal failure are listed in Table 4.4, although in practice there may be some overlap. The prerequisite for using these values is the presence of oliguria, when the presence of concentrated low-sodium urine is a reliable indication of prerenal uraemia. Dilute sodium-containing urine is characteristic of intrinsic renal failure in the presence of oliguria, but is also found in well-hydrated healthy individuals. The biochemical values for making this distinction are all invalidated by the use of diuretics, and osmolalities are invalidated by the use of X-ray contrast media.

Case 4.2

A 58-year-old man, a patient with known manic depression who was being treated with lithium, was admitted to a hospital psychiatric ward with a recent history of lethargy and confusion. On examination he was found to be very dehydrated, and the results of biochemical investigations were:

	Plasma (mmol/L)	Reference range (mmol/L)
[Urea]	16.1	2.5–6.6
[Na+]	197	132–144
[K+]	3.6	3.3–4.7
[Glucose]	6.2	

Urine osmolality (mmol/kg)
209

Comments on Case 4.2

The value for the calculated plasma osmolality, using the formula given on p. 16, is 423 mmol/kg. This high value accords with the findings on clinical examination. The kidneys would have been expected to be producing a very concentrated urine, and the low urinary osmolality (lower than the plasma value) indicates either that vasopressin is not being secreted (leading to diabetes insipidus), or that the kidneys are not responding to vasopressin (nephrogenic diabetes insipidus).

It was not known whether or not the patient felt thirsty, but patients with any kind of diabetes insipidus, if unable or unwilling to respond to the thirst stimulus, rapidly become dehydrated. This patient was confused. In addition, he was on lithium treatment; lithium has a narrow therapeutic : toxic ratio, and its dosage should be reviewed periodically (p. 287). Lithium is also a known cause of nephrogenic diabetes insipidus.

Case 4.3

A previously healthy 32-year-old bricklayer was admitted to hospital in shock, with severe crush injuries to his legs caused by the collapse of a wall under which he had been trapped for several hours. The following results were obtained on specimens collected three days later:

		Urine
Volume (mL/24 h)		36
[Urea] (mmol/L)		280
[Na+] (mmol/L)		62
Osmolality (mmol/kg)		330

	Plasma	Reference range
[Urea] (mmol/L)	42	2.5–6.6
[Na+] (mmol/L)	131	132–144
[K+] (mmol/L)	6.8	3.3–4.7
[Total CO$_2$] (mmol/L)	12	24–30
Osmolality (mmol/kg)	330	280–290

Comments on Case 4.3

This man has developed acute renal failure as a result of his crush injury. The combination of hypovolaemia with the release of myoglobin from the crushed muscles has caused acute impairment of renal function, with a high plasma [urea]. The plasma [K+] is increased as a result of the acute renal failure; there might also be significant K+ leakage from damaged cells contributing to this increase. The low plasma [total CO$_2$] reflects the

Continued on p. 67

Case 4.3 continued

metabolic acidosis that is a feature of acute renal failure.

The urine volume is very low, as glomerular filtration has almost completely ceased. This low volume is accompanied by a urine with a composition inappropriate for someone who is severely volume-depleted, i.e. it is dilute and contains a relatively high [Na+]. Vasopressin and aldosterone levels would both be expected to have been high in this patient, leading to urine that was both concentrated and low in [Na+].

In general terms, the formation of a urine that is both dilute and contains relatively high [Na+], in a patient with an acute increase in plasma [urea], favours an acute failure of renal function rather than prerenal uraemia (where renal function may be intrinsically normal). A urine osmolality > 500 mmol/kg and a urine [Na+] < 20 mmol/L would tend to favour a prerenal (reversible) cause for the uraemia, whereas a urine osmolality < 400 mmol/kg and a urine [Na+] > 40 mmol/L would tend to favour a renal cause for the uraemia.

Case 4.4

A 62-year-old man visited his general practitioner and complained of malaise, tiredness and weight loss over the previous six months. His only other complaint was of passing more urine than usual, especially at night, when he had to get up three or four times. He appeared pale, and was hypertensive, with a blood pressure of 182/114. Urinalysis revealed protein, but no glucose.

The results of simple initial investigations were as follows:

Analyte	Result	Reference range
Sodium (mmol/L)	129	132–144
Potassium (mmol/L)	5.4	3.3–4.7
Urea (mmol/L)	38.2	2.5–6.6
Creatinine (mmol/L)	635	55–120
Total CO_2 (mmol/L)	17	21.0–27.5
Glucose (mmol/L)	5.2	4.0–6.0
Calcium (mmol/L)	1.88	2.12–2.62
Phosphate (mmol/L)	2.38	0.8–1.4
Alkaline phosphatase (U/L)	226	40–125
Haemoglobin (g/L)	92	135–180

Comments on Case 4.4

The lengthy history suggests the onset of a slowly progressive illness, rather than an acute one. The symptoms of weight loss, tiredness and polyuria might suggest the onset of diabetes, but the lack of glycosuria, backed up by the normal random [glucose], rules this out. The results are typical of chronic renal failure. This is supported by the anaemia and the raised alkaline phosphatase (due to renal osteodystrophy), neither of which are specific findings, but which are more consistent with chronic rather than acute renal failure. Chronic renal failure is also supported by the presence of hypertension, and by the finding of small kidneys if the patient goes on to receive an abdominal ultrasound examination.

Case 4.5

A 6-year-old boy developed marked oedema over a period of a few days, and his parents had noted that his urine had become frothy. His general practitioner detected proteinuria, and arranged admission to hospital, where the following results were obtained:

Analyte	Result	Reference range
Sodium (mmol/L)	131	132–144
Potassium (mmol/L)	4.0	3.3–4.7
Urea (mmol/L)	3.4	2.5–6.6
Creatinine (mmol/L)	48	55–120
Total CO_2 (mmol/L)	27.0	21.0–27.5
Calcium (mmol/L)	1.65	2.12–2.62
Albumin (g/L)	14	36–47
Total protein (g/L)	34	63–83
Cholesterol (mmol/L)	11	
Triglyceride (mmol/L)	15	
24-hour urine protein (g)	12	

Comments on Case 4.5

The nephrotic syndrome is the combination of oedema, hypoproteinaemia and proteinuria, as seen in this child. The oedema is the consequence of the hypoproteinaemia causing a redistribution of extracellular fluid from the vascular compartment to the interstitial fluid, often exacerbated by a consequent secondary hyperaldosteronism causing sodium retention and potassium depletion. Proteins other than albumin are also depleted, including antithrombin III, immunoglobulins and complement. Conversely, some large proteins are present in high concentrations— fibrinogen and apolipoproteins being examples. These changes can predispose patients to infection and to venous thrombosis.

In nephrotic syndrome, the GFR may be low, normal or high. In the age group of this patient, the commonest cause of nephrotic syndrome is minimal change nephropathy. The GFR is often high, as reflected by the observed low urea and creatinine. These patients usually respond satisfactorily to steroids, and the prognosis is good.

CHAPTER 5

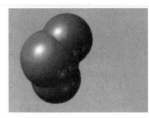

Disorders of Calcium, Phosphate and Magnesium Metabolism

Introduction, 69
Calcium balance, 69

Biological functions of calcium
   and phosphate, 69

Magnesium metabolism, 82

Introduction

Calcium[1] is the most abundant mineral in the body, there being about 25 mol (1 kg) in a 70 kg man. About 99 % of the body's calcium is present in bone, mainly as the mineral hydroxyapatite, where it is combined with phosphate. About 85 % of the body's phosphate content is in bone.

Both hypercalcaemia and hypocalcaemia are relatively common biochemical abnormalities, as are abnormalities in plasma [phosphate]. Abnormal plasma [calcium] measurements often arise from alterations in plasma [albumin], the major calcium binding protein in plasma. Other cases result from an increase or decrease in the unbound or ionized calcium. It is important to identify the latter group, since pathological levels of ionized calcium may be life-threatening and the conditions themselves are amenable to treatment.

In this chapter, the hormonal regulation of plasma [Ca^{2+}] and [phosphate] is described, followed by a consideration of the causes of hypercalcaemia and hypocalcaemia and their investigation. Abnormalities in plasma [phos-

phate] and [magnesium] are also briefly discussed.

Calcium balance

In adults, calcium intake and output are normally in balance. External balance is largely achieved through the body normally matching net absorption over 24 hours closely with the corresponding 24-hour urinary excretion; this varies with the diet. On a normal diet, urinary calcium excretion in healthy adults may overlap with the output in some patients who are stone-formers. In infancy and childhood, there is normally a positive balance, especially at times of active skeletal growth. In older age, calcium output may exceed input, and a state of negative balance then exists; this negative external balance is particularly marked in women after the menopause, and is important in the development of postmenopausal osteoporosis. In women, the mother loses calcium to the fetus during pregnancy, and by lactation.

Figure 5.1 summarizes the typical daily movements of calcium between extracellular fluid, gut, bone and kidney.

Biological functions of calcium and phosphate

In an extracellular location, calcium is a major mechanical constituent of bone. Bone itself is a

---

1 In this book, 'calcium' is used as a composite term that embraces ionized calcium, protein-bound calcium and complexed calcium, whereas 'Ca^{2+}' means that only calcium ions are being considered. The total concentration of calcium in plasma or urine is shown as plasma or urine [calcium], whereas plasma [Ca^{2+}] refers specifically and solely to the concentration of ionized calcium.

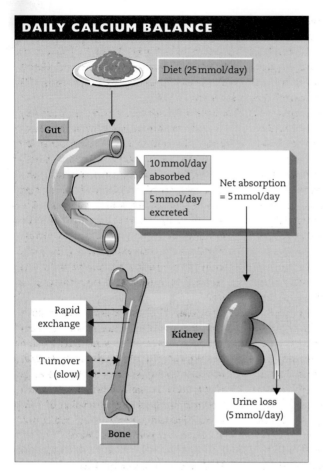

DAILY CALCIUM BALANCE

Diet (25 mmol/day)

Gut

10 mmol/day absorbed

Net absorption = 5 mmol/day

5 mmol/day excreted

Rapid exchange

Kidney

Turnover (slow)

Urine loss (5 mmol/day)

Bone

Fig. 5.1 Daily calcium balance.

specialized mineralized connective tissue containing cellular elements (bone-forming osteoblasts and bone-resorbing osteoclasts), organic matrix (type I collagen, proteoglycan, etc.) and hydroxyapatite. Calcium salts in bone have a mechanical role, but are not metabolically inert. There is a constant state of turnover in the skeleton associated with deposition of calcium in sites of bone formation and release at sites of bone resorption (about 5% per year of the adult skeleton is remodelled). Calcium in bone also acts as a reservoir that helps to stabilize extracellular fluid (ECF) [Ca^{2+}].

Maintenance of extracellular [Ca^{2+}] within narrow limits is necessary for normal excitability of nerve and muscle. An increase in [Ca^{2+}]

raises the threshold for the nerve action potential and vice versa. The ion is also required in the activation of the clotting and complement cascades.

Whilst the ECF [Ca^{2+}] is about 1 mmol/L (10^{-3} M), cytosolic [Ca^{2+}] is much lower, about 100 nmol/L (10^{-7} M). Cells possess a number of transport mechanisms for Ca^{2+} that allow maintenance of this large gradient across the cell membrane.

An increase in cytosolic [Ca^{2+}] serves as a signal for several cell processes, which include cell shape change, cell motility, metabolic changes, secretory activity and cell division. Many intercellular signals, including several hormones, bring about an increase in cytosolic [Ca^{2+}] by opening plasma membrane Ca^{2+}

channels, or by releasing intracellular stores of Ca^{2+}, or by a combination of these effects.

About 15% of phosphorus (as phosphate compounds) is present outside bone, largely in an intracellular location. In the ECF, phosphate is mostly inorganic, where it exists as a mixture of HPO_4^{2-} and $H_2PO_4^-$ at physiological pH. Intracellular phosphate has vital functions in macromolecular structure (e.g. in DNA), energy metabolism (e.g. energy-rich phosphates such as adenosine triphosphate, ATP), cell signalling and enzyme activation by phosphorylation. Intracellular phosphate is largely organic, as a component of phospholipids, phosphoproteins, nucleic acids and nucleotides (e.g. ATP).

Control of calcium metabolism

Calcium is present in plasma in three forms (Table 5.1), in equilibrium with one another. Plasma $[Ca^{2+}]$ is the physiologically important component, and is closely regulated in humans by parathyroid hormone (PTH) and 1:25-dihydrocholecalciferol (DHCC); these both act to increase plasma $[Ca^{2+}]$ and hence plasma [calcium]. The body's responses to a fall in plasma $[Ca^{2+}]$, in terms of changes in PTH and 1:25-DHCC production, are shown in Figure 5.2. Growth hormone, glucocorticoids (e.g. cortisol), oestrogens, testosterone and thyroid hormones (T4, thyroxine and T3, triiodothyronine) also influence calcium metabolism.

Parathyroid hormone (PTH)

Parathyroid hormone is the principal acute regulator of plasma $[Ca^{2+}]$. Plasma PTH levels exhibit a diurnal rhythm, being highest in the early hours of the morning and lowest at about 9 a.m. The active hormone is secreted in response to a fall in plasma $[Ca^{2+}]$, and its actions are directed to increase plasma $[Ca^{2+}]$. An increase in plasma $[Ca^{2+}]$ suppresses PTH secretion.

On bone, PTH stimulates bone resorption by osteoclasts, with a requirement for osteoblasts to mediate this effect. Biochemical measures of both increased osteoblast activity (e.g. increased plasma alkaline phosphatase activity) and increased osteoclast activity (e.g. raised urinary hydroxyproline and deoxypyridinoline excretion) may be evident. In severe hyperparathyroidism, radiological demineralization may be seen, including subperiosteal resorption of the terminal phalanges, bone cysts and pepper skull.

On the kidney, PTH increases the distal tubular reabsorption of calcium. It also reduces proximal tubular phosphate reabsorption and promotes activity of the 1α-hydroxylation of calcidiol (see below). Renal loss of HCO_3^- also increases, which may lead to a mild metabolic acidosis. Formation of 1:25-DHCC indirectly increases the absorption of calcium from the small intestine.

1:25-Dihydroxycholecalciferol (1:25-DHCC, or calcitriol)

Most vitamin D_3 (cholecalciferol) is synthesized by the action of ultraviolet light on 7-dehydrocholesterol precursor in the skin. Vitamin D_3 is also present naturally in food (a rich source is fish oils), whilst vitamin D_2 (ergosterol) is added to margarine.

Endogenous synthesis of vitamin D_3 is

CALCIUM IN PLASMA	
Calcium component	Percentage of plasma [calcium]
Ionised calcium, Ca^{2+}	50–65
Calcium bound to plasma proteins	30–45
Calcium complexed with citrate, etc.	5–10

Table 5.1 The components of calcium in plasma.

CALCIUM HOMEOSTASIS

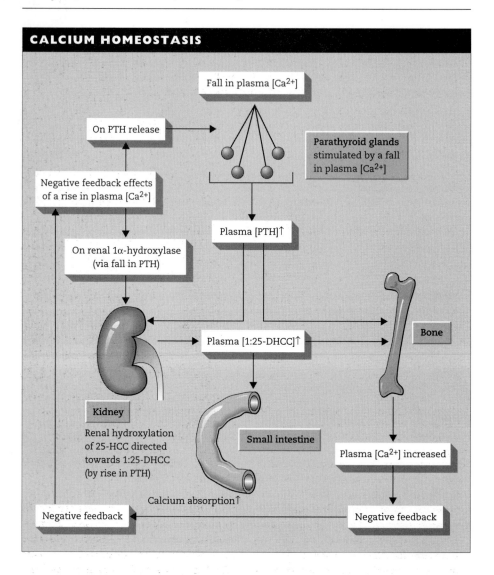

Fig. 5.2 Calcium homeostasis in man, showing the main hormonal responses to a fall in plasma [Ca²⁺], and indicating the places where the negative feedback mechanism operates if plasma [Ca²⁺] becomes high. The effect of PTH on the renal tubules, causing increased reabsorption of calcium, is not shown.

important. Vitamin D deficiency can develop if exposure to sunlight is inadequate, or because of inadequate dietary intake, but is usually a result of the combined effects of these two factors. In the body, vitamin D_3 and vitamin D_2 undergo two hydroxylation steps before attaining full physiological activity (Fig. 5.3):

25-Hydroxylation. This occurs in the liver, with the production of 25-hydroxycholecalciferol (25-HCC, or calcidiol). Other inactive metabolites are formed, but excreted in the bile. The main form of vitamin D circulating in the plasma is 25-HCC, bound to a specific transport protein; it is carried to the kidney for further metabolism. Plasma [25-HCC] shows marked seasonal variation, with levels highest in summer.

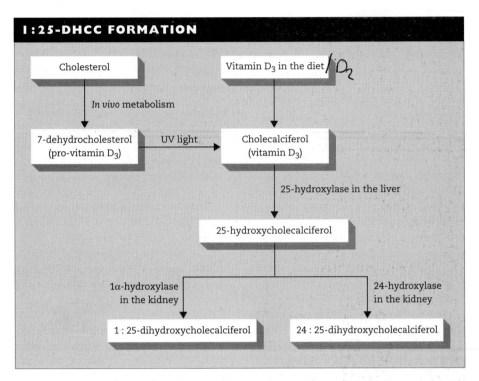

Fig. 5.3 The formation of 1:25-dihydroxycholecalciferol (1:25-DHCC), the most active form of vitamin D_3, from pro-vitamin D_3 (normally the main source of the vitamin in man) and from dietary vitamin D_3. Vitamin D_2 (ergosterol) undergoes similar hydroxylations. By the action of ultraviolet (UV) light, pro-vitamin D_3 is converted in the dermis into pre-vitamin D_3 (not shown) in which the B-ring of the steroid skeleton has been opened; pre-vitamin D_3 then rearranges spontaneously to give vitamin D_3. The factors that influence the hydroxylation of 24-HCC in the direction of 1:25 DHCC or 24:25 DHCC are described in the text.

1α-Hydroxylation of 25-HCC. This takes place in the kidney, with the production of 1:25-DHCC, biologically the most active naturally occurring derivative of vitamin D. The kidney also contains other hydroxylases, such as 24-hydroxylase, which converts 25-HCC to 24:25-dihydroxycholecalciferol (24:25-DHCC). Renal 1α-hydroxylation is increased by low plasma [phosphate], high [PTH] and where there is a tendency to hypocalcaemia, whatever the cause. The reverse circumstances direct metabolism of 25-HCC towards the formation of 24:25-DHCC, which has no clearly established physiological function.

The principal action of 1:25-DHCC is to induce synthesis of a Ca^{2+}-binding protein in the intestinal epithelial cell necessary for the absorption of calcium from the small intestine. Deficiency of 1:25-DHCC leads to defective bone mineralization. Maintenance of both ECF $[Ca^{2+}]$ and ECF [phosphate] by 1:25-DHCC may be a key factor in normal mineralization.

Calcitonin

Although calcitonin can decrease plasma $[Ca^{2+}]$ by reducing osteoclast activity and decreasing renal reabsorption of calcium and phosphate, its actions are transient, and chronic excess or deficiency is not associated with disordered calcium or bone metabolism. Its use as a tumour marker is discussed elsewhere (p. 96).

Investigation of abnormal calcium metabolism

Measurement of plasma calcium and albumin, inorganic phosphate and alkaline phosphatase, sometimes PTH and vitamin D metabolites, underlie the diagnosis of most disorders of calcium metabolism.

Plasma calcium (reference range, 2.12–2.62 mmol/L)

Most laboratories only measure plasma [calcium] routinely, even though the physiologically important fraction is plasma [Ca²⁺].

Effects of plasma [albumin]. Because albumin is the principal binding protein for calcium, a fall in plasma [albumin] will lead to a fall in bound calcium and a decrease in total [calcium] (and vice versa). The unbound plasma [Ca²⁺], the physiologically important fraction, will be maintained at normal levels by PTH. Hence, a low or high plasma [calcium] should always alert the clinician to measure plasma [albumin] to avoid misdiagnosis of hypocalcaemia or hypercalcaemia,

respectively. This is illustrated in Figure 5.4. The plasma [calcium] (in mmol/L) can be approximately 'corrected' to take account of an abnormal albumin (in g/L) using a formula such as:

$$\text{'Corrected'} \left[\text{calcium}\right] = \text{measured} \left[\text{calcium}\right] + 0.02 \times \left(40 - \left[\text{albumin}\right]\right)$$

Effects of plasma H⁺. In acidosis, the protonation of albumin reduces its ability to bind calcium, leading to an increase in unbound [Ca²⁺] and vice versa, without any change in total [calcium]. Thus, hyperventilation with respiratory alkalosis can reduce plasma [Ca²⁺], with the development of tetany. In chronic states of acidosis or alkalosis, PTH acts to readjust the plasma [Ca²⁺] back to normal.

Plasma phosphate (reference range, 0.8–1.4 mmol/L)

Plasma [phosphate] shows considerable diurnal variation, especially following meals;

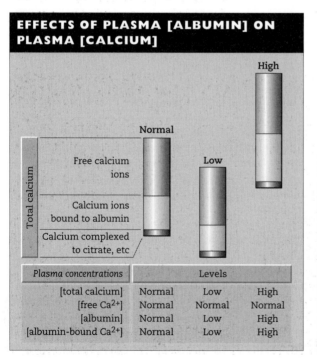

EFFECTS OF PLASMA [ALBUMIN] ON PLASMA [CALCIUM]

Plasma concentrations	Levels		
[total calcium]	Normal	Low	High
[free Ca²⁺]	Normal	Normal	Normal
[albumin]	Normal	Low	High
[albumin-bound Ca²⁺]	Normal	Low	High

Fig. 5.4 The effects of changes in plasma [albumin] on the distribution of calcium between free and albumin-bound calcium ions, and the consequent effects on plasma [total calcium]; plasma [free Ca²⁺] is unaltered. Of calcium in plasma, 50–65 % is normally present in the free, ionized form and 30–45 % bound to albumin, with the remaining 5–10 % consisting of calcium complexed with organic ions (e.g. citrate).

the reference range relates to the fasting state. Different ranges should be used for different age groups. About 85% of plasma phosphate is free and 15% protein bound.

A plasma [phosphate] below 0.4 mmol/L may be associated with widespread cell dysfunction and even death. Muscle pain and weakness, including respiratory muscle weakness, associated with a raised creatine kinase, are possible. Urgent phosphate supplementation is required. Dietary deficiency is unusual (phosphate occurs widely in food), but antacids may bind phosphate. Movement of phosphate into the cell occurs with metabolic and respiratory acidosis. Hypophosphataemia in diabetic ketoacidosis may be worsened when insulin is administered (insulin promotes cellular uptake of glucose and phosphate). Hyperalimentation or re-feeding starved patients is also accompanied by cellular utilization of phosphate and the potential for serious hypophosphataemia in the absence of appropriate supplementation. The causes of hypophosphataemia and hyperphosphataemia are listed in Table 5.2.

Table 5.2 Causes of hyperphosphataemia and hypophosphataemia.

Alkaline phosphatase

Reference ranges for plasma alkaline phosphatase activity are very method-dependent. For physiological reasons, there are also considerable variations in this enzyme's activity in childhood, adolescence and pregnancy (p. 103).

The bone isoenzyme of alkaline phosphatase activity is increased in plasma from patients with diseases in which there is increased osteoblastic activity, e.g. hyperparathyroidism, Paget's disease, rickets and osteomalacia, and carcinoma with osteoblastic metastases.

Hypercalcaemia

Increased plasma [Ca^{2+}] is a potentially serious problem that can lead to renal damage, cardiac arrhythmias and general ill health. The clinical features are listed in Table 5.3. The commonest causes (Table 5.4) are primary hyperparathyroidism and malignant disease.

Potentially misleading increases in plasma [calcium], in which plasma [Ca^{2+}] is normal, often result from abnormal calcium binding, due to raised plasma [albumin]. This is often due to faulty or non-standardized venepuncture technique (p. 88).

CAUSES OF HYPER- AND HYPOPHOSPHATAEMIA

Hyperphosphataemia		Hypophosphataemia	
Increased intake	Intravenous therapy Phosphate enemas	Decreased intake/absorption	Vitamin D deficiency (see also below) Malabsorption Oral phosphate binders
Reduced excretion	Acute/chronic renal failure		Primary PTH excess
	Low PTH or resistance to PTH	Increased excretion	Secondary PTH excess (e.g. vitamin D deficiency)
	Vitamin D toxicity		Postrenal transplant Re-feeding starved patients
Redistribution	Tumour lysis Rhabdomyolysis	Redistribution	Hyperalimentation Recovery from diabetic ketoacidosis
	Heat-stroke		Alkalosis (respiratory)

Primary hyperparathyroidism

Autonomous overproduction of PTH occurs typically from a single, parathyroid adenoma. Diffuse hyperplasia (all four glands) or, rarely, parathyroid carcinoma may be responsible.

The excess PTH leads to a raised $[Ca^{2+}]$, with the potential for clinical problems (Table 5.3). Both plasma [calcium] and [albumin] should be measured, and may need to be repeated, since the hypercalcaemia can be intermittent. Plasma [phosphate] is sometimes low as a result of the phosphaturic effect of PTH, though this is not a reliable finding. A mild metabolic acidosis may be present, since PTH increases urinary HCO_3^- losses. Some patients develop bony problems as a consequence of the high plasma [PTH], especially if the problem becomes chronic. Markers of increased osteoblast and osteoclast activity may be increased (p. 80). Table 5.5

Table 5.4 The causes of hypercalcaemia.

HYPERCALCAEMIA: CLINICAL FEATURES

Neurological symptoms (inability to concentrate, depression, confusion)
Generalized muscle weakness
Anorexia, nausea, vomiting, constipation
Polyuria with polydipsia
Nephrocalcinosis, nephrolithiasis
ECG changes (shortened Q–T interval), with bradycardia, first-degree block
Pancreatitis, peptic ulcer

Table 5.3 Clinical consequences of high $[Ca^{2+}]$.

summarizes the results of first-line chemical tests for the investigation of suspected hyperparathyroidism.

PTH assay

The definitive diagnosis depends largely on finding hypercalcaemia accompanied by a high or normal (i.e. unsuppressed) serum [PTH].

HYPERCALCAEMIA: CAUSES

Category	Examples
Common	
Parathyroid disease	Hyperparathyroidism, primary and tertiary; multiple endocrine neoplasia syndromes, MEN I and MEN IIa
Malignant disease	Lytic lesions in bone: myeloma, breast carcinoma
	PTHrP: carcinoma of lung, oesophagus, head and neck, renal cell, ovary and bladder.
	Ectopic production 1,25-DHCC by lymphomas.
Uncommon	
Endogenous production of 1,25-DHCC	Sarcoidosis and other granulomatous diseases
Excessive absorption of calcium	Vitamin D overdose (including self-medication); milk–alkali syndrome
Bone disease	Immobilisation
Drug-induced	Thiazide diuretics, lithium
Miscellaneous (mostly rare)	
	Familial hypocalciuric hypercalcaemia, alone or as part of MEN I or MEN IIa syndromes
	Hypercalcaemia in childhood (p. 257)
	Thyrotoxicosis
	Addison's disease
Artefact	Poor venepuncture technique (excessive venous stasis)

HYPERPARATHYROIDISM: CHEMICAL TESTS

Plasma or serum	Comments
Calcium	If increased [calcium], supports the diagnosis
Albumin	Should be performed as a check on plasma [calcium]
Phosphate (fasting)	If decreased [phosphate], supports the diagnosis
Alkaline phosphatase	If enzymic activity increased, supports the diagnosis
Total CO_2	If decreased, supports the diagnosis
Creatinine and/or urea	Simple tests of renal function, needed in all patients with suspected abnormalities of calcium metabolism

Table 5.5 'First-line' chemical tests for investigating suspected hyperparathyroidism.

Modern immunometric assays for PTH are sensitive, and are specifically designed to measure only the intact PTH molecule (serum intact PTH (reference range, 10–55 ng/L)). If a parathyroid adenoma or other parathyroid abnormality is not found in any of the usual sites, blood can be collected from veins draining other regions before the operation is completed. Measurement of serum [PTH] in these regional blood specimens may help in planning further surgery. A sestamibi parathyroid imaging scan may also be useful.

Management of primary hyperparathyroidism

In view of the technical difficulty often associated with parathyroid surgery, it is not unusual for the operation to be deferred in patients with asymptomatic hyperparathyroidism if their plasma [calcium] is less than 3.0 mmol/L. As symptoms may develop insidiously, these patients must be followed up with regular further measurements of plasma [calcium] and careful clinical reassessment. Indications for parathyroidectomy include: the presence of symptoms; a urine calcium excretion over 9 mmol/24h; cortical radial bone density over 2 SD below normal; reduced creatinine clearance (if no other cause identified); age under 50 years. In general, it is advisable to proceed to parathyroidectomy early rather than late.

After parathyroidectomy, plasma [calcium] falls rapidly, and it should be measured several times on the first postoperative day and at least daily for the next few days. If the plasma [calcium] falls below normal, calcium gluconate should be given and treatment with 1:25-DHCC or 1α-hydroxycholecalciferol (1α-HCC) should be started.

Multiple endocrine neoplasia (MEN) syndromes. Primary hyperparathyroidism may be one of the abnormalities in the so-called MEN syndrome. Three types of MEN syndrome have been described, all of them familial. Further details are discussed elsewhere (p. 201).

Hypercalcaemia of malignancy

Several factors are responsible for the hypercalcaemia of malignancy. These vary, depending on the type of tumour and on whether or not there are bone metastases:

1 Solid tumours that have metastasized to bone may cause hypercalcaemia by paracrine activation of osteoclasts. The tumour cells may also increase bone resorption directly.

2 Some solid tumours (e.g. carcinoma of the lung, head and neck), in the absence of bony metastases, may give rise to hypercalcaemia. An important factor in this humoral hypercalcaemia of malignancy is PTH-related protein (PTHrP), a peptide with marked sequence homology with PTH that also acts through the PTH receptor. True ectopic production of PTH appears to be rare.

3 In multiple myeloma, hypercalcaemia appears to result from the release of local cytokines that promote local bone resorption. Lymphomas may also cause hypercalcaemia.

Other causes of hypercalcaemia

The history of the patient's illness, the findings on clinical examination, and various investigations as suggested by the provisional diagnosis, will usually mean that the other conditions (Table 5.4) can be recognized. These will be briefly considered here.

Vitamin D excess. Increased plasma [1:25-DHCC] and hypercalcaemia may result from excessive vitamin D intake or if overdosage with 25-HCC, 1α-HCC or 1:25-DHCC occurs. Measurement of serum [25-HCC] or [1:25-DHCC] confirms the diagnosis.

Sarcoidosis. About 10–20% of patients with sarcoidosis may have hypercalcaemia, often only intermittently. More often, they have hypercalciuria. Increased conversion of 25-HCC to 1:25-DHCC by sarcoid tissue macrophages is responsible (with increased intestinal absorption of calcium).

Milk–alkali syndrome. Milk consumption may be excessive in patients with symptoms of peptic ulceration; calcium intake is correspondingly increased. If this is accompanied by excessive intake of alkali (e.g. $NaHCO_3$), as an antacid, hypercalcaemia may develop. The alkali is thought to reduce urinary calcium excretion and to be important in the pathogenesis of the condition.

Tertiary hyperparathyroidism. This description refers to the development of parathyroid hyperplasia as a complication of previously existing secondary hyperparathyroidism (p. 179). This diagnosis needs to be considered in patients with renal failure or intestinal malabsorption if they develop hypercalcaemia that is not attributable to treatment with vitamin D or one of its hydroxylated derivatives (usually 1α-HCC or 1:25-DHCC). Plasma [calcium] is almost always increased and serum [PTH] inappropriately high. Unlike primary hyperparathyroidism, however, fasting plasma [phosphate] may be increased, especially if tertiary hyperparathyroidism develops in a patient with renal failure.

Other bone-related causes. Causes other than malignant disease include Paget's disease in association with immobilization.

Endocrine disorders. Hypercalcaemia has been reported occasionally in association with hypoadrenalism, phaeochromocytoma and thyrotoxicosis.

Drugs. A mild degree of hypercalcaemia may develop during treatment with thiazide diuretics; these interfere with renal calcium excretion. Long-term lithium therapy may also be a cause, possibly by stimulating PTH secretion.

Familial hypocalciuric hypercalcaemia (FHH). This uncommon disorder is transmitted by an autosomal dominant gene. Patients with FHH mostly have lifelong hypercalcaemia without symptoms, but unaccompanied by the hypercalciuria that would normally be expected under these circumstances. The problem is believed to arise because the high plasma [Ca^{2+}] is sensed as 'normal', with normal plasma [PTH]. The condition should always be considered, since surgery is unnecessary. Measurement of urinary calcium excretion may be helpful.

Hypocalcaemia

If potentially misleading hypocalcaemia due to decreased plasma [albumin] is first excluded, the hypocalcaemia must be pathological and must result from a decrease in plasma [Ca^{2+}].

Tetany is the symptom that classically suggests the presence of a low plasma [Ca^{2+}]. It may occur in any of the conditions listed in Table 5.6, and may also be caused by a rapid fall in plasma [H^+] (e.g. acute respiratory alkalosis produced by hyperventilation or intravenous infusion of $NaHCO_3$). Occasionally it is due to a low plasma [Mg^{2+}] in the absence of low plasma [Ca^{2+}], and rarely it is due to a sudden increase in plasma [phosphate]. Neuropsychiatric symptoms and cataract are other possible consequences of hypocalcaemia (Table 5.7).

The commonest pathological cause of hypocalcaemia is defective calcium absorption due to inadequate plasma levels of 1:25-DHCC.

HYPOCALCAEMIA: CAUSES

Category	Examples
Hypoproteinaemia	Low plasma [albumin] (p. 87)
Renal disease	Hydroxylation of 25-HCC impaired.
Inadequate intake of calcium	Deficiency of calcium or vitamin D, or of both; intestinal malabsorption (p. 132)
Hypoparathyroidism	Autoimmune, post-surgical, Mg deficiency, infiltrative disease
Pseudohypoparathyroidism	Target organ resistance to PTH
Neonatal hypocalcaemia	P. 253
Acute pancreatitis	Calcium soaps in the abdominal cavity?

Table 5.6 The causes of hypocalcaemia.

HYPOCALCAEMIA: CLINICAL FEATURES

Enhanced neuromuscular irritability (positive
  Chvostek's sign and Trousseau's sign);
  tetany
Numbness, tingling (fingers, toes, circumoral)
Muscle cramps (legs, feet, lower back)
Seizures
Irritability, personality changes
ECG changes (prolonged Q–T interval)
Basal ganglia calcification; subcapsular
  cataracts (esp. with low PTH)

Table 5.7 Clinical consequences of
hypocalcaemia.

Vitamin D deficiency

Deficiency of 1:25-DHCC may result from lack
of vitamin D or failure at any stage in its conversion to 1:25-DHCC (Fig. 5.3); rarely, the
action of 1:25-DHCC is defective at the receptor level. In malnutrition, the effects of vitamin
D deficiency are accentuated by inadequate
dietary calcium.

Defective absorption of calcium leads ultimately to a low plasma $[Ca^{2+}]$ accompanied by
increased PTH secretion in response to the
low ECF $[Ca^{2+}]$ (i.e. secondary hyperparathyroidism). Plasma [phosphate] is often low,
partly through impaired absorption, but also as
a result of the secondary hyperparathyroidism

(renal disease is an exception). Plasma alkaline
phosphatase activity is often increased,
reflecting increased osteoblastic activity. However, its measurement is of limited diagnostic value in childhood, because of the
marked physiological variations in activity that
normally occur in this age group. Urinary
calcium excretion is nearly always low or very
low.

Confirmation of the diagnosis of vitamin D
deficiency depends on measurement of serum
[25-HCC] or (less widely available) serum
[1:25-DHCC]. Serum [25-HCC] assays provide a reasonable indication of the overall
vitamin D status of the patient if renal function
is normal and renal 1α-hydroxylase activity
can be assumed to be normal. There is a seasonal variation in serum [25-HCC] that can
make interpretation of single results difficult.
Measurement of serum [25-HCC] is also of
value in monitoring patients who are being
treated for vitamin D deficiency by dietary
supplementation.

The main causes of hypocalcaemia due to
lack of vitamin D or of disturbances of its
metabolism will be briefly considered here:

1 *Nutritional deficiency of vitamin D.* Poor diet,
inadequate exposure to sunlight, or a combination of these, can lead to vitamin D deficiency
with development of hypocalcaemia and
osteomalacia (see section on 'biochemical
bone disease', p. 80). This has largely been
eliminated in developed countries with vitamin
D supplementation of food, but the elderly are
still at risk (as they may be immobile indoors

with an inadequate diet). Cultural and geographical factors are probably important in the susceptibility to vitamin D deficiency of the immigrant Asian community in Northern Europe.

2 *Malabsorption of vitamin D.* This may be due to coeliac disease, or occur as a result of fat malabsorption due to pancreatic disease, biliary obstruction, or as a complication of gastric or intestinal surgery (e.g. intestinal bypass or resection). Biliary obstruction is much more likely to lead to vitamin D deficiency (through malabsorption) than the theoretical possibility of 25-HCC deficiency in parenchymal liver disease.

3 *Renal disease.* Destruction of the renal parenchyma leads to loss of 1α-hydroxylase activity, reduced formation of 1:25-DHCC and consequent malabsorption of calcium. Plasma [phosphate] is likely to be high in renal failure, and this may interfere with the 1α-hydroxylation step.

Specific deficiency of 1α-hydroxylase may be the cause of hypocalcaemia in vitamin D-resistant rickets, type I, a rare inherited disorder. In vitamin D-resistant rickets, type II, there is end-organ unresponsiveness to 1:25-DHCC.

Hypoparathyroidism

Primary hypoparathyroidism is rare. The combination of a reduced plasma [calcium] and an increased [phosphate] in a patient who does not have renal disease suggests the diagnosis of hypoparathyroidism; plasma alkaline phosphatase activity is usually normal. Measurement of serum [PTH] confirms the diagnosis; it is reduced to below 10 ng/L, and is sometimes undetectable even by the most sensitive assays.

Failure to secrete PTH may be a complication of surgery, or it may be familial or sporadic in origin. Also, the parathyroid glands may be destroyed by an auto-immune process, or as a result of infiltration by carcinoma of the thyroid or other neoplasms. Occasionally, the parathyroid glands are suppressed as a result of magnesium deficiency; normal magnesium levels are necessary for PTH release.

Pseudohypoparathyroidism is a rare but interesting condition, in which the end-organ receptors in the bone and kidneys fail to respond normally to PTH. Patients with pseudohypoparathyroidism have increased serum [PTH].

Other causes of hypocalcaemia are listed in Table 5.6.

Biochemical bone diseases

Generalized defects in bone mineralization, frequently associated with abnormal calcium or phosphate metabolism, are sometimes grouped together under the term 'biochemical or metabolic bone diseases'. The most common are osteoporosis, rickets and osteomalacia, and Paget's disease.

In many examples of metabolic bone disease, patients show features of two or more of these conditions, and it can be difficult to define the pathological process fully, even with the aid of radiological examination and bone biopsy. Results of chemical investigations (Table 5.8) must be interpreted in relation to all the available evidence. For example, in renal osteodystrophy, a combination of osteomalacia, hyperparathyroidism and other metabolic abnormalities contributes to the metabolic bone disease. Various other conditions, often rare, may produce generalized bone disease, with or without biochemical changes.

It is sometimes useful to assess bone formation or bone resorption. The plasma bone isoenzyme of alkaline phosphatase (ALP) is a measure of osteoblast activity. A bone-specific protein, osteocalcin, also reflects osteoblast activity. Measures of osteoclast activity depend upon the quantitation of breakdown products of the collagen matrix, usually the so-called pyridinium cross-links (derived from the amino acids that cross-link the mature collagen) measured in a timed urine specimen.

Rickets and osteomalacia

Patients who have vitamin D deficiency or disturbed metabolism of vitamin D are all liable to suffer from the bone disease osteomalacia or, in children, from rickets. These patients have

METABOLIC BONE DISEASE: CHEMICAL INVESTIGATIONS

Diagnosis	Calcium	Phosphate (fasting)	PTH	Alkaline phosphatase	Ca++
Hyperparathyroidism					
Primary	↑ (or N)	↓ or N	↑ or N*	N or ↑	↑ (or N)
Secondary	↓ or N	↑ or N	↑	↑ or N	N
Tertiary	↑ or N	↑ or N	↑	↑ or N	↑
Rickets and osteomalacia					
Deficient intake	↓ or N	↓ or N	↑ (or N)	↑	N (or ↓)
Renal failure	↓ or N	↑ or N	↑	↑	N
Fanconi syndrome†	↓ or N	↓ or N	N	↑	N
Osteoporosis	N	N	N	N	N
Paget's disease	N (or ↑)	N	N	↑	N

N, normal; ↑, increased; ↓, decreased. N* indicates that, with sensitive PTH assays, plasma [PTH] is sometimes within the reference range, i.e. it is inappropriately high in primary hyperparathyroidism and not suppressed, as would normally be expected, in the presence of hypercalcaemia. † Included as an example of proximal renal tubular defects.

Table 5.8 Metabolic bone disease: chemical investigations on blood specimens.

bone pain, with local tenderness, and may have a proximal myopathy. Skeletal deformity may be present, particularly in rickets. Mineralization of osteoid is defective, with absence of the calcification front.

Other causes of rickets or osteomalacia, unrelated to vitamin D deficiency or defects in its metabolism, have also been described. An inherited defect in the tubular reabsorption of phosphate, hypophosphataemic vitamin D–resistant rickets, leads to similar bone deformities, but without muscle weakness; there is a low plasma [phosphate] and phosphaturia. In Fanconi's syndrome (p. 58), tubular phosphate loss may also lead to low plasma [phosphate] associated with rickets or osteomalacia.

Hypophosphatasia is a hereditary disease in which vitamin D–resistant rickets is the most prominent finding. Tissue and plasma alkaline phosphatase activities are usually low, and excessive amounts of phosphoryl ethanolamine are present in the urine.

Osteoporosis

This is a very common disorder that affects about one in four women. It is characterized by low bone mass and susceptibility to vertebral, forearm and hip fractures in later life. Results of routine chemical investigations are usually all normal.

Table 5.9 lists some of the risk factors for the development of osteoporosis. The diagnosis should exclude primary hyperparathyroidism, thyrotoxicosis, corticosteroid excess, multiple myeloma and hypogonadism.

Paget's disease

This is a common disorder of bone, affecting up to 5 % of the population over 55 years old in the United Kingdom. Bone turnover is focally increased, with disordered bone remodelling. Plasma [calcium] and [phosphate] are usually normal, although hypercalcaemia can develop, especially as a result of immobilization. The increased bone turnover leads to a high plasma alkaline phosphatase activity and an increase in indices of osteoclast activity.

Renal osteodystrophy

The pathophysiology of renal osteodystrophy

OSTEOPOROSIS: RISK FACTORS

Unmodifiable
  Age (1.4–1.8-fold increase per decade)
  Genetic (Caucasians & Orientals > Blacks & Polynesians)
  Sex (female > male)
Modifiable (environmental)
  Nutritional calcium deficiency
  Physical inactivity
  Smoking
  Alcohol excess; drugs (e.g. glucocorticoids, anticonvulsants)
Modifiable (endogenous)
  Endocrine (oestrogen or androgen deficiency, hyperthyroidism)
  Chronic diseases (gastrectomy, cirrhosis, rheumatoid arthritis)

Table 5.9 Risk factors for osteoporosis.

is complex. The bone changes in it are varied, and derive from one or more of the following mechanisms:

1 *Vitamin D metabolism.* There is ineffective conversion of 25-HCC to 1:25-DHCC due to loss of renal 1α-hydroxylase. This causes defective calcium absorption and osteomalacia in adults, or rickets in children. It may be corrected by treatment with 1α-HCC or 1:25-DHCC.

2 *Phosphate retention.* There is increased plasma [phosphate], and this, by complexing with Ca^{2+} and combined with defective calcium absorption, tends to make plasma [Ca^{2+}] fall. This leads to secondary hyperparathyroidism, which tends to restore plasma [phosphate] and plasma [calcium], towards normal. Phosphate retention can further inhibit the renal 1α-hydroxylase. Osteitis fibrosa, if it develops, may require parathyroidectomy.

3 *Phosphate binders.* Failure of the secondary hyperparathyroidism to maintain normal plasma [phosphate] as renal disease progresses leads to treatment of patients with oral phosphate binders, usually aluminium hydroxide. Excess absorption of aluminium may cause

osteomalacia and dialysis dementia. Plasma [aluminium] should be measured periodically.

4 *Dialysis fluid composition.* The fluid [calcium] must be carefully controlled; if it is too low, osteoporosis often develops. If fluid [calcium] is too high, extraskeletal calcification may occur. Care is also needed to ensure that dialysis fluid [aluminium] is sufficiently low.

In order to control and treat these various abnormalities, all patients with chronic renal failure require biochemical monitoring. Plasma creatinine, urea, Na^+, K^+, total CO_2, albumin, calcium and phosphate concentrations and alkaline phosphatase activity should all be measured regularly. The main object of treatment with 1α-HCC or 1:25-DHCC is to increase plasma [calcium] to normal and to reverse bone disease due to parathyroid overactivity. If treatment is successful, serum PTH falls to normal. When treatment is first started, it may be difficult to adjust the dose of 1α-HCC or 1:25-DHCC satisfactorily, and hypercalcaemia, possibly with extraskeletal calcium deposition, may occur if too much is given.

Magnesium metabolism

Magnesium is the second most abundant intracellular cation. It is essential for the activity of many enzymes, including the phosphotransferases. Bone contains about 50% of the body's magnesium; a small proportion of the body's content is in the ECF.

Dietary intake of magnesium is normally about 12 mmol (300 mg) daily. Green vegetables, cereals and meat are good sources. Significant amounts are contained in gastric and biliary secretions. Factors concerned with the control of magnesium absorption have not been defined, but may involve active transport across the intestinal mucosa by a process involving vitamin D. Renal conservation of magnesium is at least partly controlled by PTH and aldosterone. When the dietary intake is restricted, renal conservation mechanisms are normally so efficient that depletion, if it develops at all, only comes on very slowly.

Plasma [magnesium] is normally kept within narrow limits, which implies close homeostatic control. Marked alterations in the body's content can occur with little or no change detectable in plasma [magnesium]. In this respect, magnesium is very like potassium. The plasma [magnesium] may be normal although a state of intracellular depletion exists.

Hypomagnesaemia and magnesium deficiency

Magnesium deficiency (Table 5.10) rarely occurs as an isolated phenomenon. Usually it is accompanied by disorders of potassium, calcium and phosphorus metabolism. It may therefore be difficult to identify signs and symptoms that can be specifically attributed to magnesium deficiency. However, muscular weakness, sometimes accompanied by tetany, cardiac arrhythmias and central nervous system abnormalities (e.g. convulsions), may all be due to magnesium deficiency.

Magnesium deficiency should be suspected in patients with hypocalcaemia or hypokalaemia who fail to respond to treatment of these abnormalities. Plasma [magnesium] is usually below 0.5 mmol/L in patients with symptoms directly attributable to magnesium

Table 5.10 Magnesium deficiency.

deficiency; its level should be measured before treatment with magnesium salts is instituted.

Plasma [magnesium] may not reflect the true state of the body's reserves, particularly in chronic disorders. Other tests have been advocated (e.g. erythrocyte [magnesium], muscle [magnesium], magnesium loading tests), but there is no general agreement on the best test to use. Urinary excretion of magnesium is relatively easy to measure, and it is useful in distinguishing renal losses of magnesium from the other causes of hypomagnesaemia and magnesium deficiency. Renal excretion of magnesium often falls below 0.5 mmol/24 h in nonrenal causes of magnesium deficiency.

Hypermagnesaemia

This is most often due to acute renal failure or the advanced stages of chronic renal failure. Its presence is readily confirmed by measuring plasma [magnesium]. There may be no symptoms. However, if plasma [magnesium] exceeds 3.0 mmol/L, nausea and vomiting, weakness and impaired consciousness may then develop, but these symptoms may not necessarily be caused solely by the hypermagnesaemia.

Hypermagnesaemia may rarely be caused by intravenous injection of magnesium salts, and adrenocortical hypofunction may cause a slight increase in plasma [magnesium].

MAGNESIUM DEFICIENCY	
Causes	Examples
Abnormal losses	
GI tract	Prolonged aspiration, persistent diarrhoea, malabsorptive disease, fistula, jejuno-ileal by-pass, small-bowel resection
Urinary tract	
Renal disease	Renal tubular acidosis, chronic pyelonephritis, hydronephrosis
Extrarenal	Conditions that modify renal function (e.g. primary and secondary hyperaldosteronism, diuretics, osmotic diuresis)
	Conditions affecting transfer of magnesium from cells to bone (e.g. primary and tertiary hyperparathyroidism, ketoacidosis)
Reduced intake	If severe and prolonged, protein-energy malnutrition
Mixed aetiology	Chronic alcoholism, hepatic cirrhosis

KEY POINTS

1 Calcium is the most abundant body mineral, largely present in bone. In addition to this major mechanical function, extracellular calcium is necessary for normal neuromuscular function, blood clotting and complement activation. Intracellular calcium is a key signal for many important cellular events (contraction, motility, secretion, cell division).

2 About 50 % plasma calcium is bound to albumin, the rest being mostly ionized (the physiologically active fraction). Changes in plasma [albumin] may alter plasma total [calcium] without any pathological change in the ionized fraction [Ca^{2+}].

3 Parathyroid hormone (PTH) is a key regulatory hormone of plasma [Ca^{2+}]. A fall in [Ca^{2+}] stimulates PTH, which increases Ca^{2+} release from bone, renal reabsorption of Ca^{2+} and loss of phosphate in the urine. 1,25-dihydrocholecalciferol (DHCC) is essential for intestinal absorption of calcium (and phosphate) and the longer-term maintenance of plasma [Ca^{2+}] and [phosphate].

4 True hypercalcaemia (increase in [Ca^{2+}]) is most commonly due to primary hyperparathyroidism or malignant disease. True hypocalcaemia (decrease in [Ca^{2+}]) is most often the result of low 1,25-DHCC levels (vitamin D deficiency, malabsorption, renal disease), less often to hypoparathyroidism.

5 Defects in bone mineralization (biochemical bone disease) include rickets and osteomalacia, renal osteodystrophy (both associated with abnormalities in [Ca^{2+}] and [phosphate]) and osteoporosis and Paget's disease (typically without effect on these measurements).

6 Magnesium deficiency is usually associated with other electrolyte deficiencies. Hypermagnesaemia is most often found in acute or chronic renal failure.

Case 5.1

A 47-year-old secretary was admitted as an emergency with left-sided ureteric colic. She had had one similar episode three years before, when she had passed a small calculus spontaneously. In addition, she had been receiving treatment with cimetidine for the previous six months, for dyspepsia.

Physical examination only revealed slight tenderness in the left loin and on palpating the abdomen. Side-room tests on urine showed a trace of blood, and a plain X-ray of the abdomen showed a small opacity in the line of the left ureter. Blood investigations were performed, with the following results:

Plasma analysis	Results	Reference range	Units
[Creatinine]	150	55–120	μmol/L
[Na+]	141	132–144	mmol/L
[K+]	4.2	3.3–4.7	mmol/L
[Total CO_2]	20	24–30	mmol/L
Urea	8.1	2.5–6.6	mmol/L
[Albumin]	40	36–47	g/L
[Calcium]	3.49	2.12–2.62	mmol/L
[Phosphate]	0.60	0.8–1.4	mmol/L
ALP activity	160	40–125	U/L

What was the likely cause of this patient's urinary calculi? What further chemical investigations would you have requested in order to confirm the diagnosis? What treatment would you have instituted after initiating these further investigations?

Comments on Case 5.1
The most likely diagnosis is primary hyperparathyroidism; the history of recurrent renal calculi and peptic ulceration are highly suggestive, and strongly supported by the results for the plasma calcium, phosphate and

Continued on p. 85

Case 5.1 *continued*

alkaline phosphatase measurements, and by the presence of a mild metabolic acidosis.

The diagnosis in this patient was confirmed by measuring serum [PTH]; results for this analysis are most readily interpreted if the blood specimen is collected at a time when the plasma [calcium] is increased, i.e. before any calcium-lowering treatment is instituted. This patient's plasma [calcium] was sufficiently high to warrant urgent attempts to lower it, after an intravenous urogram had been performed to make sure that the calculus was not causing obstruction. Treatment would consist of fluids to correct dehydration, and might require a loop diuretic (frusemide). This patient then proceeded to parathyroidectomy for removal of a solitary adenoma.

Case 5.2

A 64-year-old retired shop assistant with Crohn's disease (regional ileitis) had had her condition well controlled by means of oral prednisolone until two or three months before her regular follow-up out-patient appointment. Latterly, she had had severe pain in the back, and radiological examination showed a compression fracture of the fourth lumbar vertebra. Chemical investigations on a blood specimen gave the following results:

Plasma analysis	Results	Reference range	Units
[Albumin]	26	36–47	g/L
[Calcium]	1.72	2.12–2.62	mmol/L
[Phosphate, fasting]	0.8	0.8–1.4	mmol/L
ALP activity	170	40–125	U/L
[Total protein]	50	63–83	g/L
[Creatinine]	110	55–120	μmol/L
[Urea]	5.8	2.5–6.6	mmol/L
[Na$^+$]	136	132–144	mmol/L
[K$^+$]	3.5	3.3–4.7	mmol/L
[Total CO$_2$]	21	24–30	mmol/L

Comment on these results. What further investigations might be indicated?

Comments on Case 5.2

The plasma [calcium] is low, and lower than can be accounted for in terms of the low plasma [albumin]. The combination of a low plasma [calcium] with a low normal plasma [phosphate] and elevated alkaline phosphatase activity is consistent with a diagnosis of osteomalacia. The low plasma [total protein] and [albumin], and the low [total CO$_2$], indicative of a mild metabolic acidosis, suggest that chronic diarrhoea with intestinal malabsorption could be the cause of the osteomalacia.

A diagnosis of osteomalacia can be confirmed by bone biopsy. However, this is seldom required if the history is suggestive and the results of chemical investigations and radiological examination (generalized rarefaction of bones, Looser's zones) are characteristic. Measurement of 25-HCC in plasma might be considered worthwhile, and responses to a therapeutic trial of vitamin D might be helpful as a means of making a diagnosis of osteomalacia retrospectively.

CHAPTER 6

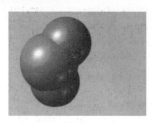

Abnormalities of Proteins in Plasma

Role of plasma proteins, 86
Methods of investigating
  plasma proteins, 86

Plasma proteins and disease, 86
The immunoglobulins, 91

Tumour markers, 95

Plasma contains over 300 proteins. Many of these have a specific biochemical role; organic disease may result when their concentration in plasma is reduced. Other plasma proteins, including most enzymes and tumour markers, have no known function in blood, and arise as a result of cell death or tissue damage.

In this chapter, the functions and diagnostic roles of a number of the clinically more important plasma proteins are described.

Role of plasma proteins

Many proteins in plasma have a specific role to play and carry out a wide range of functions, including:

1 Maintenance of colloid osmotic pressure – mainly a function of albumin.

2 Transport functions, carried out by various carrier proteins (Table 6.1).

3 Defence reactions – functions that depend on:

(a) Immunoglobulins, synthesized in the lymphoreticular system.

(b) The complement system.

4 Coagulation and fibrinolysis. This involves some of the proteins circulating in plasma, and others liberated from damaged cells or tissues (e.g. platelets).

Some diseases may affect most plasma proteins, e.g. if there is malnutrition or loss of blood. In other diseases, only certain specific proteins are affected.

Methods of investigating plasma proteins

Chemical and immunological methods are available that can quantify the concentration of a specific plasma protein with a high degree of specificity. Less commonly, electrophoresis is used to provide a semiquantitative estimate of the pattern of serum proteins expressed. Electrophoresis separates the proteins into five broad fractions – albumin, α_1-globulins, α_2-globulins, β-globulins and γ-globulins (Fig. 6.1); each of the globulin fractions consists of a mixture of several proteins (Table 6.2). Serum protein electrophoresis has limited diagnostic value, and the measurement of specific proteins using immunoassay methods is most commonly used.

Plasma proteins and disease

A summary of the proteins commonly measured in clinical practice is given in Table 6.2. Most diseases that alter plasma protein concentrations do so by affecting their volume of distribution or their rates of synthesis, catabolism or excretion. In some patients, more than one of these factors may be operating.

Total protein

Many laboratories have stopped measuring plasma or serum [total protein], as a fall in the

TRANSPORT FUNCTIONS OF PLASMA PROTEINS

Carrier proteins	Carrier functions
Pre-albumin	Retinol (vitamin A), T4 and T3
Albumin	Inorganic constituents of plasma (e.g. calcium)
	Free fatty acids
	Hormones (e.g. T4 and T3)
	Excretory products (e.g. unconjugated bilirubin)
	Drugs and other toxic substances
Hormone-binding proteins	Corticosteroids, sex hormones and thyroid hormones each have their own specific binding proteins
Metal-binding proteins	Copper (by ceruloplasmin); iron (by transferrin)
Apolipoproteins	Lipids (transport of essential metabolites)

Table 6.1 Examples of the transport functions of plasma proteins.

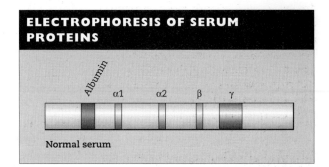

Fig. 6.1 Separation of serum proteins by electrophoresis.

concentration of one protein may be masked by a coincident or compensatory increase in another, e.g. a fall in plasma [albumin] can be masked by an increase in plasma [immunoglobulins]. Situations that give rise to changes in the concentration of [total protein] are as given for albumin (Table 6.3). Total protein may also be influenced as a result of changes in plasma [immunoglobulins].

Albumin

Albumin (M_r 66 kDa) has two main functions:

Oncotic pressure. Albumin is quantitatively the most important contributor towards maintaining the colloid oncotic pressure of plasma, and hypoalbuminaemia may lead to the development of oedema.

Transport. Albumin acts as a non-specific transport vehicle for many substances (Table 6.1).

Hypoalbuminaemia

This condition may be due to physiological or pathological causes, but artefact due to taking a blood sample from a site close to an intravenous infusion should always be considered (Table 6.3).

Pathological causes include:

• *Reduced synthesis,* due to liver disease (p. 113), malnutrition, and intestinal malabsorptive disease (p. 131), if these are severe and prolonged.

• *Altered distribution,* due to increased capillary permeability, which enables plasma to leak into the extravascular compartment (e.g. severe burns), or to serous effusion (e.g. ascites), when there is sequestration of proteins.

• *Increased catabolism,* as a result of injury (e.g. major surgery or trauma), infection, or malignant disease.

PLASMA PROTEINS

Proteins and their electrophoretic mobility	Principal function(s)	Used in the detection or investigations of disease
Pre-albumin	Unknown (has some transport functions)	Malnutrition, liver disease, effects of trauma
Albumin	Colloid oncotic pressure, transport functions	Malnutrition, malignancy, liver, kidney and GI disease
α_1-Globulins		
α_1-Fetoprotein	Unknown	Neural tube defects, also as a tumour marker
α_1-Protease inhibitor (API)	Antiprotease	API deficiency
Prothrombin	Blood clotting	Coagulation screen; also as a liver function test
α_2-Globulins		
Ceruloplasmin	Copper transport	Wilson's disease
Haptoglobin	Haemoglobin binding	Haemolytic disorders
α_2-Macroglobulin	Antiprotease, transport functions	Proteinuria (e.g. selectivity investigations)
Thyroxine-binding globulin	T4 and T3 transport	Thyroid disease
β-Globulins		
C-reactive protein	Body's defence mechanisms	Nonspecific test that may be used instead of the ESR
β_2-Microglobulin	Body's defence mechanisms	Monitoring myeloma, renal failure
Transferrin	Iron transport	Iron deficiency
γ-Globulins		
Immunoglobulins (IgG, IgA, IgM, etc.)	Body's defence mechanisms	Liver disease, infections, auto-immune disease, paraproteinaemias, etc.

Table 6.2 Examples of plasma proteins commonly measured for the diagnosis and monitoring of disease.

• *Abnormal losses.* The liver can normally replace albumin losses of up to 5 g/day. Greater losses (which may involve losses of other proteins besides albumin) may occur in nephrotic syndrome (p. 63), gastrointestinal tract disease and in burns or certain skin diseases.

• *Overhydration,* which is usually iatrogenic.

Hyperalbuminaemia

Increased plasma [albumin] is found in dehydration and excessive stasis during venepuncture.

Hereditary abnormalities

Analbuminaemia is a rare disorder in which plasma [albumin] is usually less than 1.0 g/L.

However, there may be no symptoms or signs – not even oedema – due to compensatory increases in plasma [globulins]. Albumin normally appears as a single, fairly discrete band on serum protein electrophoresis. *Albumin variants* occur in the healthy population, and heterozygotes for some variant albumins may express two gene products, which appear as two bands. This is known as *bisalbuminaemia,* and has no pathological significance.

Acute-phase response and the acute-phase proteins

Following trauma, infection, inflammation, burns, etc., the body responds by initiating a series of mechanisms that lead to:

CAUSES OF HYPOALBUMINAEMIA

Artefact	Physiological	Pathological
Dilution of sample – sample taken from drip arm	Pregnancy Recumbency	Impaired synthesis – malnutrition, malabsorption, chronic liver disease, analbuminaemia Excessive loss – from kidney, GI tract or skin Overhydration Increased metabolism – injury

Table 6.3 Causes of hypoalbuminaemia.

ACUTE-PHASE PROTEINS

Protein	Function	Increase
C-reactive protein	Binds extracts of pneumococcal cell walls	↑↑↑↑
Anti-protease inhibitors	Protease inhibitor	↑↑↑
Ceruloplasmin	Copper transport Superoxide scavenger	↑↑↑
α_1-Acid glycoprotein	Tissue repair?	↑↑
Fibrinogen	Clotting	↑↑
Haptoglobin	Binds haemoglobin	↑

Table 6.4 Acute-phase proteins.

• Acute haemodynamic changes.

• A rapid decrease in the concentration of many plasma proteins (e.g. albumin, prealbumin and transferrin).

• An increase in the concentration of several specific proteins some hours after the injury. These proteins are the acute-phase proteins, and are listed in Table 6.4.

The cytokines and a host of vasoactive substances are important mediators of the acute-phase response (Fig. 6.2). The rapid decrease in concentration of certain proteins appears to result from loss of plasma protein into the extravascular space, due to increased vascular permeability caused by vasoactive substances, including cytokines, prostaglandins and histamine. The increase in the acute-phase plasma proteins results from increased synthesis and release, which appears to be mediated by interleukin-6. The following are all acute-phase proteins.

C-reactive protein (M_r 105 kDa)

This protein is a β-globulin, originally named after a property of serum that had been obtained from acutely ill patients, which caused the precipitation of a polysaccharide (fraction C) from pneumococcal extracts. C-reactive protein (CRP) binds strongly to certain lipids, particularly phospholipids. It seems that CRP is somehow involved in the body's response to foreign materials.

The haptoglobins

This is a group of proteins, all β_2-globulins, that bind haemoglobin to form haptoglobin–haemoglobin complexes, which are then rapidly broken down in the lymphoreticular system. This provides a mechanism whereby body iron stores can be conserved, since uncomplexed haemoglobin is filtered at the kidney and thus lost in urine. There is a genetic polymorphism for the hapto-

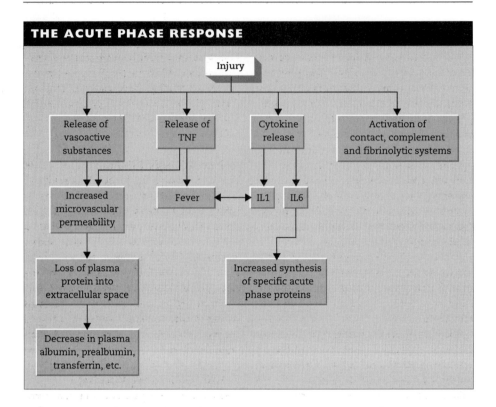

THE ACUTE PHASE RESPONSE

Fig. 6.2 The acute-phase response.

globins that leads to multiple bands on electrophoresis.

• Plasma [haptoglobin] falls whenever intravascular haemolysis is increased (e.g. in haemolytic anaemia), and free haptoglobin may then be undetectable. Decreased plasma [haptoglobin] is found also in liver disease, and rarely as a congenital abnormality.

• Plasma [haptoglobin] increases in acute infections and following trauma: haptoglobin is one of the acute-phase reactants (p. 88). It is also increased in the nephrotic syndrome.

α_1-Protease inhibitor (API)

Proteases such as trypsin, chymotrypsin, elastase and thrombin are continually being released into the blood in small amounts from a number of sources, including the pancreas, leukocytes and intestinal bacteria. API is one of several plasma proteins that inhibit the activity of these proteases, particularly neutrophil elastase, and may function to limit proteolytic activity at sites of inflammation. Interest in API principally relates to the association between certain diseases of the lung and liver and to API deficiency due to genetic polymorphism.

Clinical consequences of the genetic polymorphism of API

Many allelic genes code for API, the alleles being given the general designation Pi (protease inhibitor). The most common allele has been named M, with the usual homozygote being PiMM (the MM type). Individuals who are homozygous for the PiZ allele (i.e. who are PiZZ, the ZZ type) make up one in 3000 of the population in the United Kingdom. Individuals of the ZZ type (and SZ, who have one silent PiS allele) produce only a small amount of plasma API. They are prone to the following disorders:

• *Pulmonary emphysema.* About 1% of patients with emphysema have API deficiency, but this percentage is much higher in young patients. When associated with API deficiency, emphysema tends to manifest itself in the 20–40 age group. Smoking seems to be a strong predisposing factor for the development of the disease in these patients, possibly because particles in smoke stimulate phagocytic activity, with the local release of proteases.

• *Hepatic disorders.* Neonatal jaundice, usually presenting as a predominantly cholestatic picture, is common in type ZZ individuals. Although the jaundice may resolve, there is usually progression to hepatic cirrhosis. In about 20% of children with cirrhosis, the hepatic disorder can probably be attributed to API deficiency. In adults, cirrhosis and hepatoma are associated with the PiZ phenotype.

Phenotyping of API by isoelectric focusing is desirable in all cases in which plasma API levels are low or borderline, so that appropriate genetic counselling can be given to affected individuals or to their parents. Molecular techniques can also be used to investigate relatives of patients with API deficiency (p. 274).

Ceruloplasmin (M_r 132 kDa)

This is a copper-containing protein, an α_2-globulin with a mean concentration in plasma of 0.35 g/L. It has oxidase properties and can scavenge superoxide. It normally binds about 90% of the copper present in plasma. Plasma [ceruloplasmin] is *reduced* in Wilson's disease (p. 119), in patients with malnutrition, and in the nephrotic syndrome.

α_1-Fetoprotein (M_r 69 kDa)

This is present in the tissues and plasma of the fetus. Plasma concentration falls very rapidly after birth, but minute amounts (up to 15 µg/L) are present in plasma from adults. The functions of α_1-fetoprotein (AFP) are unclear, but it may play an immunoregulatory role during pregnancy. Measurements of AFP have two important applications:

1 *Pregnancy.* Women carrying fetuses with open neural tube defects have increased amniotic fluid and plasma [AFP], whilst women carrying a fetus with Down's syndrome will usually have decreased plasma [AFP]. Screening programmes involving measurement of maternal serum [AFP] at 16–18 weeks' gestation are now widely practised (p. 241).

2 *Tumour marker* (p. 118).

α_2-Macroglobulin (M_r 820 kDa)

This is the major α_2-globulin; it has a mean concentration of about 2.5 g/L in plasma. It binds endopeptidases such as trypsin and chymotrypsin; the resulting complexes have no endopeptidase activity. It is not known whether this antiprotease activity represents the major biological function of α_2-macroglobulin. It also has transport functions.

Plasma [α_2-macroglobulin] is *increased* greatly in the nephrotic syndrome, in some patients with cirrhosis, and in some of the collagen disorders.

β_2-Microglobulin (M_r 11.8 kDa)

This protein forms part of the human leucocyte antigen (HLA) system, and is a surface constituent of most cells. The β_2-microglobulin in plasma is mainly derived from myeloid and lymphoid cells, and is normally synthesized at a fairly constant rate. Plasma levels (mean concentration normally about 1.5 mg/L) are increased whenever there is lymphoid or myeloid proliferation.

The rate of removal of β_2-microglobulin from plasma depends on the glomerular filtration rate (GFR, p. 51), and plasma [β_2-microglobulin] is *increased* in the presence of renal failure. It may also rise in some malignant and immunological disorders. Its measurement may be of value in monitoring patients with renal failure, and in following the progress of patients with multiple myeloma.

The immunoglobulins

These are a group of structurally related proteins that function as antibodies; they are synthesized by the cells of the lymphoreticular system.

The basic immunoglobulin (Ig) molecule is made up of four polypeptide chains consisting of a pair of heavy chains (M_r 50–75 kDa each) and a pair of light chains (M_r 22 kDa each). There are five principal types of heavy chain (γ, α, μ, δ and ε) and two types of light chain (κ and λ). Every immunoglobulin can be assigned a formula that indicates its composition, according to its types of chain (e.g. $\alpha_2\lambda_2$, $\gamma_2\kappa_2$, etc.). The antigen-combining sites are between the adjacent light and heavy chains (Fig. 6.3).

The immunoglobulin classes

Three major classes of immunoglobulin (IgG, IgA and IgM) and two minor ones (IgD and IgE) have been recognized; the type of heavy chain determines the class. Table 6.5 lists several features of the major classes. Both light and heavy chains have 'constant' and 'variable' sections. The 'constant' portion varies little within each particular chain type, whereas the variable portion (which is associated with the antigen-combining site) is different for each immuno-globulin, even within a single chain type. The variable portion is responsible for the specificity of the antibody.

IgG immunoglobulins are formed particularly in response to soluble antigens such as toxins

Table 6.5 Some features of the major classes of the immunoglobulins.

and the products of bacterial lysis. They are widely distributed in the extracellular fluid (ECF), and cross the fetoplacental barrier.

IgM immunoglobulins in plasma are penta-mers of the basic immunoglobulin structure linked around a J chain polypeptide. They tend to be formed especially in response to particu-

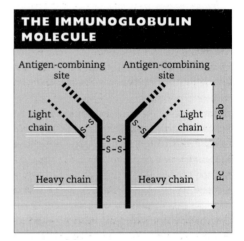

THE IMMUNOGLOBULIN MOLECULE

Fig. 6.3 The immunoglobulin molecule, which consists of two identical pairs, of heavy and light chains, held together by disulphide bonds (shown as –S–S). The molecules can be split by papain into three components; these are the two antigen-binding fragments (Fab), each of which has one binding site, and the crystallizable fragment (Fc). The variable regions of the Ig molecule are shown as interrupted lines. The heavy chains are one of five types (γ, α, μ, δ or ε), and the light chains are one of two types (κ or λ).

THE MAJOR IMMUNOGLOBULIN CLASSES

Feature	IgG	IgA	IgM
Average mol. mass	146 kDa	160 kDa	875 kDa
Plasma concentration	5.0–13.0 g/L	0.5–4.0 g/L	0.3–2.5 g/L
Light-chain type	κ or λ	κ or λ	κ or λ
Heavy-chain type	γ	α	μ
Structure of protein	$\gamma_2\kappa_2$ or $\gamma_2\lambda_2$	$\alpha_2\kappa_2$ or $\alpha_2\lambda_2$	$(\mu_2\kappa_2)_5$ or $(\mu_2\lambda_2)_5$
Plasma half-life	21 days	6 days	5 days
Immune response	Secondary	Local, secretory	Primary
Present in secretions	Trace	Yes	Trace
Transplacental passage	Yes	No	No

late antigens, such as those on the surface of bacteria. In the presence of complement, IgMs are very effective in producing lysis of these cells. Following an antigenic stimulus, IgM formation usually precedes IgG formation, and IgMs are thought to provide an early defence mechanism against intravascular spread of infecting organisms.

IgA immunoglobulins, as they occur in plasma, are monomers. However, over 50 % of IgA synthesis occurs in lymphoreticular cells under the mucosa of the respiratory and alimentary tracts. The IgA molecules are taken up here by the mucosal epithelial cells and are linked through the addition of a J chain to form an IgA dimer, e.g. $(\alpha_2\lambda_2)_2$; a secretory piece is also added that protects the molecule from proteolysis. The resulting protein, called secretory IgA, is secreted into the alimentary tract or respiratory tract, and may form part of the defence mechanism against local viral and bacterial infections.

IgD immunoglobulins are present in minute amounts in plasma. They are also often present, with monomer IgM, on the surface of B lymphocytes. Their function in plasma is unknown. However, on lymphocytes they are probably concerned with antigen recognition and with the development of tolerance.

IgE immunoglobulins include the reagins, which bind to cells such as the mast cells of the nasopharynx. In the presence of antigen (allergen), one result of the antigen–antibody reaction is the release of histamine and other amines and polypeptides from the cell, giving rise to a local hypersensitivity reaction.

Polyclonal (diffuse) hypergammaglobulinaemia

Liver disease, infection and autoimmune disease gives rise to stimulation of B cells and an increased production of γ-globulin, which on serum protein electrophoresis is revealed as a broad band (Fig. 6.1). The increase may affect all the Ig classes, or it may affect predominantly one class. The antibodies produced are heterogeneous. Quantitation of the separate Ig classes is occasionally helpful in diagnosis. In

most cases, however, the cause of the diffuse increase in plasma [total Ig] is apparent.

Multiple discrete bands (oligoclonal bands) or, rarely, a single discrete band may occur in the γ-globulin region in response to an antigenic stimulus.

Monoclonal (discrete) hypergammaglobulinaemia (paraproteinaemia)

Discrete immunoglobulin bands, visible on electrophoresis of serum, are known as paraproteins or monoclonal components. They are due to production of a single immunoglobulin or immunoglobulin fragment (e.g. light-chain or heavy-chain fragments) by a single clone of B cells. The detection of a paraprotein in blood or urine requires further investigation, to determine whether the paraproteinaemia is malignant or benign. Malignant paraproteinaemias occur in multiple myeloma (and plasmacytoma), macroglobulinaemia and other malignant lymphoid tumours (chronic lymphatic leukaemia, etc.). The prevalence of paraproteinaemia rises with age, and is about 3 % in the geriatric population.

Multiple myeloma is a disease in which there is proliferation of plasma cells and plasma cell precursors. The disorder often presents as bone pain (associated with lytic areas on X-ray), pathological fractures, or anaemia. Most myelomas produce complete Ig molecules, usually IgA or IgG, and the amount produced is often proportional to the tumour mass. Excessive amounts of Ig fragments (light chains or parts of heavy chains) are also produced in about 85 % of cases. Dimers of light chains (M_r 44 kDa) are usually found in urine, and are called 'Bence Jones' proteins. In about 10–20 % of cases of myeloma (usually the less differentiated – termed 'light-chain disease' or 'Bence Jones myeloma'), excess light chains may be the only abnormality in serum.

Waldenström's macroglobulinaemia usually follows a more prolonged course than multiple myeloma. There is proliferation of cells that resemble lymphocytes rather than plasma cells. They produce complete IgM molecules and often an excess of light chains. Increased plasma [IgM] causes increased plasma viscosity, which tends to make the circulation sluggish, and thromboses are common.

Heavy-chain disease (Franklin's disease) comprises a group of rare conditions in which heavy-chain fragments corresponding to the Fc portion of the immunoglobulins are synthesized and excreted in urine. Abnormal production of α and γ heavy chains is the most common derangement.

Benign paraproteinaemia may be transient or persistent. Paraproteins may occur transiently during acute infection and in autoimmune disease due to antigen stimulation. Stable or persistent benign paraproteinaemia may be due to a benign tumour of the B cells, but this can only be determined on follow-up (see below).

Cryoglobulins. These are immunoglobulins that precipitate when cooled to $4\,^{\circ}C$ and redissolve when warmed to $37\,^{\circ}C$; sometimes they precipitate at temperatures intermediate between $37\,^{\circ}C$ and $4\,^{\circ}C$. They occur in a number of diseases associated with hypergammaglobulinaemia, both the diffuse and the discrete forms. Their detection is of little value in determining the aetiology of the conditions in which they are formed. However, their importance lies in the fact that they may be associated with Raynaud's phenomenon. If cryoglobulin determinations are to be performed, blood needs to be collected into a warmed syringe without anticoagulant, and maintained at $37\,^{\circ}C$ until the serum for cryoglobulin investigation has been separated from the cells.

Investigation of paraproteinaemia

Chemical, haematological and radiological investigations, and lymph-node biopsy, are all of value when investigating cases of suspected paraprotelnaemla (Table 6.6).

Initial investigations

Serum protein electrophoresis shows a single discrete band, usually in the γ-globulin region but occasionally in the β-globulin or α_2-globulin region, in over 90% of patients in whom there is overproduction of complete immunoglobulin molecules; the concentrations of the other immunoglobulins may be reduced. Occasionally, a band due to the presence of light chains may be observed. Electrophoresis is the most sensitive widely available test for paraproteins; plasma must not be used, since the fibrinogen band may obscure or mimic paraproteins.

Urine protein electrophoresis on a fresh early-morning urine sample is usually needed to demonstrate Bence Jones protein; its small size (M_r 44 kDa) means that it is cleared rapidly by the kidney. If Bence Jones protein is detected, the monoclonal nature of the light chains can be confirmed by immunofixation. In multiple myeloma, the light chains are nearly always dimers of type κ or type λ, but not a mixture of the two. Most cases of myeloma and many cases of macroglobulinaemia have Bence Jones

MULTIPLE MYELOMA

Clinical features
Bone pain, fatigue, anaemia, infection, renal failure, hyperviscosity

Investigations
Diagnosis
  Paraprotein band in serum and urine.
  Lytic lesions on bone X-ray
  Bone marrow biopsy shows abnormal plasma cells
Progress and management
  Hypercalcaemia – bone involvement
  Raised creatinine and urea – impaired renal function
  Raised β_2-microglobulin – impaired renal function, tumour burden
  Low Hb – tumour burden, marrow depression
  Low non-paraprotein Igs – predisposition to infection

Table 6.6 Clinical features and investigations in multiple myeloma.

proteinuria. In light-chain disease, there is Bence Jones proteinuria but usually no serum paraprotein component.

On finding a paraprotein, the most important diagnostic decision is whether the condition is benign or malignant. Chemical features that point to the condition being benign are:

1 Other immunoglobulin classes are normal.
2 Bence Jones proteinuria is absent.
3 The serum [paraprotein] is less than 10 g/L.
4 The serum [paraprotein] does not increase with time.

Further investigations

If a paraprotein is found, further chemical measurements should usually be performed, as follows:

1 *The concentration and type of paraprotein* (IgG, IgA, etc.). This should be determined, since the concentration often correlates with the tumour mass.

2 *'Normal' (i.e. non-paraprotein) Ig*. The serum concentrations of these immunoglobulins should be measured, to assess the likelihood of intercurrent infection.

3 *Plasma [β_2-microglobulin]*. This provides a good index of prognosis, presumably because plasma [β_2-microglobulin] depends on both the turnover of tumour cells and on renal function. High levels indicate a poor prognosis.

4 *Plasma [creatinine]*, to assess renal (glomerular) function. Myeloma is commonly associated with both glomerular and tubular dysfunction.

5 *Plasma [calcium]*. This is often raised due to increased release of calcium from bone. *Plasma alkaline phosphatase* activity is usually normal or only slightly raised, as osteoblastic activity is not increased in multiple myeloma.

6 *Plasma [urate]*. This may be raised due to increased cell breakdown, especially after cytotoxic therapy. Urate deposition may cause renal damage in myeloma.

7 *Haemoglobin*. Anaemia is quite common.

Many of the results of these tests will be abnormal not only in multiple myeloma but in the other paraproteinaemias, particularly in Waldenström's macroglobulinaemia.

Progress of paraproteinaemia

Both malignant and benign paraproteinaemias can be followed up by measuring serum [paraprotein], serum ['normal' immunoglobulins], and plasma [β_2-microglobulin]. These investigations may need to be repeated several times before it becomes clear whether the paraproteinaemia is benign or malignant. Monitoring the progress of benign paraproteinaemias indicates that they only rarely become malignant.

Immunoglobulin deficiencies

Inherited deficiencies of immunoglobulin synthesis

Hypogammaglobulinaemia and, rarely, *agammaglobulinaemia* are conditions in which there is defective production of IgG, IgA and IgM. Children begin to develop severe, recurrent bacterial infections when over the age of one.

Acquired deficiencies of immunoglobulin synthesis

Secondary hypogammaglobulinaemia is much commoner than the inherited deficiencies. It may occur in lymphoid neoplasia (e.g. chronic lymphatic leukaemia, Hodgkin's disease, multiple myelomatosis), in 'toxic' disorders or certain types of drug therapy, in protein-losing syndromes (e.g. nephrotic syndrome), and in prematurity and delayed maturity.

Tumour markers

Tumours may secrete a wide range of substances into blood, including hormones, enzymes and tumour antigens, which are collectively referred to as tumour markers. Table 6.7 lists the tumour markers that are in common use.

Tumour markers can be used in a number of ways, including:

Monitoring treatment and detecting recurrence of disease. These are the most useful roles for tumour markers. An example of how sequential measurements of a tumour

TUMOUR MARKERS

Malignancy	Marker	Monitoring and follow-up	Aiding diagnosis	Prognosis	Screening
Choriocarcinoma	HCG	Yes	Yes	Yes	Yes
Colorectal	CEA	Yes			
Germ cell	HCG	Yes	Yes	Yes	
Germ cell	AFP	Yes	Yes	Yes	
Hepatoma	AFP	Yes	Yes		Yes
Lung (small cell)	NSE	Yes			
Myeloma	Paraprotein	Yes	Yes	Yes	
Ovarian	CA-125	Yes	Yes		
Prostatic	PSA	Yes	Yes		
Thyroid, medullary	Calcitonin	Yes	Yes		Yes
Thyroid, follicular	Thyroglobulin	Yes			

Table 6.7 Tumour markers commonly used in clinical practice.

USE OF CEA IN MONITORING

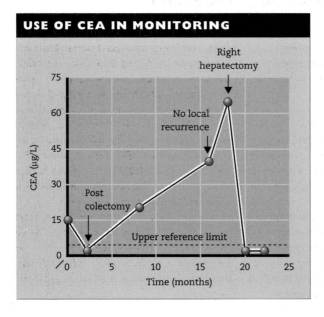

Fig. 6.4 Carcinoembryonic antigen (CEA) levels in a 68-year-old man who presented with a colonic tumour.

marker can be used to monitor treatment is shown in Figure 6.4.

Diagnosis. Tumour markers provide an aid to diagnosis, but only when used in conjunction with clinical and radiological evidence. Often, tumour marker concentrations may be increased in clinical conditions not associated with malignancy.

Screening. Tumour markers are of little value in screening for asymptomatic disease, but in some specific instances may be used to screen high-risk groups. Examples include measuring [calcitonin] after pentagastrin stimulation (p. 201) to screen close relatives of patients with medullary carcinoma of the thyroid, and human chorionic gonadotrophin (hCG), which is used to screen for choriocarcinoma in women who have had a hydatidiform mole.

Prognosis. Tumour markers can only be used for prognosis on the few occasions when the plasma concentration correlates with tumour mass. For example, hCG is used in choriocarcinoma, IgG in paraproteinaemia, and AFP and hCG in testicular tumours.

Examples of tumour markers used in clinical practice

Germ-cell tumours. Patients presenting with a lump in the testes or a malignancy of unknown origin should have plasma [AFP] and [hCG] measured. If raised due to secretion by the tumour, these measurements can also be used to monitor treatment. However, only about 75 % of non-seminomatous germ-cell tumours and a minority of patients with seminoma or dysgerminoma secrete these markers.

Choriocarcinoma. About 50% of cases of choriocarcinoma follow a hydatidiform mole pregnancy, and hCG is used to screen these women. hCG is also used to assess prognosis and response to treatment.

Ovarian cancer. Measurements of the cancer antigen CA-125 are used to monitor treatment and during follow up in patients with non-germ cell ovarian tumours. CA-125 measurements may also aid diagnosis, but measurements do not appear to be of value in prognosis or screening.

Prostatic cancer. Prostatic acid phosphatase measurements were once widely used as a marker for prostatic cancer, but it is now recognized that the glycoprotein prostate-specific antigen (PSA) is a superior marker. Serum PSA rises with age, and levels are also increased in benign prostatic hypertrophy, lower urinary tract infections and after trauma to the prostate. Screening of the general population is not recommended, partly because of the above-mentioned overlap with non-neoplastic disorders, but more importantly because of uncertainties about the efficacy of various treatment strategies for early prostatic cancer. Most PSA circulates in plasma bound to α_1-antichymotrypsin, but a small fraction circulates unbound to any protein (free PSA). Patients with prostatic cancer appear to have a higher ratio between α_1-antichymotrypsin–PSA complex and free PSA than patients with benign hypertrophy; this may be of diagnostic value.

PSA is of value in monitoring the response to therapy.

Gastrointestinal cancer. Endocrine tumours of the GI tract and hepatoma are covered in Chapters 8 and 9.

Carcinoembryonic antigen (CEA) is used to monitor non-endocrine tumours of the GI tract, particularly colorectal cancer. Measurements of plasma [CEA] do not have the sensitivity or specificity required for use as a screening test, and should never be used in isolation to establish a diagnosis of cancer. CEA is detectable in the serum of normal people, and levels may be mildly raised in many non-malignant diseases. The main indication for measuring plasma [CEA] is in monitoring for recurrence of the disease, but this knowledge often has little effect on the outcome.

Small-cell lung cancer. Neurone-specific enolase (NSE) is used to monitor response to treatment and detect early recurrence. The measurement of NSE is neither sufficiently sensitive nor specific to be used for screening or diagnosis.

KEY POINTS

1 Albumin is the protein with the highest concentration in plasma. Hypoalbuminaemia may be caused by reduced synthesis in the liver, altered distribution, increased catabolism, abnormal losses, or overhydration.

2 Following trauma, infection, etc., there is an acute-phase response, with increased plasma [C-reactive protein], [fibrinogen], [haptoglobin], [ceruloplasmin] and [α_1-protease inhibitor] and decreased concentrations of some other plasma proteins, including albumin.

3 Individuals who are homozygous for the Pi^z allele of α_1-protease inhibitor are more likely to develop pulmonary emphysema and hepatic disease.

4 Measurement of α-fetoprotein in maternal serum and amniotic fluid is used for screening for fetal neural tube defects.

5 On serum electrophoresis, a discrete immunoglobulin band (paraprotein) is highly suggestive of multiple myeloma, particularly if Bence Jones protein is detected in urine.

6 Tumour markers are of value in monitoring treatment and detecting recurrent disease. They are usually of little value in screening for asymptomatic disease, or in determining the prognosis.

Case 6.1

A 23-year-old man was admitted to hospital with fulminant hepatorenal failure. He was jaundiced, with marked abnormalities in his liver function tests. There was also clear evidence of intravascular haemolysis. He had been experiencing vague abdominal discomfort over the past three years, and over that time his liver function tests had been normal with the exception of alanine aminotransferase, which was found to be consistently elevated at 80 U/L (reference range 10–35 U/L).

Abdominal ultrasound showed a picture consistent with cirrhosis, with no evidence of biliary obstruction. Blood cultures, antimitochondrial and antinuclear antibodies were negative, as were tests for hepatitis B surface and core antibodies. There was no history of drug abuse, and paracetamol was not detected in the serum.

A liver biopsy revealed inflammatory and fatty changes, and stained heavily for copper. Serum ceruloplasmin was slightly decreased at 140 mg/L (reference range 150–600 mg/L).

What is the likely diagnosis? How would you confirm this?

Comments on Case 6.1

The man has Wilson's disease (p. 119). The diagnosis was confirmed by finding a decreased plasma [ceruloplasmin] of 140 mg/L (reference range 150–600 mg/L). The usual clinical manifestations of the disease are caused by excessive copper deposition, particularly in the liver and brain. The biochemical defect is present at birth, but symptoms typically appear in older children, adolescents and young adults. Most patients present with hepatic or neurological dysfunction. The haemolysis is thought to be due to the sudden release of copper from the liver, which damages the erythrocytes. About 30 % of patients present with features of chronic hepatitis. Most, but not all patients have Kayser–Fleischer rings. About 15 % of patients with active hepatic involvement have normal serum ceruloplasmin concentrations; this is thought to be due to hepatic inflammation, which leads to an increase in ceruloplasmin production as part of the acute-phase response that may be sufficient to bring values into the reference range.

Patients presenting with fulminant hepatic failure usually die unless a liver transplant can be performed. In other patients, treatment with a low copper diet and penicillamine to chelate and increase urinary copper excretion usually leads to a good prognosis.

Case 6.2

A 70-year-old man complained to his doctor of back pain that he had had for several months, and of feeling generally unwell. He appeared pale and he was tender over the lumbar spine.

His urine contained protein (1 g/L) and his erythrocyte sedimentation rate (ESR) was very high (90 mm in the first hour). The following abnormalities were reported:

Plasma analysis	Result	Reference range	Units
Albumin	32	36–47	g/L
Calcium	2.72	2.12–2.62	mmol/L
Alkaline phosphatase	90	40–110	U/L
Creatinine	180	55–120	mmol/L
Total protein	84	63–83	g/L
IgA	<0.4	0.5–4.0	g/L
IgG	37	5.0–13	g/L
IgM	<0.2	0.3–2.5	g/L

How would you interpret these results, and what further chemical investigations would you request in this patient?

Comments on Case 6.2

Serum and urine protein electrophoresis would both be indicated. The serum pattern showed a discrete band in the γ-globulin region, with marked reduction of the other immunoglobulins, and urine electrophoresis revealed the presence of Bence Jones protein, subsequently identified as of the λ type. The diagnosis of multiple myeloma was confirmed on X-ray examination (which demonstrated osteolytic lesions in the skull, vertebral column, ribs and pelvis) and by the finding of atypical plasma cells in the bone marrow.

Hypercalcaemia is present in about 30 % of patients with multiple myeloma, and about 50 % show some evidence of impaired renal function at the time of presentation; this is associated with a poor prognosis.

Case 6.3

A 73-year-old man presented to his doctor, complaining of back pain and increasing problems with passing urine. The following results from chemical tests were found:

Plasma analysis	Result	Reference range	Units
Prostate-specific antigen	70	<4	mg/L
Albumin	38	36–47	g/L
ALP activity	200	40–125	U/L
ALT activity	35	10–40	U/L
Bilirubin total	10	2–17	mmol/L
GGT activity	35	10–55	U/L

What is the likely diagnosis?

Comments on Case 6.3

The man is likely to have metastatic prostatic cancer. Although there is overlap in the levels of PSA seen in men with benign prostatic hypertrophy and prostatic cancer, the high levels of PSA found in this patient are usually seen only in patients with metastatic disease.

The elevated ALP in the presence of normal γ-glutamyl transferase and other liver function tests also suggest metastatic spread to bone.

Examination of the prostate per rectum disclosed an enlarged and hard prostate, and tissue obtained during a transurethral resection demonstrated the presence of tumour.

Case 6.4

A 50-year-old lecturer presented to his doctor, complaining of tiredness, abdominal discomfort and poor appetite. He had worked in Africa in the past, where he had contracted hepatitis B and had become a carrier. On examination, he was jaundiced and his liver was enlarged. Urine was positive for both bilirubin and urobilinogen.

The following results were found:

Plasma analysis	Result	Reference range	Units
Albumin	34	36–47	g/L
ALP activity	400	40–125	U/L
ALT	150	10–40	U/L
Bilirubin total	60	2–17	mmol/L
GGT activity	150	10–55	U/L
α_1-fetoprotein	3000	Not detectable	kU/L

What is the likely diagnosis?

Comments on Case 6.4

The patient has a primary hepatocellular carcinoma. This is a rare malignancy in the developed world, but common in China, South-East Asia and parts of Africa as a result of the high incidence of hepatitis B in these regions. Chronic carriers of the virus have an increased risk of developing the malignancy. The liver function tests show a mixed pattern of cholestasis, probably arising from the tumour, and hepatitis, arising from the chronic hepatitis. The very high concentration of α_1-fetoprotein is highly suggestive of hepatocellular carcinoma, but levels of up to about 500 kU/L can be found in some patients with nonmalignant hepatobiliary disease.

CHAPTER 7

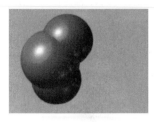

Plasma Enzyme Tests in Diagnosis

Release of enzyme from
  cells, 101
Selecting plasma enzyme
  tests, 101

Examples of clinically
  important plasma
  enzymes, 102

Biochemical tests in myocardial
  infarction, 105

Most of the enzyme tests used in diagnosis depend on the very high concentration of enzyme within the cell relative to that in plasma. Consequently, cellular damage resulting from disease or trauma often results in measurable increases in enzyme activity in plasma as the enzyme is released from the damaged cell. Furthermore, the pattern of enzyme release is largely determined by the tissue of origin of the enzyme, thus aiding diagnosis – particularly in liver disease and in myocardial infarction.

In this chapter we discuss:

1 The factors determining enzyme release and selection of enzyme tests.
2 Some enzymes and isoenzymes commonly used in diagnosis – lactate dehydrogenase (LD), creatine kinase (CK), the transaminases, amylase, alkaline phosphatase (ALP) and γ-glutamyl transferase.
3 Disease resulting from abnormal or deficient enzymes – Scoline apnoea and cholinesterase.
4 Use of enzyme tests in myocardial infarction.

Release of enzyme from cells

Changes in plasma enzyme activity are nearly always due to increases in the rate of release of enzymes into the circulation, most commonly caused by:

1 *Necrosis or severe damage to cells*, usually caused by ischaemia or toxins.
2 *Increased rate of cell turnover* during active growth, tissue repair, or in cancer.
3 *Increased concentrations of enzymes within cells*, usually as a result of induction by disease or drugs.
4 *Duct obstruction.* Enzymes normally present in exocrine secretions (e.g. amylase) may be regurgitated into the blood if the normal route of outflow is obstructed.

The rate of removal of different clinically important enzymes from the circulation, mainly by uptake into the cells of the lymphoreticular system, varies from a few hours to a few days.

Selecting plasma enzyme tests

The most important diagnostic questions are:
1 Has tissue damage occurred, and if so, what is its extent? This will determine the sensitivity of the test, which will largely depend on the tissue : plasma ratio of enzyme activity, which for most enzymes of clinical value lies between 1000 : 1 and 10 000 : 1.
2 Which tissues have been damaged? This is often a major problem, since few enzymes are tissue-specific. The difficulty may sometimes be overcome by the use of isoenzymes or enzyme combinations.

3 How does plasma enzyme activity change during the course of the disease? This depends on its rate of release into and removal from the circulation.

Enzyme units

Plasma enzyme measurements are usually made in terms of *activity* or of *concentration*. These usually, but not always, parallel one another.

Catalytic activity is measured in terms of reaction rates. The *international unit (IU) of enzyme activity* is defined as 'that amount of enzyme which, under given assay conditions, will catalyse the conversion of 1 mmol of substrate per minute'. However, since reaction conditions are not always standardized, reference values must be obtained from the laboratory performing the test. For simplicity in a general text like this, we have adopted a pragmatic approach, and usually express enzyme results in relation to the upper reference value for the method of measurement.

> ## Examples of clinically important plasma enzymes

Many of the enzymes considered below exist in the body in more than one form. *Isoenzymes* are proteins that possess similar catalytic activity, but which show genetically determined differences in their structure and in certain other properties (e.g. electrophoretic mobility, stability to heat). When an enzyme is released from damaged tissue, the isoenzyme pattern of the organ may be reflected by a corresponding change in the pattern detectable in plasma. Isoenzyme studies may thus help to localize the tissue of origin of an increased plasma enzyme activity.

Lactate dehydrogenase (LD)

Lactate dehydrogenase is widely distributed in the body, and human tissues contain five major proteins with lactate dehydrogenase activity, each having different electrophoretic mobility

and different physical and chemical properties. These differences enable the laboratory to distinguish two main patterns of LD isoenzymes in plasma in disease. Following release from myocardium or red or white blood cells, the anodal or so-called 'heart-specific' isoenzymes are present in serum, whereas the cathodal isoenzymes are released from the liver when that organ is damaged.

Creatine kinase (CK)

There are three principal CK isoenzymes, each comprising two polypeptide chains, either B or M; these give the dimers BB, MB and MM.

1 *Skeletal muscle* has a very high total CK content; over 98% normally comprises CK-MM, less than 2% CK-MB. CK-MB may rise to 5–15% in some patients with muscle disease, and also in athletes in training.

2 *Cardiac muscle* also has a high CK content. It comprises 70–80% CK-MM and 20–30% CK-MB. As a general rule, cardiac muscle is the only tissue with more than 5% CK-MB.

3 Other organs, such as brain, contain less CK, often CK-BB. However, CK-BB rarely appears in plasma and is not of diagnostic importance. Plasma normally contains more than 95% of its CK as CK-MM.

Plasma CK is valuable in the diagnosis of myocardial infarction and some muscle diseases (see below). Increases, sometimes large, may occur after trauma or surgical operations, intramuscular injections, in comatose patients, diabetic ketoacidosis, acute renal failure and hypothyroidism, and after prolonged muscular exercise, especially in unfit individuals.

Creatine kinase isoforms

The CK-MM released from tissue contains two intact polypeptide chains, each with a terminal lysine. A carboxypeptidase in plasma splits off the terminal lysine from each chain in turn, with resulting changes in electrophoretic mobility, but not in activity. These different forms of CK are called *isoforms,* and are usually termed CK-MM3 (as released from muscle), CK-MM2 (the hybrid) and CK-MM1 (with both lysine residues removed). After myocardial infarction, there is a very early absolute and relative increase in CK-MM3. Technical difficulties have precluded general use of the measurements.

Creatine kinase and muscle disease

Plasma CK, aspartate aminotransferase (AST), LD and alanine aminotransferase (ALT) activities may be increased in muscle disease. However, plasma total CK is usually the measurement of choice, irrespective of the aetiology of the disorder, since it is increased in the greatest number of cases and shows the largest changes.

Muscular dystrophy. In Duchenne-type dystrophy, high plasma CK activity is present from birth, before the onset of clinical signs. During the early clinical stages of the disease, very high activities are usually present, but these tend to fall as the terminal stages of the disease are reached. Smaller CK increases are present in other forms of muscular dystrophy. About 75% of female carriers of the Duchenne dystrophy gene have small increases in plasma CK activity.

Malignant hyperpyrexia. This is a rare but serious disorder, characterized by raised body temperature, convulsions and shock following general anaesthesia. Many of the patients show evidence of myopathy. Extremely high plasma CK activities are seen in the acute, postanaesthetic stage, but smaller increases often persist and can also be detected in the relatives of affected patients. Preoperative screening of plasma CK is not a reliable way of detecting patients liable to develop malignant hyperpyrexia, and should be limited to those patients with a family history of anaesthetic deaths or of malignant hyperpyrexia.

Miscellaneous muscle diseases. CK is variably increased in various myopathies, including that due to alcohol. It is also raised in polymyositis.

Neurogenic muscle disease. Plasma CK activity is usually normal in peripheral neuritis, poliomyelitis and motor neurone disease.

The aminotransferases
Aspartate aminotransferase (AST)

This is present in most tissues, but especially in skeletal and cardiac muscle, liver and kidney. It is mainly used in the investigation of patients with suspected myocardial infarction (p. 106) and liver disease (p. 113).

Alanine aminotransferase (ALT)

This is also widely distributed. Its concentration in most tissues is considerably less than that of AST, but in the liver the activities of the two enzymes are about the same. ALT activity is most often measured as one of a group of 'liver function tests' as a measure of hepatocellular damage (p. 113), since it is more liver-specific than AST.

Alkaline phosphatase (ALP)

This is the generic name for a group of enzymes that display maximum activity in the pH range 9.0–10.5. They are widely distributed, different tissues possessing one (occasionally more) characteristic and analytically distinguishable forms. Liver, bone, placenta and intestine are clinically important sources of plasma ALP activity. It is possible to determine the tissue of origin of increased alkaline ALP activity in serum by electrophoresis, immunoassay, or other methods.

The precise biochemical role of ALP is not known. In many tissues, it is attached to cell membranes, suggesting an association between ALP activity and membrane transport. In the liver, for example, activity is localized on those parts of the cell membrane of the parenchymal cell adjoining the biliary canaliculus and the sinusoid.

Physiological changes in activity

Plasma ALP activity may be significantly increased (compared with adult reference values) for entirely physiological reasons in:

Normal pregnancy. Release of ALP from the placenta may cause its total activity in plasma to rise in the second and third trimesters to about twice normal adult levels.

Infancy and childhood. The upper reference value here is as much as three or four times the adult value. This increase is a direct result of the intensive osteoblastic activity associated with normal bone growth (e.g. at puberty), since osteoblasts secrete ALP.

Meals containing fat. These may cause transient small increases in plasma intestinal ALP activity. Blood for ALP measurements should preferably be collected from patients who have not eaten recently.

Changes in activity due to disease

Alkaline phosphatase is commonly used in the investigation of patients with liver and bone disease. Most laboratories include ALP in their standard grouping of 'liver function tests' (p. 110); its activity is often greatly increased whenever there is cholestasis, whereas hepatocellular damage causes relatively little increase.

In bone disease, plasma ALP activity is raised when there is increased osteoblastic activity, as in Paget's disease, hyperparathyroidism, rickets and osteomalacia (Chapter 5). The uses of these measurements as tumour markers are discussed on p. 95.

γ-Glutamyl transferase (GGT)

This enzyme, sometimes called gamma-glutamyl transpeptidase, is found mainly in the kidney, liver, biliary tract and pancreas. The form of the greatest diagnostic importance occurs in the liver and, as with ALP, it is associated with the cell membrane adjoining the biliary canaliculus.

In liver disease, plasma GGT activity generally increases in parallel with alkaline phosphatase, i.e. it rises most when there is cholestasis. However, it tends to be raised more than ALP in other disorders affecting the liver, such as hepatocellular damage. Hepatic synthesis of the enzyme is also induced by alcohol and by several drugs (e.g. the antiepileptics), thereby causing plasma GGT to rise. Its activity is not raised in bone disease, and plasma GGT can therefore help to identify the tissue of origin of a raised plasma ALP activity.

α-Amylase (amylase)

Large amounts of amylase are present in the pancreas and salivary glands, and smaller amounts in other tissues. Salivary and pancreatic isoenzymes (both have M_r 45 kDa) are partially filtered from plasma at the glomerulus. These isoenzymes can be differentiated by immunological or electrophoretic methods, or by using an inhibitor (a wheat protein) that preferentially inhibits nonpancreatic isoenzymes of amylase.

Plasma amylase measurements are mostly used to help diagnose acute intra-abdominal conditions (p. 127).

Cholinesterase (ChE)

There are two principal ChEs: (1) the enzyme that is synthesized in the liver and present in plasma (formerly known as pseudocholinesterase), and (2) acetylcholinesterase, which is present at nerve endings and in the erythrocytes, but not in plasma (formerly known as 'true' cholinesterase).

Plasma ChE is of particular value in the diagnosis of patients with Scoline apnoea and organophosphorus insecticide poisoning (p. 291), but changes also occur in other conditions (Table 7.1).

Scoline apnoea

Some patients exhibit prolonged apnoea, lasting several hours, after succinylcholine (Scoline, suxamethonium) administration. This drug is normally hydrolysed by plasma ChE. Over 50% of patients sensitive to Scoline have genetically determined abnormalities in the ChE enzyme protein. At least four allelic genes are involved:

$E_1{}^u$ codes for the *usual* form of ChE, present in over 95% of the population in the United Kingdom.

$E_1{}^a$ codes for an *atypical* ChE that is resistant to inhibition by dibucaine.

$E_1{}^f$ codes for an atypical ChE that is resistant to inhibition by fluoride.

LOW PLASMA CHOLINESTERASE

Category of cause	Examples
Physiological reasons	Infancy, third trimester of pregnancy
Inherited abnormality	Scoline sensitivity (ChE variants)
Acquired abnormality	
(a) Liver disease	Impaired protein synthesis
(b) Industrial poisoning	Organophosphorus insecticides
(c) Drug effects	Oral contraceptives, monoamine oxidase inhibitors, cytotoxic drugs

Table 7.1 Causes of low plasma cholinesterase activity.

$E_1{}^s$ codes for a silent protein that has little or no ChE activity.

Most individuals with abnormal variants have low plasma ChE activity, but the only reliable way of demonstrating the variants is by means of inhibitor studies. Dibucaine and fluoride are the two most widely used inhibitors. For example, the normal enzyme ($E_1{}^u E_1{}^u$) is inhibited by about 80% by dibucaine – giving it a dibucaine number (DN) of 80 – whereas the most common abnormal ChE homozygote ($E_1{}^a E_1{}^a$) that can cause severe Scoline apnoea is only about 20% inhibited by dibucaine (DN= 20). In a similar fashion, using other inhibitors as well as dibucaine, it is possible to determine the probable genotype of most individuals and thus their likely susceptibility to Scoline. It is important to recognize these abnormalities of plasma ChE, since affected relatives can then be traced, and anaesthetists can be warned not to use Scoline.

Biochemical tests in myocardial infarction

After myocardial infarction, a number of intracellular proteins are released from the damaged cells. The proteins of major diagnostic interest include:
- Enzymes, such as CK, CK-MB, AST and LD (or 'heart-specific' LD)
- Myoglobin
- Troponin I and troponin T

The enzymes will be considered in the greatest detail here, since they are the most commonly used indices of myocardial damage.

Time-course of enzyme changes

After a myocardial infarction, the time-course of plasma enzyme changes always follows the same general pattern (Fig. 7.1). After an initial 'lag' phase of at least three hours, during which activities remain normal, they rise rapidly to a peak between 18 and 36 hours. Activities then return to normal at rates that depend on the half-life of each enzyme in plasma. The rapid rise and fall of CK-MB activity and the relatively prolonged rise of LD activity should be particularly noted.

Thrombolytic therapy

In patients treated with thrombolytic agents, the general pattern of plasma enzyme activity changes shown in Figure 7.1 is slightly modified. Following successful thrombolytic therapy (e.g. with streptokinase), there is a 'washout' of enzymes from the infarcted area, and plasma enzyme activities rise rapidly to reach an early peak, at 10–18 hours.

Optimal times for blood sampling

In most patients, a minimum of two samples is advisable (and usually sufficient).

1 A 'baseline', admission sample, with which to compare subsequent results.

2 A sample taken between 12 and 24 hours after the onset of symptoms (Table 7.2).

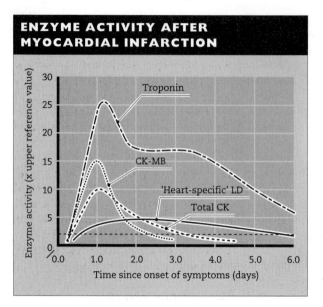

ENZYME ACTIVITY AFTER MYOCARDIAL INFARCTION

Fig. 7.1 Patterns of enzyme activity in the first few days after an uncomplicated myocardial infarction. Urea-stable lactate dehydrogenase (LD) is an example of so-called 'heart-specific' LD. Troponin, which is not an enzyme is also shown.

MYOCARDIAL INFARCTION: PLASMA ENZYME CHANGES

Enzyme	Abnormal activity detectable (h)	Peak value of abnormality (h)	Duration of abnormality (days)
CK-MB isoenzyme	3–10	12–24	1.5–3
Total CK	5–12	18–30	2–5
AST	6–12	20–30	2–6
'Heart-specific' LD	8–16	30–48	5–14

Table 7.2 Time-course of plasma enzyme activity changes after myocardial infarction.

Except for the occasional patient seen for the first time two days or more after the episode, in whom LD measurements might still be useful, it is very rarely of any value to take samples for plasma enzyme studies after 48 hours from the onset of symptoms that suggest a diagnosis of myocardial infarction.

Selection of enzyme tests

Plasma CK (possibly with CK-MB) measurements are requested most often; less often,

total LD or 'heart-specific' LD may be requested, particularly if more than 36 hours have elapsed since the episode of chest pain.

CK-MB isoenzyme

CK-MB is a more sensitive and specific test for myocardial damage than total CK. However, its transient rise and the lack of reliability of some methods have weighed against its general introduction as the first-line test for myocardial infarction in all laboratories. In the following circumstances, however, plasma CK-MB measurements (preferably by a mass measurement method) are strongly indicated:

1 When *very early* evidence of infarction is

required (less than eight hours from the onset of symptoms).

2 When investigating *postoperative* or *traumatized* patients for suspected myocardial infarction. In these patients, plasma CK-MB remains normal in the absence of myocardial damage, whereas AST, total CK and LD activities are often increased in plasma for noncardiac causes.

3 In patients suspected of having had a *second infarct* within a few days of the first. It is easier to show that a second rise in plasma enzyme activity has occurred if the activity of the enzyme that is being measured rises and falls rapidly after the previous incident involving myocardial damage (Fig. 7.1).

4 When concurrent release of CK-MM is likely (e.g. after an intramuscular injection).

Enzyme tests and the electrocardiogram

We recommend measurement of plasma enzyme tests, normally CK and a 'heart-specific' LD on all patients suspected of having had a myocardial infarction within the previous 48 hours. (Depending on local availability, a policy based on the use of troponin measurements also has much to recommend it; see below). In many patients, this might seem unnecessary, since the electrocardiogram (ECG) often provides unequivocal evidence of infarction. However, it is possible to misinterpret ECG traces, especially in the presence of arrhythmias, and the ECG is by no means always abnormal in patients who have recently had a myocardial infarction. In addition, enzyme measurements can provide an indication of infarct size, and thus prognosis.

Plasma enzymes and the ECG are complementary in the investigation of patients with suspected myocardial infarction. Used appropriately and correctly interpreted, the tests compare as shown in Table 7.3. If both types of investigation are performed correctly, few wrong diagnoses of myocardial infarction should be made.

Non-enzyme tests in myocardial infarction

Troponin T and *troponin I* are components of the contractile complex of muscle, and although they are mainly insoluble, there is a soluble fraction. Cardiac-specific forms can be recognized, and these are currently the most sensitive and specific indices of myocardial damage available.

In general, although the initial rise in cardiac troponins after myocardial infarction occurs at about the same time as CK and CK-MB, this rise continues for longer than for most of the enzymes, possibly because of later release of 'insoluble' protein from the infarcted muscle. Because of the inherent sensitivity of the tests for myocardial damage, increases are seen in some patients with angina, as well as those with infarcts. Cardiac troponin measurements are particularly useful in excluding the diagnosis of myocardial damage, particularly after 12 hours following chest pain or other symptoms, and in patients who are likely to have concurrent cardiac and skeletal muscle damage.

Myoglobin is also a sensitive index of myocardial damage, and it rises very rapidly after the event at about the same rate as CK-MB. However, it is nonspecific, since it is raised following any form of muscle damage.

MYOCARDIAL INFARCTION: PLASMA ENZYMES VS. ECG		
	Sensitivity (%)	Specificity (%)
Electrocardiogram	70	100
Plasma enzymes	95	90

Table 7.3 Comparable value of plasma enzyme tests and electrocardiography in the investigation of patients with suspected myocardial infarction.

KEY POINTS

1 Enzymes are present in high concentration in cells, and are released following tissue damage, increased cell turnover, or induction.
2 Enzyme release is modified by intracellular location, and enzymes are eliminated from plasma at different rates.
3 The pattern of enzymes present in plasma generally reflects that of the damaged tissue.
4 In liver disease, alanine aminotransferase (ALT) and aspartate aminotransferase (AST) are greatly raised in hepatocellular damage; alkaline phosphatase (ALP) and γ-glutamyl transferase (GGT) are raised in cholestatic disease.
5 In myocardial infarction, enzymes—in particular CK and CK-MB—usually become raised after a lag period of 4–6 hours after the onset of symptoms, reach a peak at 18–30 hours, and have returned to normal within 3–7 days.

Case 7.1

A 66-year-old man had experienced central chest pain on exertion for some months, but in the afternoon of the day prior to admission had had a particularly severe episode of the pain lasting for about an hour. On admission the following morning, he was noted to be pale, but there were no other abnormalities on examination. The ECG was normal, but plasma enzymes taken at that time were as follows:

Enzyme	Result (IU/L)	Reference range (IU/L)
Creatine kinase (CK)	150	30–200
Aspartate aminotransferase (AST)	45	10–35
Lactate dehydrogenase (LD)	2500	230–460

Comment on these results. Is there evidence that this man has had a myocardial infarct?

Comments on Case 7.1
There is no evidence other than the symptoms of central chest pain to suggest a myocardial infarct. The abnormal LD result can be discounted, since following myocardial infarction, AST and CK during the period 18–30 hours after onset of chest pain would be expected to show an even larger rise than LD. Further investigations revealed that the patient had a macrocytic megaloblastic anaemia, which responded to vitamin B_{12} treatment. The raised plasma LD activity is a regular finding in this condition, and is due to release of enzyme from immature red cells in the bone marrow (ineffective erythropoiesis).

Case 7.2

A 59-year-old man attended his doctor's surgery complaining of weight loss. Further questioning revealed a recent alteration in bowel habit. No positive physical signs were seen, but investigations revealed a positive faecal occult blood and the following test results:

Test	Result	Reference range
Bilirubin	16 mmol/L	2–17 mmol/L
Alanine aminotransferase	30 IU/L	10–40 IU/L
Alkaline phosphatase	310 IU/L	40–100 IU/L
γ-Glutamyl transferase	190 IU/L	10–55 IU/L
Albumin	38 g/L	36–48 g/L

Comment on these results.

Comments on Case 7.2

The history and positive faecal occult blood suggest the possibility of a carcinoma of the lower bowel. The biochemical tests—raised alkaline phosphatase and GGT—suggest localized area(s) of cholestasis in the liver causing induction and release of these enzymes from the affected area, but not sufficiently to affect bilirubin excretion from the unaffected areas.

CHAPTER 8

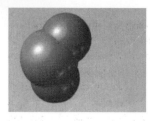

Liver Disease

Structure of the liver, 110
Liver function tests, 110

The place of chemical tests in
    the diagnosis of liver disease,
    114

Biochemistry of specific liver
    diseases, 117
Specific disorders, 118

The liver plays a key role in intermediary metabolism, including the synthesis of carbohydrates, lipids and many proteins. It exchanges substances with the plasma, adding some for distribution in the body and removing others, often with subsequent metabolism. The liver is the organ mainly responsible for the detoxification of many drugs and carcinogens; it also secretes bile salts.

Liver disease is relatively common, and the measurement of serum levels of bilirubin, hepatic enzymes and albumin, as well as the prothrombin time, provide simple tests to determine whether disease is present and give some guidance as to its nature.

This chapter outlines the principles governing the use and interpretation of the common liver function tests.

Structure of the liver

Only about 60% of the cells in the liver are hepatocytes (Fig. 8.1); the remainder are endothelial (Kupffer) cells lining the hepatic sinusoids (30%) and vascular and supporting tissue cells (10%).

The *functional unit* of each liver acinus consists of the portal tract, surrounded by radiating cords of hepatocytes. Blood enters the acinus via the portal tract and passes along the sinusoids towards the central vein. Hepatocytes in the periportal area, zone 1, receive relatively well oxygenated blood, whereas the hepatocytes surrounding the central vein, zone 3, receive blood that has lost much of its oxygen and exchanged other substances with the cells of zones 1 and 2. Cells in zone 3 are the most susceptible to anoxia and to injury by a wide range of toxic substances.

Cells in zone 1 have relatively high concentrations of the enzymes usually measured in blood for diagnostic purposes (e.g. alkaline phosphatase and the aminotransferases), whilst cells in zone 3 are relatively deficient in these enzymes. This may help to explain why some patients with centrilobular liver damage may have normal plasma enzyme activities.

Liver function tests

Most laboratories perform a standard group of tests (Table 8.1), which do not assess genuine liver function but are useful for:
- Detecting the presence of liver disease.
- Placing the liver disease in the appropriate broad diagnostic category. This then allows the selection of further, more expensive and time-consuming investigations such as ultrasound, computed tomography (CT) scanning, endoscopy and liver biopsy.
- Following the progress of liver disease.

Hepatic anion transport: bilirubin

Measurements of bilirubin in blood and urine are usually used to assess hepatic anion transport, although many other anions, including bile salts, are also transported by the liver. Understanding the mechanisms by which bilirubin is formed and removed greatly helps in the diagnosis of patients with jaundice or liver disease, since abnormal levels of bilirubin in blood can occur in patients in whom there is no liver disease.

Bilirubin production and metabolism

The pathway of bilirubin production and excretion is shown in Figure 8.2.

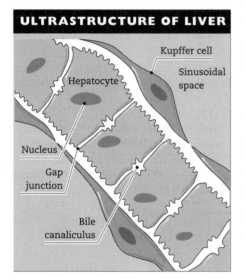

ULTRASTRUCTURE OF LIVER

Kupffer cell

Sinusoidal space

Hepatocyte

Nucleus

Gap junction

Bile canaliculus

Fig. 8.1 The ultrastructure of the liver. The liver ultrastructure mainly consists of hepatocytes and Kupffer cells (part of the reticuloendothelial system). The bile canaliculus is formed by the plasma membrane of two hepatocytes.

Production

About 80% of bilirubin formed each day from haem arises from red cells. The remaining 20% comes from red cell precursors destroyed in the bone marrow ('ineffective erythropoiesis'), and from other haem proteins such as myoglobin, the cytochromes and peroxidase. Iron is removed from the haem molecule, and the porphyrin ring is opened to form bilirubin.

Transport in plasma and hepatic uptake

Bilirubin is insoluble in water and is carried in plasma bound to albumin, and is thus not filtered at the glomerulus unless there is glomerular proteinuria. On reaching the liver, the bilirubin is taken into the hepatocyte by a specific carrier mechanism.

Conjugation of bilirubin and secretion into bile

In the endoplasmic reticulum of the hepatocyte, the enzyme *bilirubin UDP-glucuronyltransferase* conjugates bilirubin with glucuronic acid to produce bilirubin glucuronides which are water soluble and readily transported into bile. Secretion of bilirubin glucuronides into bile occurs against a high concentration gradient; a carrier-mediated energy-dependent process is probably involved.

Further metabolism of bilirubin in the gut

Bilirubin glucuronides are degraded by bacterial action, mainly in the colon, to a mixture of colourless water-soluble compounds collectively termed urobilinogen. These compounds

Table 8.1 Routine groups of liver function tests (examples of widely performed groups of plasma measurements).

ROUTINE LIVER FUNCTION TESTS	
Standard group of tests	Property being assessed
Plasma [albumin], prothrombin time	Protein synthesis
Plasma [bilirubin (total)]	Hepatic anion transport
Plasma enzyme activities	
ALT, AST	Hepatocellular integrity
ALP, GGT	Presence of cholestasis

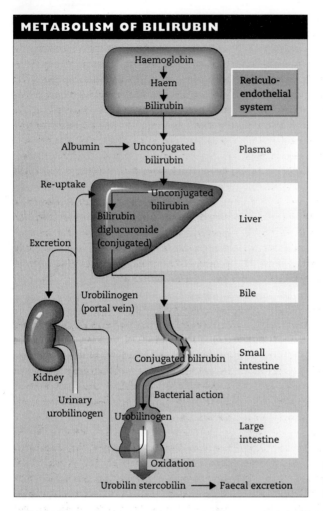

Fig. 8.2 The formation and metabolism of bilirubin and its excretion into the intestine.

oxidize to brown compounds known as urobilins and stercobilins.

Urobilinogen is mostly excreted in the faeces, but a small percentage is absorbed and carried to the liver in the portal blood supply, i.e. it undergoes an *enterohepatic circulation*. Most of this urobilinogen is cleared by the liver, but a proportion escapes clearance and is filtered at the kidney and appears in urine, where it can be detected using side-room tests (p. 298).

Measurements of plasma bilirubin

Normally, more than 95 % of bilirubin in plasma is unconjugated, but in liver disease the conjugated form may predominate. For most purposes, the measurement of plasma [total bilirubin] (i.e. the sum of the unconjugated and conjugated forms) is sufficient, especially when results are interpreted in relation to the patient's history, findings on clinical examination, and the results of side-room tests on urine specimens for urobilinogen and bilirubin. Occasionally, it may be helpful to measure plasma [conjugated bilirubin] and plasma [unconjugated bilirubin] separately.

Hepatocellular damage: aminotransferase measurements

Soluble cytoplasmic enzymes and, to a lesser

extent, mitochondrial enzymes are released into plasma in hepatocellular damage. The measurement of the activity of alanine aminotransferase (ALT) or aspartate aminotransferase (AST) in plasma provide a sensitive index of hepatocellular damage. Plasma ALT measurements are more liver-specific than AST. AST has both cytoplasmic and mitochondrial isoenzymes, and tends to be released more than ALT in chronic hepatocellular disease (e.g. cirrhosis). The aminotransferases are mainly located in the periportal hepatocytes, and they do not give a reliable indication of centrilobular liver damage. As with all tests based on the release of enzymes from damaged tissue, there is a lag period of some 24 hours from the initiation of tissue damage to the first appearance of increased enzyme levels in the plasma.

Cholestasis: alkaline phosphatase and γ-glutamyl transferase

Some enzymes, such as alkaline phosphatase (ALP) and γ-glutamyl transferase (GGT), are normally attached, or 'anchored', to the biliary canalicular and sinusoidal membranes of the hepatocyte. For this reason, ALP and GGT tend to be released into plasma in only small amounts following hepatocellular damage. However, they are released in much greater amounts when there is cholestasis, since their synthesis is induced and they are rendered soluble – due, at least in part, to the presence of high hepatic concentrations of bile acids.

Changes in the activities of GGT and ALP often parallel each other in cholestatic liver disease. Plasma GGT has the advantage of being more liver-specific, as plasma ALP may also be increased due to release from bone in bone disease.

Hepatic protein synthesis

The measurement of certain plasma proteins provides an index of the liver's ability to synthesize protein.

Albumin

In chronic hepatocellular damage, there is impaired albumin synthesis. Plasma [albumin] falls – providing, in the later stages, a fairly good index of the progress of the disease. In acute liver disease, however, there may be little or no reduction in plasma [albumin], as the biological half-life of albumin is about 20 days and the fractional clearance rate is therefore low. Factors other than impaired hepatic synthesis may lead to a decreased plasma [albumin]. These include loss of albumin into the extravascular compartment, ascites, increased degradation and poor nutritional status (p. 87).

Ascites. Increased portal venous pressure, a low plasma colloid oncotic pressure and Na^+ retention due to secondary hyperaldosteronism combine to cause ascites in cirrhotic patients. This often develops when plasma [albumin] falls below 30 g/L.

Coagulation factors

In liver disease, the synthesis of prothrombin and other clotting factors is diminished, leading to an increased *prothrombin time*. This may be one of the earliest abnormalities seen in patients with hepatocellular damage, since prothrombin has a short half-life (approximately six hours).

Deficiency of *fat-soluble vitamin K*, due to failure of absorption of lipids, may also cause a prolonged prothrombin time. In vitamin K deficiency, the coagulation defect can often be corrected by parenteral administration of vitamin K, but this has no effect in hepatocellular damage.

Immunoglobulins

Plasma immunoglobulin (Ig) measurements are of little value in liver disease, because the changes are of low specificity. In most types of cirrhosis, plasma [IgA] is often increased, whilst in primary biliary cirrhosis, plasma [IgM] increases greatly. In chronic active hepatitis, plasma [IgG] tends to be most increased.

Serological tests

Antimitochondrial antibodies are present in over 95% of patients with primary biliary cirrhosis, and anti-smooth muscle antibodies are found in about 50% of patients with chronic active hepatitis.

Disordered metabolism

Patients with severe liver disease may have:

- Significant *decreases in plasma [urea]*, due to failure of the liver to convert amino acids and NH_3 to urea. These changes occur late in the disease. Note that there are other causes of a low plasma [urea] (Table 4.2, p. 54).
- *Hypoglycaemia* due to impaired gluconeogenesis or glycogen breakdown, or both.
- Raised concentrations of all the *plasma lipid fractions,* if cholestasis is present. An abnormal lipoprotein that contains high concentrations of phospholipid, *lipoprotein X*, is present in plasma in nearly all cases of cholestasis.

The place of chemical tests in the diagnosis of liver disease

The jaundiced patient

Jaundice is due to hyperbilirubinaemia, and becomes clinically apparent when the plasma [bilirubin] exceeds about 50 μmol/L, although smaller degrees of hyperbilirubinaemia may be of diagnostic significance.

Measurements of plasma [bilirubin] give a quantitative index of the severity of the jaundice, whilst plasma enzyme activity measurements and side-room tests (p. 115) on fresh urine specimens, for bilirubin and urobilinogen, usually allow the cause of jaundice to be defined as prehepatic, hepatocellular, or

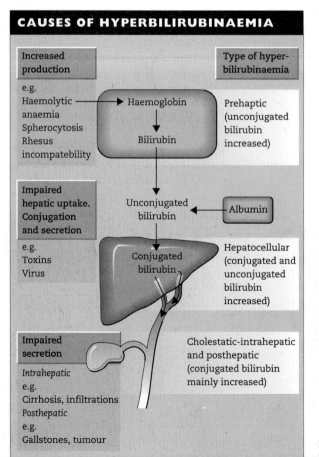

CAUSES OF HYPERBILIRUBINAEMIA

Increased production	Type of hyper-bilirubinaemia
e.g. Haemolytic anaemia Spherocytosis Rhesus incompatebility	Prehaptic (unconjugated bilirubin increased)
Impaired hepatic uptake. Conjugation and secretion	
e.g. Toxins Virus	Hepatocellular (conjugated and unconjugated bilirubin increased)
Impaired secretion	Cholestatic-intrahepatic and posthepatic (conjugated bilirubin mainly increased)
Intrahepatic e.g. Cirrhosis, infiltrations Posthepatic e.g. Gallstones, tumour	

Haemoglobin → Bilirubin → Unconjugated bilirubin ← Albumin → Conjugated bilirubin

Fig. 8.3 Types and causes of hyperbilirubinaemia.

cholestatic (Fig. 8.3). Appropriate further tests can then be requested (Table 8.2).

Investigations of the jaundiced patient often use the strategy shown in Figure 8.4.

Prehepatic hyperbilirubinaemia

This is due to over-production of bilirubin causing increased plasma [unconjugated bilirubin]. It occurs in:

- Haemolytic anaemia.
- Haemolytic disease of the new-born, due to rhesus incompatibility.
- Ineffective erythropoiesis (e.g. pernicious anaemia).
- Bleeding into the tissues (e.g. sports injuries).
- Rhabdomyolysis.

Hepatocellular hyperbilirubinaemia

This can arise from:

- *Hepatocellular damage* caused by infective agents, drugs and toxins.
- *Cirrhosis* – usually as a relatively late complication.
- *Low activity of bilirubin UDPglucuronyltrans-*

ferase in congenital deficiency (Gilbert's syndrome and Crigler–Najjar syndrome; see below), premature infants (the enzyme normally develops at about full term), or competitive inhibition of the enzyme by drugs (e.g. due to novobiocin). This leads to increased plasma [unconjugated bilirubin].

Cholestatic hyperbilirubinaemia

Cholestasis may be intrahepatic or extrahepatic. In both, there is conjugated hyperbilirubinaemia and bilirubinuria.

Intrahepatic cholestasis commonly occurs in:

- Acute hepatocellular damage (e.g. due to infectious hepatitis).
- Cirrhosis.
- Intrahepatic carcinoma (most commonly secondary).
- Primary biliary cirrhosis.
- Drugs (e.g. methyltestosterone, phenothiazines).

Extrahepatic cholestasis is most often due to:

- Gallstones.
- Carcinoma of the head of the pancreas.
- Carcinoma of the biliary tree.
- Bile duct compression from other causes.

The congenital hyperbilirubinaemias

These are all due to inherited defects in the mechanism of bilirubin transport metabolism.

Table 8.2 Bilirubin and urobilinogen measurements (examples of results in various conditions).

BILIRUBIN AND UROBILINOGEN IN JAUNDICE

	Urine tests (side-room)		Plasma [bilirubin]	
Condition	Urobilinogen	Bilirubin	Total* (μmol/L)	Conjugated
Healthy individuals	Trace	Nil	2–17	About 5%
Gilbert's syndrome	Trace	Nil	<50	Below 5%
Haemolytic diseases	Increased	Nil	<60	Below 5%
Hepatitis				
Prodromal	Increased	Detectable	<35	Raised
Icteric stage	—Undetectable	Present	<250	Much raised
Recovery stage	Detectable	Falling	Falling	Falling
Biliary obstruction	—Undetectable	Present	<400	Much raised

*Values for plasma [total bilirubin] are included so as to give indications of the order of severity of the hyperbilirubinaemia that may be observed in the various conditions listed.

INVESTIGATION OF JAUNDICE

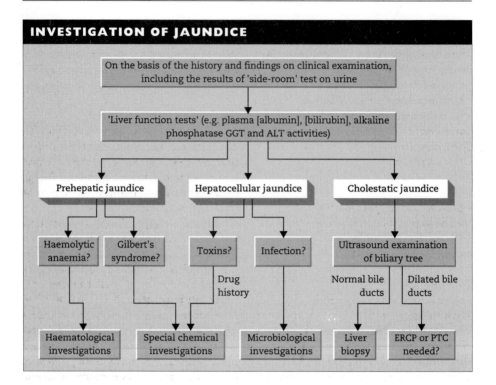

On the basis of the history and findings on clinical examination, including the results of 'side-room' test on urine

'Liver function tests' (e.g. plasma [albumin], [bilirubin], alkaline phosphatase GGT and ALT activities)

Prehepatic jaundice

Hepatocellular jaundice

Cholestatic jaundice

Haemolytic anaemia?

Gilbert's syndrome?

Toxins?

Infection?

Ultrasound examination of biliary tree

Drug history

Normal bile ducts

Dilated bile ducts

Haematological investigations

Special chemical investigations

Microbiological investigations

Liver biopsy

ERCP or PTC needed?

Fig. 8.4 The investigation of jaundice. Endoscopic retrograde cholangiopancreatography (ERCP) or percutaneous transhepatic cholangiography (PTC) may be needed whenever the cause of dilated bile ducts is uncertain.

Gilbert's syndrome

This familial autosomal dominant trait is probably present in 2–3% of men; it is two to seven times more common in men than women. The unconjugated hyperbilirubinaemia is usually asymptomatic, and plasma [bilirubin] fluctuates, higher levels tending to occur during intercurrent illness. Most patients have a plasma [bilirubin] less than 50 μmol/L, but higher levels are not uncommon. Other commonly performed tests of 'liver function' are normal, and there is no bilirubinuria.

Gilbert's syndrome is caused by decreased expression of bilirubin UDPglucuronyltrans-ferase, due to a mutation in the regulatory portion of the gene.

Gilbert's syndrome can most easily be differentiated from the mild degree of hyperbilirubinaemia in haemolytic anaemia by haematological investigations. Sometimes this differentiation is made by observing the effects on plasma [bilirubin] of a *reduced energy intake* (1.67 MJ/day; 400 kcal/day), particularly a reduction in the intake of lipids, for 72 hours. This results in at least a doubling of plasma [unconjugated bilirubin] in patients with Gilbert's syndrome, whereas in normal individuals it does not rise above 25 μmol/L.

Fasting plasma [bile acids] are normal in Gilbert's syndrome, but raised in hyperbilirubinaemia due to liver disease.

Crigler–Najjar syndrome

This rare condition, due to low activity of bilirubin UDP-glucuronyltransferase, gives rise to severe hyperbilirubinaemia in neonates, leading to kernicterus and often to early death.

Dubin–Johnson syndrome and Rotor's syndrome

These rare disorders are characterized by a benign conjugated hyperbilirubinaemia, accompanied by bilirubinuria. In both, there is a defect in the transfer of conjugated bilirubin into the biliary canaliculus. Urinary coproporphyrins are normal in patients with the Dubin–Johnson syndrome, but increased in Rotor's syndrome.

Biochemistry of specific liver diseases

Acute liver disease

Acute hepatitis

This is usually caused by viruses or toxins. There is often a pre-icteric phase when increases in plasma ALT and AST activities and in urobilinogen in urine occur. By the time clinical jaundice appears, plasma ALT and AST activities are usually more than six times, and occasionally more than 100 times, the upper reference value. The stools may be very pale, due to impaired biliary excretion of bilirubin, and urobilinogen then disappears more or less completely from the urine. Alkaline phosphatase (ALP) activity is usually only slightly increased, up to about twice the upper reference value, but it may be considerably raised in cases (relatively uncommon) in which there is a marked cholestatic element, as occurs in acute alcoholic hepatitis.

Acute viral hepatitis usually resolves quickly, and chemical indices of abnormality revert to normal within a few weeks. However, chronic persistent hepatitis occurs in a few patients, in whom plasma aminotransferase activities may remain high for months.

Poisoning and drugs

Findings similar to those in acute viral hepatitis are observed in patients with hepatocellular toxicity due to drugs (e.g. paracetamol overdose (p. 288), halothane jaundice, carbon tetrachloride poisoning). Drugs such as chlorpromazine may produce cholestasis, with increased plasma ALP and GGT, whilst phenytoin, barbiturates and ethanol induce GGT synthesis without necessarily causing liver damage.

Cholestatic liver disease

Both extrahepatic and intrahepatic obstruction commonly cause cholestasis. The distinction between the two is often clinically important from the point of view of further investigation and treatment, but it can rarely be made by chemical tests.

Plasma [bilirubin] is often greatly increased, and there is marked bilirubinuria; urobilinogen often becomes undetectable in urine. Plasma ALP and GGT activity is considerably increased, often to more than three times the upper reference values, but plasma ALT and AST activities are usually only moderately raised. In long-standing cholestatic jaundice, hepatic protein synthesis may be impaired and plasma alkaline phosphatase activity may start to fall as a result, and even return to normal; this emphasizes the importance of performing a baseline set of investigations as early as possible in patients with liver disease.

Plasma ALP and GGT activities may be markedly increased in patients with partial biliary obstruction, due to local obstruction in one of the smaller biliary ducts, such as often occurs in both primary and secondary carcinoma of the liver. Partial biliary obstruction may have little or no effect on the capacity of the liver to excrete bilirubin, so there may be no evidence of jaundice in these patients, at least initially; bilirubin excretion in the other parts of the liver may be able to compensate fully for the sector affected by the local biliary obstruction.

Chemical features that may help to distinguish cholestasis from hepatocellular damage are summarized in Table 8.3. These are 'typical' findings, and many cases do not follow these patterns exactly. The distinction between intrahepatic and extrahepatic cholestasis is usually made by radiological investigations – e.g. endoscopic retrograde

HEPATOCELLULAR DAMAGE AND CHOLESTASIS

Investigation	Hepatocellular damage		Cholestasis
	Acute	Chronic	
Albumin	N or ↓	N, ↓ or ↓↓	N or ↓
Bilirubin (total)	N, ↑ or ↑↑	N or ↑	N* ↑ or ↑↑
Aminotransferases	↑↑ or ↑↑↑	N or ↑	↑
Alkaline phosphatase	N or ↑	N or ↑	↑↑
GGT	N or ↑	N or ↑	↑↑
Immunoglobulins	N or ↑	↑ (Note 1)	↑ (Note 2)
Lipoprotein X	Not present unless there is cholestasis		Present
Prothrombin time (PT)	N or ↑	N or ↑	N or ↑
Effect of parenteral vitamin K on PT	None	None	May correct PT

N normal; ↑ increased; ↑↑ much increased and ↑↑↑ very much increased; ↓ decreased, ↓↓ much decreased. N* indicates that plasma [bilirubin] is often normal when cholestasis is localized, as it often is with secondary deposits in the liver.

Notes
1. Plasma [IgA] is particularly increased in cirrhosis, and plasma [IgG] in chronic active hepatitis.
2. Plasma [IgM] is increased in primary biliary cirrhosis.

Table 8.3 Hepatocellular damage and cholestasis (plasma or serum measurements that may help to differentiate between these conditions).

cholangiopancreatography (ERCP), ultrasound, or computed tomography (CT) scanning – or by liver biopsy.

Specific disorders

Infiltrations of the liver

The liver parenchyma may be progressively disorganized and destroyed in patients with primary or secondary carcinoma, amyloidosis, the reticuloses, tuberculosis, sarcoidosis and abscesses. These diseases often lead to partial biliary obstruction, with the associated chemical changes described above. Plasma [α_1-fetoprotein] (AFP) is often greatly increased in hepatoma (p. 91).

Cirrhosis of the liver

Alcoholism, viral hepatitis and prolonged cholestasis are the most frequent known causes of cirrhosis in Britain, but in half the cases no obvious cause is found. Less often, cirrhosis is associated with metabolic disorders such as Wilson's disease (see below), cystic fibrosis (p. 255), API deficiency (p. 90), haemochromatosis (p. 180), or galactosaemia (p. 161).

Mild or latent cirrhosis. In mild cases, no clinical abnormalities may be apparent, due to the reserve functional capacity of the liver. Plasma GGT measurements provide a sensitive means of detecting mild cirrhosis, but most heavy drinkers (many of whom do *not* have cirrhosis of the liver) have raised plasma GGT activities; these usually fall within two months of stopping drinking. Marked abnormalities in liver function tests are rarely present.

Severe cirrhosis. The following clinical features may occur, either alone or in combination: haematemesis, ascites and acute hepatic decompensation, often fatal. Jaundice may develop, plasma [albumin] falls and the prothrombin time becomes abnormal. Clinical deterioration accompanied by prolonged prothrombin time, a generalized amino aciduria, increased plasma [NH_3] and reduced plasma [urea] may herald the development of acute hepatic failure.

Copper in liver disease

The liver is the principal organ involved in copper metabolism. The amount it contains is maintained at normal levels by excretion of copper in bile and by incorporation into ceruloplasmin (p. 91). The liver's copper content is increased in Wilson's disease, primary biliary cirrhosis, prolonged extrahepatic cholestasis, and intrahepatic bile duct atresia in the neonate.

Wilson's disease (hepatolenticular degeneration) is a rare, hereditary, autosomal recessive disorder with a prevalence of about one in 30 000. The defective gene encodes a protein involved in the hepatobiliary excretion and renal reabsorption of copper. Copper is deposited in many tissues, including the liver, brain, eyes and kidney. Symptoms are mainly due to liver disease and to degenerative changes in the basal ganglia. Plasma [ceruloplasmin] is nearly always low, but it is not clear how this relates to the aetiology of Wilson's disease.

The diagnosis may be suspected from the family history or on clinical grounds, such as liver disease in patients less than 20 years old, or characteristic neurological disease. Kayser–Fleischer rings, due to the deposition of copper in the cornea, can be detected in most patients. The following chemical tests may be valuable:

• Plasma [ceruloplasmin]. This is usually less than 200 mg/L (reference range, 250–450 mg/L).

• Plasma [copper]. This is usually less than 12 μmol/L (reference range, 12–26 μmol/L).

• Urinary copper output. This is always more than 1.0 μmol/24 h (normally below 0.5 μmol/24 h).

• Liver [copper] is always greater than 250 μg/g dry weight (reference range 50–250 μg/g dry

weight). This is the most sensitive test, but it involves liver biopsy.

These tests are not 100 % specific for Wilson's disease. For example, plasma [ceruloplasmin] may occasionally be low in severe cirrhosis, and urinary copper output and liver [copper] may be raised in biliary cirrhosis. However, urinary copper output is valuable for case-finding among relatives, since a normal result virtually excludes Wilson's disease.

Abnormalities of other chemical tests are often present in Wilson's disease. There is usually evidence of renal tubular damage, with a generalized (overflow) amino aciduria, glycosuria and phosphaturia and, in advanced cases, renal tubular acidosis.

Alcoholic liver disease

Chronic over-indulgence in ethanol is a common cause of hepatic cirrhosis. Ethanol is metabolized by alcohol dehydrogenase, catalase and an NADP-dependent microsomal P450-dependent enzyme oxidizing system. The relative importance of these enzymes varies, depending on the blood [ethanol] and on the length of any period of chronic overindulgence.

The diagnosis of alcohol abuse is difficult, but the following tests may be of value:

• GGT and mean cell volume (MCV) of erythrocytes. Alcohol induces the synthesis of GGT by the liver, but as a single test for the recognition of chronic alcohol abuse, plasma GGT lacks sensitivity. The diagnostic value of plasma GGT measurements can be increased by measuring the mean cell volume (MCV) of erythrocytes as well, and the finding of both a slight macrocytosis and an increased plasma GGT activity provides probably the best routinely available combination of measurements for detecting alcohol abuse.

• Carbohydrate-deficient transferrin (CDT). In patients with alcohol-induced liver disease, transferrin in plasma has a reduced carbohydrate (sialic acid) content. Plasma [CDT] is increased in about 90 % of patients who drink more than 60 g alcohol per day.

• Blood ethanol.

Ascites

Liver disease is the commonest cause of ascites. If a diagnostic paracentesis is performed, the appearance of the fluid (blood-stained, bile-stained, milky, etc.) should be noted, and fluid [total protein] should be determined.

Transudates and exudates

Ascites with a fluid [protein] less than 30 g/L is called a *transudate*. It is usually associated with noninfective causes such as uncomplicated cirrhosis, in which there is a combination of back-pressure effects and low plasma [albumin].

However, fluid [protein] may be greater in some of these patients, and 30 g/L is not a reliable diagnostic cut-off point.

Ascites with a fluid [protein] much in excess of 30 g/L is called an *exudate*. It usually indicates the presence of infective conditions such as tuberculous peritonitis, or malignant disease or pancreatic disease. If pancreatic disease is thought to be the cause, fluid amylase activity should be measured; a serosanguinous fluid with a high amylase activity will help to confirm the diagnosis. If hepatoma is suspected, plasma and ascitic fluid [AFP] may both be considerably increased.

KEY POINTS

1 Bilirubin, alanine aminotransferase (ALT), alkaline phosphatase (ALP), γ-glutamyl transferase (GGT), albumin (and sometimes the prothrombin time) are often requested as a group of tests to determine whether liver disease is present and to give some indication of aetiology. Normal results do not exclude liver disease.

2 In jaundiced patients, unconjugated hyperbilirubinaemia is usually due to haemolysis or Gilbert's syndrome. Bilirubin is absent from the urine and urinary [urobilinogen] is increased in haemolysis.

3 In conjugated hyperbilirubinaemia and in some patients in whom liver damage is insufficient to cause hyperbilirubinaemia, large increases in ALT suggest hepatocellular damage, caused by drugs, toxic agents or infection. On the other hand, marked elevations in GGT and ALP suggest cholestasis. Chemical tests do not distinguish intrahepatic from posthepatic cholestasis.

4 Plasma [albumin] provides a fairly good index of the progress of chronic liver disease, but is of less value in acute liver disease, due to its half-life of about 21 days. The prothrombin time provides a better index of rapid progression of liver damage.

Case 8.1

A 13-year-old boy was taken by his mother to see their general practitioner because he had been feeling hot for the previous two days and had been complaining that his muscles ached. He had eaten little for the previous two days. On examination, the doctor found that the boy was pyrexial (38.4 °C) and appeared jaundiced.

There was no abdominal pain or tenderness, lymphadenopathy, or enlargement of the spleen or liver. Side-room tests on urine showed that the urobilinogen was within normal limits, and there was no detectable bilirubin in the specimen. The doctor requested liver function tests, which were as follows:

Continued on p. 121

Case 8.1 *continued*

Plasma analysis	Result	Reference range	Units
[Albumin]	45	36–47	g/L
ALP activity	180	40–125	U/L
ALT activity	30	10–40	U/L
[Bilirubin, total]	60	2–17	µmol/L
GGT activity	35	10–55	U/L

Five days later, the boy had recovered. He had no fever and his jaundice had gone, but plasma [bilirubin] was still elevated at 30 mmol/L, as was the alkaline phosphatase activity at 175 U/L. The reticulocyte count and other haematological investigations had all been normal on both occasions. What is the most likely diagnosis, and how would you explain the abnormal results among the liver function tests?

Comments on Case 8.1
This patient has Gilbert's syndrome. This was revealed when he developed a flu-like illness and went off his food. Caloric restriction in these patients can be used as a test to unmask the latent mild hyperbilirubinaemia. The absence of bilirubin in the urine showed that the hyperbilirubinaemia was due to increased plasma [unconjugated bilirubin], and the normal reticulocyte count excluded haemolytic anaemia as the cause.

The raised alkaline phosphatase activity is expected in a child of this age entering puberty (p. 000). The plasma GGT activity was normal, which helped to confirm this explanation.

Case 8.2

A 40-year-old housewife complained to her general practitioner of generalized severe itching during the previous nine months. She had no other symptoms, and she said that her alcohol consumption was small (two to three units per week). On clinical examination, she was slightly jaundiced, and bilirubin was detected in the urine on side-room testing. The results of liver function tests were as follows:

Plasma analysis	Result	Reference range	Units
[Albumin]	38	36–47	g/L
ALP activity	450	40–125	U/L
ALT activity	60	10–40	U/L
[Bilirubin, total]	60	2–17	µmol/L
GGT activity	150	10–55	U/L

Comments on Case 8.2
This patient has cholestatic jaundice. Her pruritus is caused by the retention of bile salts. The presence of serum antimitochondrial antibodies in high titre indicated that the diagnosis was primary biliary cirrhosis, one of the causes of intrahepatic cholestasis. Retention of bile salts within the liver is liable to cause hepatocellular damage, which could account in this patient for the increased plasma ALT activity.

Case 8.3

A general practitioner was called to see
a 21-year-old female student who had been
complaining of a flu-like illness for two days.
The illness had become worse, with symptoms
of fever, vomiting and abdominal tenderness in
the right upper quadrant. On examining the
patient, the doctor found that she was pyrexial
and jaundiced. The liver was enlarged and
tender. On questioning her, the doctor found
that she had recently returned from a long
holiday in Asia.

A sample of urine appeared dark, and using
side-room tests it was found that bilirubin was
present and urobilinogen was increased. A
blood sample was taken for liver function tests,
the results of which were:

Plasma analysis	Result	Reference range	Units
[Albumin]	40	36–47	g/L
ALP activity	190	40–125	U/L
ALT activity	560	10–40	U/L
[Bilirubin, total]	110	2–17	mmol/L
GGT activity	60	10–35	U/L

What is the most likely diagnosis?

Comments on Case 8.3

The results and presenting features are
characteristic of hepatitis caused by an
infective agent. The presence of bilirubin in
the urine showed that there was a conjugated
hyperbilirubinaemia, and the markedly
elevated plasma ALT activity and increased
urinary urobilinogen indicated that the
jaundice was hepatocellular in origin.

Both plasma ALP activity and GGT were
slightly elevated, indicating that there was
some degree of intrahepatic cholestasis.

Possible causes could include hepatitis A,
hepatitis B, hepatitis C or Epstein–Barr virus. In
this case, the serum contained a high titre of
antibodies to hepatitis A.

Case 8.4

A 68-year-old retired labourer presented
complaining of loss of weight, tiredness and
loss of appetite. He had lost 19 kg during the
previous three months, but had been eating
normally up until three weeks previously. He
had experienced no pain, but on questioning
admitted to drinking moderately for most of his
life. He also stated that he had been passing
dark urine for some time and that his stools
were quite pale.

The examination showed a tired, thin man
with jaundice. There was a palpable mass in the
right upper quadrant of the abdomen, with no
tenderness. The results of liver function tests
were:

Plasma analysis	Result	Reference range	Units
[Albumin]	32	36–47	g/L
ALP activity	632	40–125	U/L
ALT	55	10–40	U/L
[Bilirubin, total]	90	2–17	mmol/L
GGT activity	200	10–55	U/L

Continued on p. 123

Case 8.4 continued

Side-room tests on urine showed the presence of bilirubin, and urobilinogen was undetectable. Faecal occult blood was positive. α-Fetoprotein in plasma was not increased.

What is the most likely diagnosis?

Comments on Case 8.4

The pale stools, presence of bilirubin and lack of urobilinogen in the urine, accompanied by high plasma activities of ALP and GGT, suggest that the patient has cholestatic jaundice. The abdominal mass and positive faecal occult blood suggest that a tumour of the biliary tract or the pancreas may be responsible. Hepatoma was unlikely, as α-fetoprotein was negative.

Ultrasound showed a large abdominal mass and dilated intrahepatic and extrahepatic bile ducts. A CT scan suggested that there was a tumour at the head of the pancreas that was obstructing the common bile duct.

CHAPTER 9

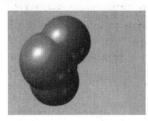

Gastrointestinal Tract Disease

Stomach, 124
The pancreas, 126

Small intestine, 127

The investigation of
malabsorption, 131

Malabsorption is a common clinical problem that may be due to disease of any part of the gastrointestinal (GI) tract, pancreas and liver. Gastric and duodenal ulceration, ulcerative colitis and Crohn's disease are other important causes of morbidity, and carcinoma is a major cause of mortality. Chemical tests now play a relatively minor part in the investigation of patients with GI tract disease. Microbiological investigations, radiological investigations, endoscopy, and biopsy procedures have more to offer.

The chemical tests that have proved most valuable and reliable for the investigation of particular conditions are given in Table 9.1. This chapter will briefly discuss the principles and problems associated with their use.

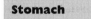

Stomach

Peptic ulcer

Most disorders of gastric function are best assessed initially using radiological investigations and endoscopy. Most peptic ulcers are associated with *Helicobacter pylori* infection. This organism can be present in the gastric mucosa, and can stimulate local acid production by converting urea into ammonia and CO_2. In the few patients who present with atypical or recurrent peptic ulceration that is resistant to treatment with H_2 antagonists and antibiotics to eradicate *H. pylori,* chemical tests to quantify plasma [gastrin] and gastric acid

secretion in response to hormonal stimuli may be of value.

Gastrin is a polypeptide released by specialized cells in the antral and duodenal mucosa. It is a potent stimulator of gastric acid production. Measurement of plasma [gastrin] and the pentagastrin test may be required to confirm achlorhydria or determine whether gastric acid hypersecretion is caused by a gastrinoma (Zollinger–Ellison syndrome, see below).

Pentagastrin test

Pentagastrin is a pentapeptide with the four C-terminal amino acids identical to those of gastrin. Like gastrin, it stimulates acid production strongly. The pentagastrin test measures gastric acid production under basal conditions and after maximal stimulation by pentagastrin. Details of the performance of the test vary between hospitals, and the local laboratory should be consulted.

The pentagastrin test may be of value in:

• The investigation of patients with suspected gastrinoma (see below).

• Differentiating superficial gastritis, in which acid output is mildly reduced, from atrophic gastritis, in which there is achlorhydria even after pentagastrin stimulation, as occurs in pernicious anaemia (except in the rare juvenile form).

• The investigation of gastric hypertrophy detected by endoscopy. Reduced acid secretion is found in giant hypertrophic gastritis (Ménétrier's disease), but secretion is

TESTS OF GI FUNCTION

Condition to be investigated	Chemical investigations
Peptic ulcer	
Zollinger–Ellison syndrome	Pentagastrin test, plasma [gastrin]
Acute pancreatitis	Plasma amylase activity
Chronic pancreatitis	
Direct (invasive) tests	Secretin/CCK-PZ test
Indirect tests	BT-PABA/[^{14}C]-PABA test, fluorescein dilaurate test
Intestinal malabsorption	
Carbohydrate absorption	Xylose absorption test
Amino acid transport	Urine chromatography
Fat absorption	Faecal fat excretion, triglyceride breath test
Bacterial colonization	Urinary indican excretion, [^{14}C]-xylose breath test
Verner–Morrison syndrome	Plasma [VIP]
Carcinoid syndrome	Urinary 5-hydroxyindoleacetic acid

Table 9.1 The principal examples of chemical tests described in this chapter for the investigation of GI tract disease.

Plasma gastrin

Plasma [gastrin], after an overnight fast, should be measured in patients with persistent, recurrent or multiple peptic ulceration in whom the provisional diagnosis is gastrinoma and in whom a high acid secretion has already been demonstrated. Gastrin is very labile, and requires special conditions for its collection and transport.

Plasma [gastrin] is reduced in diseases causing hyperacidity (e.g. duodenal ulcer), except in gastrinoma, where levels are usually increased. However, increased fasting plasma [gastrin] is not by itself diagnostic of gastrinoma, since it also occurs where there is achlorhydria or hypochlorhydria, which may be due to gastritis, treatment with H_2 antagonists or omeprazole, pernicious anaemia or previous vagotomy. Increased plasma [gastrin] may also be found in patients with hypercalcaemia or G-cell hyperplasia, or following gastric surgery, as a result of which the antral mucosa may have become isolated from gastric contents.

Zollinger–Ellison syndrome

This syndrome is due to a gastrinoma, i.e. neoplasia of either pancreatic gastrin-producing cells or gastric gastrin-producing cells, the former being the more common site. Increased gastrin production leads to chronic hypersecretion of gastric acid, which in turn causes peptic ulceration and sometimes diarrhoea and fat malabsorption. The steatorrhoea is thought to be due to high [H^+] in the intestinal lumen; this inhibits the action of pancreatic lipase. In some patients, an isolated simple duodenal ulcer or diarrhoea may be the presenting feature.

The diagnosis is often made by finding a grossly elevated fasting plasma [gastrin], usually greater than 200 ng/L, and by excluding other causes of a raised level. However, up to 30% of patients with a gastrinoma may have normal or only slightly increased plasma [gastrin], and studies of acid secretion probably represent the most important diagnostic test in these patients (Fig. 9.1).

In patients with a gastrinoma, the results of the pentagastrin test usually show the following:

increased if hypertrophic, hypersecretory gastropathy is the cause.

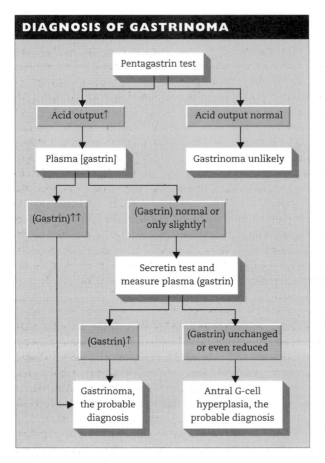

DIAGNOSIS OF GASTRINOMA

Pentagastrin test

→ Acid output↑

→ Acid output normal

Plasma [gastrin]

Gastrinoma unlikely

(Gastrin)↑↑

(Gastrin) normal or only slightly↑

Secretin test and measure plasma (gastrin)

(Gastrin)↑

(Gastrin) unchanged or even reduced

Gastrinoma, the probable diagnosis

Antral G-cell hyperplasia, the probable diagnosis

Fig. 9.1 The investigation of patients in whom a provisional diagnosis of gastrinoma (Zollinger–Ellison syndrome) has been made. Note that patients must not be taking drugs that interfere with the secretion of gastrin or of acid before these tests (e.g. H_2 antagonists).

- Resting juice is usually more than one litre, containing at least 100 mmol/L HCl.
- There is usually a high basal output of gastric H^+ (greater than 15 mmol/h), and pentagastrin causes little further stimulation; the basal secretion rate is often over 60% of the peak acid output.

About 15% of patients with gastrinoma have only slightly raised plasma [gastrin] and acid secretion. There may be similar findings in patients with antral G-cell hyperplasia. After injection of secretin, there is usually a twofold increase in plasma [gastrin] in patients with gastrinoma, while no change occurs in patients with G-cell hyperplasia.

The pancreas

Acute pancreatitis

Acute pancreatitis is commonly associated with gallstones or alcoholism; vascular and infective causes have also been recognized. Confirmation of the clinical diagnosis mainly depends on plasma amylase activity measurements. Plasma [calcium] may fall considerably in severe cases of acute pancreatitis, but sometimes not for a few days; it probably falls as a result of the formation of insoluble calcium salts of fatty acids in areas of fat necrosis.

Plasma amylase

Amylase in plasma arises mainly from the pancreas (P-isoamylase) and the salivary glands (S-isoamylase). Plasma P-isoamylase activity is a more sensitive and more specific test than total amylase for the detection of acute pancreatitis, but total plasma amylase activity is most often measured and is usually, but not always, greatly increased in acute pancreatitis. Plasma amylase activities greater than ten times normal are virtually diagnostic of acute pancreatitis. Maximum values of more than five times the upper reference limit are found in about 50% of cases; but are not pathognomonic of acute pancreatitis, since similarly high values sometimes occur in the afferent loop syndrome, mesenteric infarction and acute biliary tract disease, as well as in acute parotitis. Smaller and more transient increases may occur in almost any acute abdominal condition (e.g. perforated peptic ulcer), or after injection of morphine and other drugs that cause spasm of the sphincter of Oddi. Moderate increases have also been reported in patients with diabetic acidosis. In patients with acute pancreatitis, plasma amylase activity usually returns to normal within three to five days.

Macro-amylasaemia. In this rare disorder, part of the plasma amylase activity circulates as a high molecular weight form which, unlike normal amylase, is not cleared by the kidney. The diagnosis may be made when the increased plasma amylase activity is found to be persistent and accompanied by a normal urinary amylase activity.

Chronic pancreatitis

Impaired secretion of pancreatic enzymes may not occur until the disease is advanced, but may then give rise to malabsorption, especially steatorrhoea. Various methods involving either *direct* measurements on pancreatic fluid following duodenal intubation or *indirect* measures, without the need for intubation, have been described. The chemical function tests have proved of limited value, and radiology and endoscopy are usually the preferred investigations.

Indirect tests

BT-PABA/[¹⁴C]-PABA test and fluorescein dilaurate tests. These tests rely on the principle that pancreatic enzymes release *p*-aminobenzoic acid (PABA) from *N*-benzoyl-L-tyrosyl *p*-aminobenzoic acid (BT-PABA), or fluorescein from fluorescein dilaurate. The PABA or fluorescein so released is absorbed, partially metabolized, excreted into the urine, and measured. In the PABA test, both BT-PABA and a tracer dose of [¹⁴C]-PABA are given orally, and the administered and urinary ratios for the [¹⁴C] label and [PABA] calculated. In the fluorescein dilaurate test, the amount of fluorescein excreted following oral administration of fluorescein dilaurate is compared with that excreted following oral administration of fluorescein on the following day.

Direct test

The secretin/CCK-PZ test. The patient is intubated, and the pancreatic secretion of bicarbonate and of amylase or trypsin following stimulation with intravenous secretin and cholecystokinin-pancreozymin (CCK-PZ) is measured. Local laboratories should provide details of the performance of the test.

Abnormal results are obtained in most cases of chronic pancreatitis, enzymatic activity and $[HCO_3^-]$ tending to fall before there is any obvious reduction in the volume of juice. Results are also abnormal in some cases of pancreatic carcinoma; although all three variables (enzymatic activity, $[HCO_3^-]$ and volume) may be affected, a low volume of juice is a particularly marked feature of pancreatic carcinoma when the tumour is at the head of the pancreas and producing obstruction. Tumours in the tail of the pancreas do not give rise to abnormal results.

Small intestine

In small-intestinal disease, absorptive function may be diminished, and permeability (via intercellular junctions) is often increased. Chemical tests are available that assess absorptive function and intestinal permeability, but the availability of jejunal biopsy has greatly reduced the need to perform such tests for diagnostic purposes. These tests may be used to monitor the response to therapy (e.g. the response of patients with coeliac disease to a gluten-free diet).

Tests of carbohydrate absorption

Xylose absorption test

D-Xylose, a pentose, is normally absorbed rapidly from the small intestine and excreted in the urine; little is metabolized in the liver. It can be used to test the intestine's ability to absorb monosaccharides. There is no standard proto- col for performing the xylose absorption test, therefore it is necessary to consult the labora- tory for details of the local procedure, and for information on how to interpret the results.

In one common form of the test, a 5 g dose of xylose is given to the patient after an overnight fast, and the patient must not eat during the test. The response is best assessed on the basis of serum or blood [xylose] one or two hours after ingestion. Urine excretion is sometimes measured over a five-hour period, but blood measurements are preferable, as they are independent of renal function; they also avoid the difficulties of ensuring complete, accurately timed urine collections.

Impaired absorption and excretion of xylose occurs in patients with disease of the small intestine. Low values may also be observed in patients who have bacterial colonization of the small intestine, since the bacteria may metabolize xylose. Low urinary values occur in patients with renal disease, due to impaired excretion of xylose; blood or serum [xylose] must be measured if the patient's plasma [urea] exceeds 8 mmol/L.

Tests of intestinal permeability

Intestinal permeability can be assessed by giving [^{51}Cr]-EDTA (100 mCi) by mouth and then collecting urine for 24 hours. Increased urinary excretion of [^{51}Cr]-EDTA occurs in intestinal disease. Glomerular function should

be assessed before performing this test, as its interpretation depends on there being normal glomerular function.

Disaccharidase deficiency

Disaccharidase deficiency may be exhibited as intolerance to one or more of the disaccha- rides – lactose, maltose or sucrose. The defect may be congenital or acquired. Disaccharidase activity can be measured in small-intestinal mucosa biopsy specimens. This is the most reliable way of specifically diagnosing small- intestinal disaccharidase deficiency.

Amino acid absorption

Certain specific disorders of amino acid trans- port affect both intestinal and renal epithelial transport. In Hartnup disease (p. 58), there is impaired transport of neutral amino acids, and deficiency of some essential amino acids (espe- cially tryptophan) may occur. In cystinuria (p. 50), the basic amino acids and cystine are affected; however, there is no associated nutri- tional defect, despite the fact that lysine is an essential amino acid. These disorders are inves- tigated by examining the pattern of amino acids excreted in the urine by chromatography.

Fat absorption

Efficient digestion and absorption of fat requires both effective solubilization of fats and lipolysis, followed by the absorption of hydrol- ysed products across the jejunum. Bile salts play an important role in lipid absorption. Primary bile acids are formed in the liver, con- jugated with glycine and taurine, and secreted into bile. Together with phospholipids, bile salts form micelles, which render dietary fats soluble; bile salts also promote the action of pancreatic lipase and co-lipase. The micelles also solubilize the products of lipolysis and allow them to be absorbed.

During absorption of a fat-containing meal, bile acids must be present in the upper small intestine in concentrations sufficient to allow the formation of micelles. The bile salts are mostly reabsorbed in the terminal ileum by an active process, and are transported back to the liver, where they are re-excreted in bile, thus completing an enterohepatic circulation. Insufficient bile acids may give rise to malabsorption of fat (Table 9.2).

Fat-soluble vitamins (A, D, E and K) share absorptive mechanisms with other dietary lipids. Malabsorption of fat-soluble vitamins, which is most commonly manifest as vitamin D deficiency (p. 72), occurs in conditions causing fat malabsorption.

Determination of fat absorption
Faecal fat
In the simplest form of the test, all faecal specimens passed over a five-day period are collected and sent to the laboratory. The specimens are combined, and the total fat content is estimated. Important drawbacks of the test are the difficulty (even under the best conditions) of ensuring complete five-day collections of faeces, and the inherently unpleasant nature of the test.

Provided fat intake does not exceed 100 g/day, the normal faecal fat excretion by healthy individuals is up to 5 g/24 h. It may be increased in patients with hepatobiliary disease, pancreatic disease and in patients with intestinal mal-

absorption. In pancreatic disease, faecal fat excretion is only increased when pancreatic function has fallen to less than 10% of normal.

Triglyceride breath test
This test avoids the difficulties and unpleasantness of collecting faeces over several days. Following digestion and absorption of an oral dose of $[^{14}C]$-triolein (the marker is in the fatty acid component), part of the fatty acid is metabolized to $^{14}CO_2$, which is then excreted in expired air. A high $^{14}CO_2$ excretion is associated with normal fat absorption, whereas $^{14}CO_2$ excretion is low in patients with fat malabsorption (Fig. 9.2).

Bacterial colonization of the small intestine
The small intestine is usually virtually sterile. However, when there is stasis (e.g. blind loop, stricture) or a colonic fistula or, occasionally, when immune mechanisms are impaired, anaerobic bacteria colonize the intestine. This often causes fat malabsorption, due at least partly to deconjugation of bile acid conjugates by the bacteria. Vitamin B_{12} deficiency may also develop, due to its consumption by the bacteria.

Diagnosis of bacterial colonization of the small intestine requires intubation for the

Table 9.2 Malabsorption due to insufficient bile salts.

MALABSORPTION CAUSED BY INSUFFICIENT BILE SALTS

Reason for bile salt insufficiency	Examples of causes of the insufficiency
Impaired synthesis of bile acids	Cirrhosis of the liver
Impaired delivery of bile acids to the intestine (due to obstruction to the outflow of bile)	Gallstones, carcinoma of the head of the pancreas
Impaired delivery of bile acids to the enterohepatic circulation	
(a) Impaired absorption of bile acid conjugates from the terminal ileum	Ileal disease (e.g. Crohn's disease), resection of the terminal ileum
(b) Impaired ability of the liver to clear bile acid conjugates from the portal blood and to secrete them again into the bile	Cholestasis associated with hepatic cirrhosis
Splitting of bile acid conjugates in the upper small intestine (reducing their effective concentration at the site of fat absorption)	Bacterial colonization of the upper small intestine (the 'stagnant gut syndrome')

BREATH TESTS

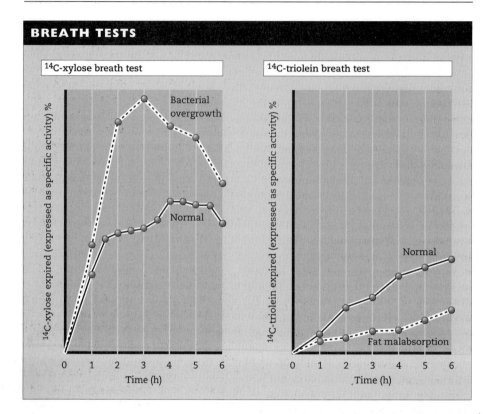

Fig. 9.2 Examples of results obtained using breath tests.

collection of specimens, on which microbiological procedures are then performed. However, some non-invasive tests have been devised for detecting the possible presence of bacterial colonization.

Urinary indican

Unabsorbed tryptophan is metabolized by the intestinal flora to indoles; these are absorbed, metabolized in the liver to indicans, and excreted in the urine. Urinary indican excretion may be increased when there are abnormal amounts of tryptophan in the colon due to disease of the small intestine, or when there is bacterial colonization of the small intestine, or when there is a tryptophan transport defect

(e.g. Hartnup disease, p. 58). In the absence of severe steatorrhoea, a urinary indican excretion of more than 200 mg/24 h is indicative of bacterial colonization.

Breath tests

The $[^{14}C]$-xylose breath test depends on the ability of anaerobic bacteria to metabolize $[^{14}C]$-xylose with the production of $^{14}CO_2$, which is then absorbed from the intestine, transported to the lungs and excreted in the expired air. Some $^{14}CO_2$ is normally produced by the liver as a result of metabolism of $[^{14}C]$-xylose, following absorption, but increased $^{14}CO_2$ production is associated with bacterial colonization. After oral administration of $[^{14}C]$-xylose, abnormally increased breath $^{14}CO_2$ occurs within the first 60 minutes in 85% of patients with bacterial colonization

(Fig. 9.2). However, if gastric emptying is delayed, the increase in $^{14}CO_2$ excretion may not become abnormal for three hours.

Terminal ileal function

Bile salts and vitamin B_{12} are absorbed in the terminal ileum, and tests are available that assess the absorption of these compounds. The Schilling test is used to assess vitamin B_{12} absorption, and is usually performed in haematology laboratories. The test is abnormal in patients with pernicious anaemia and in patients with disease of the terminal ileum.

Reabsorption of water and inorganic constituents

About 8 L of intestinal secretions are produced each day, and if these are not largely reabsorbed, deficiency states rapidly develop. Reabsorption takes place mainly in the jejunum and ileum, but also in the colon. Acute and severe disturbances may occur in patients following surgery, especially operations on the GI tract, and losses of K^+ often become very large.

Nonsurgical intestinal causes of electrolyte imbalance include severe diarrhoea (e.g. due to cholera, in which there is a defect of Na^+ reabsorption in the jejunum).

Table 9.3 Examples of the ways in which GI diseases cause malabsorption.

The investigation of malabsorption

Efficient digestion and absorption require the stomach, pancreas, hepatobiliary system and small intestine all to be functioning normally. Severe defects in the function of any one of these organs may cause intestinal malabsorptive disease; the patient may complain of diarrhoea or weight loss. The causes of carbohydrate, protein and amino acid, and lipid malabsorption are summarized in Table 9.3. Most of these have been referred to in this chapter, but a few are considered elsewhere in this book.

Clinical diagnosis

Firstly, it is important to consider the history of the patient's illness and the findings on physical examination, and to formulate a provisional diagnosis and list the differential diagnoses.

• *Pancreatic disease* may cause malabsorption of protein, fat or carbohydrate, due to deficiency of digestive enzymes.
• *Biliary disease* may cause malabsorption of fat and fat-soluble vitamins, due to lack of bile acids.
• *Intestinal mucosal disease* may affect digestion or transport, or both, of many dietary constituents, and reabsorption of bile acids. The effects may be general, or relatively specific.

MALABSORPTION: CAUSES

Dietary constituent	Disease of the GI tract	Why malabsorption may occur
Polysaccharides	Chronic pancreatitis	Amylase deficiency
Disaccharides	Intestinal mucosal defect	Disaccharidase deficiency
Proteins	Chronic pancreatitis	Pancreatic peptidase deficiency
Amino acids	Intestinal mucosal defect	Specific amino acid transport abnormalities
Lipids	Chronic pancreatitis	Lipase and/or co-lipase deficiency
	Insufficient bile salts	Micelle formation impaired
	Gastrinoma	High intestinal $[H^+]$ inhibits pancreatic lipase
	Abetalipoproteinaemia	Transfer of lipids to plasma impaired

Note: In addition to the above, any generalized intestinal disease is liable to cause malabsorption of all dietary constituents.

• *Bacterial colonization of the small intestine* may cause a functional deficiency of bile acids, and so interfere with absorption of fats. It may also interfere with the digestion of protein or absorption of amino acids, and decrease the availability of water-soluble vitamins.

Initial investigations

Microbiological examination, including stool microscopy and culture, should always be performed before chemical tests are requested whenever an infectious cause of a GI disorder needs to be excluded.

A *faecal specimen* should be inspected; this may suggest that the patient has steatorrhoea. The specimen should also be tested for occult blood.

Preliminary chemical investigations on blood specimens should include plasma [albumin] and other 'liver function tests'. Preliminary haematological investigations (haemoglobin, full blood count, vitamin B_{12} and folate) should also be performed.

Further investigations

Radiology (e.g. barium meal, barium enema), *endoscopy* (e.g. gastroscopy, duodenoscopy, endoscopic retrograde cholangiopancreatography, colonoscopy) and *mucosal biopsy* (e.g. duodenal biopsy) may be indicated. They may define the site of an anatomical abnormality, and are more reliable in this respect than most of the organ-directed chemical tests considered in this chapter.

Faecal fat (or alternative tests of fat absorption) may be abnormal whenever there is malabsorption. However, in general, severe fat malabsorption is only encountered in pancreatic and small-intestinal disease. Several other chemical abnormalities may occur in association with intestinal malabsorption, and require appropriate investigation and treatment. These include:

• *Vitamin* deficiency.
• *Defects in calcium absorption* that may cause rickets or osteomalacia.
• *Malabsorption of iron.* This may cause iron-deficiency anaemia. Mixed deficiencies of vitamin B_{12}, folate and iron may also occur.
• *Malabsorption of protein.* Reduction in plasma [albumin] most often results, but hypogammaglobulinaemia may be marked.

Carcinoid tumours and the carcinoid syndrome

Carcinoid tumours arise in the gut or in tissues derived from the embryological foregut (e.g. thyroid, bronchus). The commonest sites are the terminal ileum and the ileocaecal region. The tumours produce vasoactive amines which, because of the venous drainage of the tumours, are usually carried directly to the liver and there inactivated. Symptoms are only likely to occur either when the tumour has metastasized to the liver, or when the tumour drains into the systemic circulation (e.g. bronchial adenoma of the carcinoid type).

Most carcinoid tumours secrete excessive amounts of 5-hydroxytryptamine (5-HT: serotonin), which is metabolized and excreted in urine as 5-hydroxyindoleacetic acid (5-HIAA). 'Atypical carcinoids' contain excessive amounts of 5-hydroxytryptophan (5-HTP) and relatively little 5-HT; they may also secrete histamine. Whereas only about 1% of dietary tryptophan is normally metabolized to 5-HTP, 5-HT and 5-HIAA, in the carcinoid syndrome as much as 60% of dietary tryptophan is metabolized along this hydroxyindole pathway.

The *carcinoid syndrome* is usually associated with tumours of the terminal ileum and extensive secondary deposits in the liver. The main presenting features include flushing attacks, abdominal colic and diarrhoea, and dyspnoea, sometimes associated with asthmatic attacks. Valvular disease of the heart is often present. Carcinoid tumours can give rise to severe hypoproteinaemia and oedema, even in the absence of cardiac complications. There may also be signs of niacin deficiency, due to major diversion of tryptophan metabolism away from the pathway leading to niacin production (p. 143). Some carcinoid tumours produce

ACTH or ACTH-like peptides, and may cause Cushing's syndrome (p. 208) in the absence of the symptoms commonly associated with the carcinoid syndrome.

Chemical investigation of 5-HT metabolism

Measurement of 5-HIAA excretion in a 24-hour urine specimen is the most widely performed investigation; the output is usually greatly increased.

Bananas and tomatoes contain large amounts of 5-HT; they should not be eaten the day before or during the urine collection.

Table 9.4 Examples of gastrointestinal peptides.

Timing of urine collection. If attacks are frequent, the time of starting the collection is unimportant. If attacks are less often than daily, the patient should be instructed to wait and begin the collection when the next attack occurs.

GI hormones and Verner–Morrison syndrome

A number of GI hormones with various hormonal and local effects have been identified (Table 9.4). Excess amounts of these GI peptides are secreted by rare tumours. These tumours can often be identified by finding raised levels of the corresponding peptide in plasma. For example, in the Verner–Morrison syndrome, hypersecretion of VIP causes severe watery diarrhoea and hypokalaemia.

GI PEPTIDES

Peptide and GI location	Probable functions
Gastric antrum and duodenum	
Gastrin (in cells called G cells)	Stimulates gastric H^+ production. Also trophic to the gastric mucosa
Duodenum and jejunum	
Secretin	Stimulates water and HCO_3 secretion from the pancreas
Cholecystokinin (CCK)*	Stimulates secretion of enzymes by the pancreas, and contraction of the gallbladder
Glucose-dependent insulinotrophic peptide (GIP)†	Stimulates postprandial release of insulin, inhibits gastric acid secretion.
Motilin	Stimulates intestinal motor activity
Pancreas	
Pancreatic polypeptide	Inhibits enzyme release from the pancreas, and relaxes gallbladder
Ileum and colon	
Enteroglucagon	Increases small-intestinal mucosal growth and slows the rate of intestinal transit
All areas of the GI tract	
Vasoactive intestinal peptide (VIP)*	Secretomotor actions, also vasodilatation, and relaxation of intestinal smooth muscle

* CCK and VIP are examples of peptides found both in the GI tract and in the CNS.
† GIP is also known as gastric inhibitory polypeptide.

KEY POINTS

1 Chemical tests play a relatively minor role in the investigation of patients with suspected gastrointestinal disorders.

2 Plasma [gastrin] is raised in about 70 % of patients with gastrinoma, whilst abnormal acid secretion is demonstrable in most patients. A raised [gastrin] is also found in patients with achlorhydria and hypochlorhydria.

3 Plasma amylase activities more than ten times normal are virtually diagnostic of acute pancreatitis, and values greater than five times normal are suggestive of the disease. Moderate increases in plasma amylase occur in many acute abdominal conditions.

4 None of the chemical tests for pancreatic disease are entirely satisfactory.

5 Faecal fat is an unreliable measure of fat malabsorption unless a complete five-day collection can be ensured. In pancreatic disease, faecal fat excretion will only increase when pancreatic function has fallen to less than 10 % of normal.

6 Urinary 5-hydroxyindoleacetic acid (5-HIAA) excretion is usually greatly increased in patients with the carcinoid syndrome.

Case 9.1

A 47-year-old man had recently presented as an emergency case with haematemesis. Endoscopy demonstrated multiple healed gastric and duodenal ulcers, with two active ulcers in the pylorus. He had a long history of peptic ulceration, and had been receiving H_2-antagonists for some time, with varying benefit. A fasting gastrin level was markedly elevated at 1246 ng/L (reference range up to 120 ng/L).

Is gastrinoma the likely diagnosis?

Comments on Case 9.1

The history of aggressive peptic ulceration, resistant to treatment, and the finding of multiple large ulcers raises Zollinger–Ellison syndrome as a possibility. The gastrin level is markedly elevated, but treatment with H_2 antagonists is a cause of elevated gastrin. For the test to be of any value, therapy with H_2 antagonists should be withdrawn.

Cimetidine was withdrawn, and gastric acid production was measured under basal conditions and after pentagastrin stimulation. Basal acid production was raised at 110 mmol/h, and on stimulation this only rose to 150 mmol/h. These results are consistent with Zollinger–Ellison syndrome. A repeat gastrin measurement made before the patient recommenced cimetidine therapy was markedly raised.

The finding of a raised gastrin level in the presence of high gastric acid secretion is consistent with the diagnosis of a gastrin-secreting tumour.

Using computed tomography (CT) scanning, the tumour was found in the pancreas, with no evidence of metastases. Further biochemical and imaging investigations failed to detect any other lesions associated with the multiple endocrine neoplasia (MEN) type I syndrome. The tumour was resected.

Case 9.2

A 55-year-old man presented to the gastrointestinal clinic with a two-year history of moderately severe intermittent abdominal pain radiating through to the upper back. He had also been passing bulky, foul-smelling stools.

On questioning, he admitted to having consumed half a bottle of whisky a day for a number of years. On examination, he was found to be tired and thin, with a slight degree of ankle oedema. He had mid-abdominal tenderness. Blood pressure and pulse were normal. Side-room tests showed glycosuria. A plain abdominal X-ray of the abdomen was normal. The laboratory tests showed normal urea and electrolytes, but also the following:

Continued on p. 135

Case 9.2 continued

Plasma analysis	Result	Reference range	Units
[Albumin]	30	36–47	g/L
ALP activity	200	40–125	U/L
ALT activity	32	10–40	U/L
[Bilirubin, total]	10	2–17	mmol/L
GGT activity	65	10–55	U/L
Amylase	370	50–300	U/L

What is the most likely diagnosis?

Comments on Case 9.2

The recurrent pain and probable steatorrhoea are compatible with chronic pancreatitis or pancreatic carcinoma. However, the moderately raised plasma amylase is not diagnostic of pancreatic disease, as similar levels are found in other abdominal disorders, e.g. perforated duodenal ulcer, cholecystitis.

Five-day faecal fat output was 10 g/day (normally less than 5 g/day). The increase in plasma alkaline phosphatase (ALP) activity was entirely due to the bone isoenzyme, suggesting vitamin D deficiency due to fat malabsorption. The fasting glucose level on two occasions was 12.0 mmol/L and 15.0 mmol/L.

The ultrasound examination and CT scan showed an enlarged pancreas with calcification.

The patient has chronic pancreatitis, probably caused by years of alcohol abuse. The elevated γ-glutamyl transferase (GGT) may be the result of induction of the enzyme due to excessive alcohol consumption rather than liver disease. Similarly, the low plasma albumin may be due to maldigestion of protein, but cirrhosis should also be considered.

The patient was treated with pancreatic supplements, and dietary advice was given regarding fat intake and diabetes. He was also told to stop drinking. On this treatment, the steatorrhoea regressed, the patient gained weight and the diabetes came under control.

CHAPTER 10

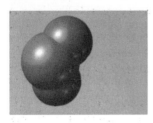

Clinical Biochemical Measurements in Nutrition

Protein-energy malnutrition
  (PEM), 136
Obesity, 137

Prinicipal dietary
  constituents, 137

Biochemical assessment of
  nutritional status, 145

In world-wide terms, nutritional disorders are responsible for much morbidity and mortality. The three main categories of nutritional disorder are *undernutrition* (which is dominated by insufficient food energy), producing the features of starvation; *malnutrition*, which is deficiency of one or more of the essential nutrients; and *obesity,* which is excessive positive energy balance. Disease is also possible as a result of nutrient excess (e.g. iron overload, alcohol excess) or the effect of potentially toxic agents in food (e.g. favism, an acute haemolytic anaemia due to sensitivity to the fava bean).

Nutritional issues, directly or indirectly, impinge upon many of the tests undertaken in clinical biochemistry. Many analytes are altered by nutritional status. For example, diet exerts important short-term effects on plasma [triglycerides], [glucose] and longer-term effects on plasma [cholesterol]. Certain inborn errors of metabolism may demand special diets, which are monitored biochemically (e.g. phenylalanine in phenylketonuria). Less obviously, diagnostic tests may only be valid if certain nutritional requirements are met. For example, faecal fat measurements are only valid if the patient is taking adequate fat intake (70–100 g daily); measurement of 5-hydroxyindoleacetic acid (5-HIAA) requires exclusion of rich sources of serotonin from the diet (p. 133); screening for hypercalciuria requires a high normal calcium intake, etc.

Laboratory measurements are also necessary in the management of patients receiving nutritional support, especially total parenteral nutrition, and in the assessment of malabsorption (e.g. faecal fat tests, xylose absorption test). Suspected nutritional deficiencies, ranging from possible iron deficiency to vitamin or trace metal deficiencies, also require specialist laboratory tests.

In this chapter, the biochemical issues related to protein-calorie malnutrition and obesity are briefly considered. This is followed by a section on the principal nutritional constituents, including the clinical significance and measurement of vitamins and trace elements. In the final section, the principles of nutritional support are discussed.

Protein-energy malnutrition (PEM)

This arises from insufficient food, anorexia, persistent vomiting or regurgitation, or malabsorption. It may also be seen where the basal metabolic rate (BMR) is increased (severe infections, thyrotoxicosis), in cancer cachexia and other illnesses. The severity of undernutrition is assessed by the body mass index (BMI), defined as weight/(height)^2 (expressed in kilograms and metres, respectively). The acceptable range of BMI is 20–25.

A range of biochemical abnormalities may be

found. Blood glucose may be low, with a corresponding increase in plasma free fatty acids and ketone bodies (with associated mild metabolic acidosis). Plasma [glucagon] and [cortisol] levels increase at the expense of a reduced [insulin]. Reverse T3 increases at the expense of normal T3. Creatinine excretion diminishes.

PEM in children leads to a spectrum of diseases. Nutritional marasmus is the childhood version of severe starvation, and is typically found where the child is weaned early onto dilute cow's milk formula. Weight is less than 60% standard, and there is often evidence of vitamin and other nutrient deficiencies, with associated chronic infections. In kwashiorkor, the diet is low in protein, but may be relatively satisfactory in carbohydrate intake (e.g. a child weaned onto diets such as yam, cassava or diluted cereal). The insulin levels may be less affected (since carbohydrate is present), with diversion of amino acids from the viscera to muscles, leading to impaired albumin synthesis by a fatty liver (with reduced lipoprotein export). The low albumin leads to the characteristic hypoalbuminaemic oedema found in this condition.

Obesity

The commonest nutritional disorder in affluent societies is defined as an excess of body fat. Obesity is stated to occur at a BMI of 30 and gross obesity at a BMI of 40 or above. In general, it arises from an excess of calorie intake over expenditure. The problem may be multifactorial, with socio-economic factors, age, sex and heredity all contributing. Occasionally, obesity is found in association with specific disorders such as hypothyroidism, Cushing's syndrome, hypogonadism, or hypopituitarism.

Biochemical measurements may all be normal, but simple obesity is associated with non-insulin-dependent diabetes mellitus (NIDDM, p. 151), hyperlipidaemia (typically, mixed), hyperuricaemia and sometimes fatty

liver with mild derangements in liver function tests.

Principal dietary constituents

Solid food itself can be considered to contain three categories of substance. The first category consists of energy (typically, as carbohydrate and fat) and nutrients, which include the essential amino acids, essential fatty acids and the 13 vitamins and 18 essential elements (in addition to carbon, hydrogen, nitrogen and oxygen) required for life. The second category includes entrapped water in food, which may often be more than half the food weight, and 'packing' as dietary fibre. In the third category is included all the other nonnutritive substances, often responsible for the colour, smell, taste of food or, indeed, its toxic qualities (e.g. gluten in wheat, responsible for gluten-sensitive enteropathy in susceptible individuals).

Carbohydrates

The major source of dietary energy is normally provided by carbohydrate, in the form of sugars (e.g. sucrose) or digestible polysaccharides; the major food polysaccharide is starch, found in cereals, root vegetables and legumes. Nondigestible polysaccharides contribute to dietary fibre. Carbohydrates are not essential nutrients, but insufficient carbohydrate intake leads to ketosis.

Fats

Dietary fat consists largely of triglycerides, with small amounts of other constituents (e.g. cholesterol). The National Food Survey (1973) showed that in Britain, on average, 42% of total energy was taken in as fat, 46% was carbohydrate and 12% was protein. Since the energy content of fat is greater than that of carbohydrate (about 9 kcal/g, compared to 4 kcal/g for protein and for carbohydrate), the *weight* of dietary fat is substantially less than for carbohydrate on this diet.

Triglycerides contain saturated or unsaturated fatty acids, or both. Saturated fats, especially those containing palmitic and myristic acids, elevate plasma [total cholesterol] and [low-density lipoprotein cholesterol], whereas unsaturated fats tend to reduce both these concentrations. Monounsaturated fatty acids (e.g. oleic acid) may exert favourable effects on lipoprotein metabolism, and may have the added beneficial effect of increasing plasma [high-density lipoprotein cholesterol]. Some long-chain, highly unsaturated fatty acids (e.g. eicosapentaenoic acid, present in fatty fish) may also be cardioprotective, reducing plasma [very low density lipoproteins] and inhibiting thrombosis.

Linoleic, linolenic and arachidonic acids comprise the 'essential' free fatty acids. They cannot be synthesized by humans, and are required for membrane synthesis and as precursors of the prostaglandins.

Proteins

Dietary protein from both animal and plant sources normally provides about 11–14% of total calories (70–100 g protein) on a 'Western' diet; the minimum requirement is 40 g of protein of good biological value (i.e. containing all the eight essential amino acids). Vegetable protein may be deficient in one or more of the eight essential amino acids, but this deficiency can be overcome by complementation, whereby a combination of cereals and legumes together provide protein of good biological value.

Trace elements

More than twenty elements are known to be essential in animal nutrition. Of these, seven are 'bulk' elements (Na, K, Ca, Mg, Cl, S and P), and the rest are referred to as trace elements, present in tissues at less than 50 mg/kg. Six of these (nickel, arsenic, vanadium, tin, silicon and fluorine) have not been shown to be associated with specific deficiency states in man, and will not be further considered. Table 10.1 lists some data about the nine that are known to be *essential* trace elements.

The clinical importance of iron, iodine and cobalt (in cobalamin) is well established. Clinical syndromes associated with deficiency of copper, selenium, zinc, chromium, manganese

Table 10.1 Trace elements essential to the human body.

TRACE ELEMENTS			
Essential trace element	Approximate total adult body content	Daily oral intake (recommended for adults)*	Plasma concentration
Chromium	<6 mg	0.1 mg	<20 nmol/L
Cobalt	1 mg	As vitamin B_{12}	<10 nmol/L
Copper	100 mg	1.2 mg	12–26 μmol/L
Iodine	10–20 mg	0.15 mg	<5 nmol/L[†]
Iron	4–5 g	Males: 10 mg	14–32 μmol/L
		Females: 10–50 mg[‡]	10–28 μmol/L
Manganese	10–20 mg	3 mg	<20 nmol/L
Molybdenum	10 mg	0.2 mg	<15 nmol/L
Selenium	15 mg	0.1 mg	<4 nmol/L
Zinc	1–2 g	7–10 mg	10–20 μmol/L

*Much smaller amounts of inorganic trace elements are required if these are being provided as part of TPN.

† The total concentration in iodine-containing compounds in plasma, mainly contained in the thyroid hormones, is 250–600 nmol/L; only 5 nmol/L is present as inorganic iodide.

‡ 10–20 mg/day in the reproductive period; 20–50 mg/day during pregnancy.

and molybdenum have all been described, and these six elements will be considered here. The effects of iodine and iron deficiency are described elsewhere (pp. 179, 191). Deficiency of *inorganic* cobalt has not been reported in man.

Deficiencies of essential trace elements usually arise in association with protein-energy malnutrition, or with other abnormal nutritional states (e.g. total parenteral nutrition, neonatal feeds, synthetic diets). Specific inherited disorders in trace element handling are rare. Excessive losses, especially in association with severe and chronic gastrointestinal (GI) diseases, may also cause deficiency.

Methods of assessing essential trace element deficiency are mostly inadequate at present; they mainly depend on blood measurements (e.g. atomic absorption spectroscopy). Plasma levels, if very low, may be useful in diagnosis and management, but smaller changes are of less significance, as they may be due to changes in concentration of the plasma proteins that bind the metals. Diagnosis is often only made retrospectively on the basis of a clinical condition likely to have given rise to deficiency, occurring in association with clinical symptoms that can be attributed to trace element lack, and which respond to treatment with the appropriate supplementation.

Copper

Copper-containing metalloproteins include ceruloplasmin, dopamine hydroxylase, tyrosinase, cytochrome C oxidase, and superoxide dismutase. Human deficiency has been reported in infants fed exclusively on cow's milk; it is characterized by an iron-resistant microcytic, hypochromic anaemia, neutropenia, skeletal fractures, and evidence of intestinal malabsorption with diarrhoea. Copper circulates in plasma over 90% bound to ceruloplasmin (p. 91); the rest is mainly bound to albumin. Wilson's disease (p. 119) and Menkes' syndrome are inherited metabolic disorders of copper transport.

Menkes' syndrome (kinky-hair disease) is a fatal, sex-linked recessive disorder in which there is cerebral and cerebellar degeneration, connective tissue abnormalities and 'kinky' hair. Both serum [copper] and [ceruloplasmin] are low, and the copper content of the liver is very low. Absorption of copper from the intestine is grossly impaired, but treatment with parenteral copper has not proved successful.

Selenium

Selenium is a component of glutathione peroxidase, which has a cellular antioxidant function. It is also an essential part of iodothyronine deiodinase (type I), the enzyme that converts thyroxine to tri-iodothyronine. For both enzymes, the coding regions of the genomic DNA contain a unique triplet that specifically codes for the insertion of selenocysteine into the primary amino acid sequence of the newly synthesized enzyme.

Selenium deficiency can be investigated by measuring plasma [selenium] or erythrocyte glutathione peroxidase activity. Difficulties in interpretation may occur because reference ranges for plasma [selenium] vary both with age and with geographical location; there is also a marked reduction (about 30%) in pregnancy. Selenium deficiency is the cause of *Keshan disease*, a cardiomyopathy affecting some areas of China. This hitherto fatal condition has been almost eliminated by prophylactic dietary supplements of selenium. A similar cardiomyopathy has been reported in a few patients on long-term total parenteral nutrition, and in other patients a skeletal muscle myopathy developed; both types of myopathy respond to treatment with selenium supplements.

Zinc

Absorption of zinc from the intestine appears to be controlled in a manner similar to iron (p. 175), with sequestration of zinc in enterocytes, as metallothionein, and transfer of some of this to the plasma; the rest is lost when the enterocytes are sloughed. Zinc is mostly transported bound to albumin, α_2-macroglobulin and transferrin. Specimens of blood for zinc measurement are affected by feeding and venous stasis;

plasma [zinc] may fall by as much as 20% after meals. The body does not store zinc to any appreciable extent in any organ; urinary excretion is fairly constant at $10\,\mu mol/24\,h$, with re-excretion into the gut being the main route for adjusting the amount excreted.

Many enzymes have been shown to contain zinc, including carbonic anhydrase, alkaline phosphatase, alcohol dehydrogenase and porphobilinogen (PBG) synthase. Additionally, zinc has a crucial role in DNA and protein synthesis.

Nutritional deficiency is relatively common in association with protein-energy malnutrition, and has been described in infants, especially in the absence of zinc supplementation, and in patients receiving total parenteral nutrition. Pregnancy, lactation, old age and alcoholism have all been reported as being associated with an increased incidence of zinc deficiency. Alcohol causes an increased loss of zinc in urine, and plasma [zinc] is lower in chronic alcoholics than in normal individuals. Zinc deficiency may also be caused by diuretics, chelating agents and anti-cancer drug treatment. Severe zinc deficiency can lead to a pustular skin rash, loss of body hair, diarrhoea and mood changes.

Marked deficiency of zinc occurs in *acrodermatitis enteropathica*, in which there is an inherited defect of zinc absorption that causes low plasma [zinc] and reduced total body content of zinc. Infants develop skin rashes and chronic diarrhoea and intestinal malabsorption. Several secondary deficiencies occur. The condition responds rapidly to oral zinc supplements, which must be continued for life.

Injury, surgery, infection and a variety of acute illnesses are often accompanied by a fall in plasma [zinc] due to the stimulation of hepatic metallothionein synthesis; this is one of the many components of the acute-phase response (p. 88). The catabolism of skeletal muscle protein after injury can also lead to increased urinary loss of zinc.

Chromium

The biologically active form of chromium, Cr^{3+},

is absorbed with low efficiency from the diet. Although its significance in metabolism is not known, chromium is involved in glucose homeostasis; a chromium complex present in brewer's yeast ('glucose tolerance factor') is able to improve glucose tolerance in some diabetics.

Malnourished infants may develop severe glucose intolerance that improves with chromium supplementation. In adults, a syndrome consisting of weight loss, peripheral neuropathy, and marked insulin-insensitive glucose intolerance has been described that improves with chromium supplementation.

Manganese

Manganese is a component of certain metallo-enzymes, and manganese ions activate a large number of other enzymes, e.g. those involved in the synthesis of glycosaminoglycans, cholesterol and prothrombin. Despite this extensive range of enzyme requirements for manganese, true deficiency in humans appears to be very rare.

Molybdenum

This is a component of xanthine oxidase and some other metallo-enzymes. Deficiency has been reported to cause xanthinuria, with low plasma [urate] and low urinary uric acid output.

Vitamins

Vitamins are all organic compounds which, as originally defined, cannot be synthesized in the human body and must be provided in the diet. They are essential for the normal processes of metabolism, including growth and maintenance of health. It is now known that the body is able to produce part or even all of its requirements for some of the vitamins, e.g. vitamin D from cholesterol and niacin from tryptophan. Table 10.2 summarizes some data concerning both water-soluble and fat-soluble vitamins.

There are five main groups of causes of a vitamin-deficiency state. These are inadequate diet, impaired absorption, insufficient utilization, increased requirement, and increased

VITAMINS

Vitamin	Outline of the principal functions	Recommended daily amounts	Some effects of deficiency
Fat-soluble vitamins			
Vitamin A (retinol)	Vision, epithelial cell function	0.7 mg (males) 0.6 mg (females)	Night blindness, keratomalacia
Vitamin D (cholecalciferol)	Intestinal absorption of calcium, bone formation	7–8.5 µg for children 5 µg for adults (10 µg pregnancy/ lactation)	Rickets and osteomalacia
Vitamin E (tocopherols)	Antioxidant, membrane stability	4–8 mg, as α-tocopherol	Haemolytic anaemia
Vitamin K (phytomenadione)	Hepatic synthesis of prothrombin	150 µg	Coagulation defects
Water-soluble vitamins			
Thiamin (vitamin B_1)	All the vitamins that comprise the group of B vitamins act	0.5 mg/1000 kcal or 1 mg (whichever is the greater)	Beri-beri, cardiac myopathy
Riboflavin (vitamin B_2)	as coenzymes or prosthetic groups for various enzymes	0.6 mg/1000 kcal or 1.2 mg (as for vitamin B_1)	Cheilosis, stomatitis
Niacin	that are important in intermediary metabolism	6.6 mg/1000 kcal or 13 mg (as for vitamin B_1)	Pellagra
Pyridoxine (vitamin B_6)	See above	2.2 mg (males) 2.0 mg (females)	Dermatitis, stomatitis, CNS symptoms
Biotin	See above	15 µg/1000 kcal (50 µg/1000 kcal in children)	Anorexia, dermatitis
Folic acid	See above	200 µg (300 µg in pregnancy)	Megaloblastic anaemia
Cyanocobalamin (vitamin B_{12})	See above	3 µg	Megaloblastic anaemia
Vitamin C (ascorbic acid)	Collagen formation	40 mg	Scurvy, anaemia

Table 10.2 The vitamins.

rate of excretion. Vitamin deficiency develops in stages:

1 *Subclinical deficiency*, in which there is depletion of body stores. These are normally relatively large in the case of fat-soluble vitamins (e.g. A and D) and vitamin B_{12}, but small in the case of the other water-soluble vitamins.

2 *Overt deficiency*, which is usually accompanied by other evidence of malnutrition (e.g. protein-energy malnutrition).

Chemical investigations help to confirm the diagnosis of some overt vitamin-deficiency diseases, and may allow the diagnosis to be made at an earlier stage. Several types of chemical test are available, only some of which will be applicable to the investigation of suspected deficiency of a particular vitamin:

1 Direct measurement of [vitamin] in whole blood, plasma, erythrocytes, leucocytes or tissue biopsy specimens.

2 Direct measurement of the vitamin or one of its major metabolites in urine.

3 Measurement in blood or urine of a metabolite that accumulates as a result of a partial or complete blockage of a metabolic pathway involving an enzyme which requires the vitamin (or derivative) as a co-factor or prosthetic group.

4 Measurements as in (3), after the pathway has been stressed by means of a loading test.

5 Enzyme co-factor saturation tests, in which the activity of the enzyme is measured *in vitro* before and after the addition of the enzyme's co-factor or prosthetic group.

6 Saturation tests, in which the patient's intake of the vitamin that is thought to be deficient is increased; the effects of the increased intake are then monitored.

It is important to note that plasma concentrations of vitamins do not necessarily reflect the vitamin status of the body. Measurements of vitamins in cells (e.g. erythrocytes, leucocytes, or tissue biopsy specimens) generally give a much better indication of the body's vitamin status. Plasma levels usually fall before cellular and tissue levels fall, but low or undetectable plasma levels can occur in the absence of deficiency. Conversely, recent dietary intake can cause the plasma concentrations of vitamins to fluctuate markedly, even in severe deficiency. However, a sustained high plasma [vitamin] usually excludes a deficiency state.

For those vitamins or their metabolites that can be measured in urine, there may be low output despite the presence of adequate tissue reserves. However, a high level of urinary excretion means that deficiency is improbable.

Deficiency of fat-soluble vitamins

Vitamin A

This vitamin is present in the diet as retinol or as β-carotene, some of which is hydrolysed in the intestine to form retinol. A rich source is liver, but leafy vegetables and some fruits provide the largest amount as β-carotene. After absorption, followed by esterification in the mucosal cells, the ester is transported in the blood by retinol-binding protein (pre-albumin, p. 87). Specific binding proteins on cell membranes are involved in the uptake of vitamin A ester from plasma into the tissues. The vitamin is stored in the liver, mainly as its ester.

The active form of vitamin A, 11-*cis*-retinal, is necessary for rod vision, and deficiency can cause night blindness. Another form, retinoic acid, induces differentiation of epithelial cells. Vitamin A deficiency predisposes to gastrointestinal and respiratory tract infections and leads to night blindness and, if severe, to keratinization of the cornea, corneal ulceration and, ultimately, blindness. Low plasma [vitamin A] has been shown to be associated with an increased risk of developing cancer.

Plasma [vitamin A] may be decreased in states of severe protein deficiency, due to lack of its carrier protein, and may then increase if the protein deficiency is corrected.

The laboratory measurement most frequently carried out is determination of plasma [vitamin A]. If the concentration is less than 0.5 μmol/l (approximately 0.5 IU/L), this supports a diagnosis of vitamin A deficiency, but provides only limited information about the state of the tissue stores. Vitamin A absorption tests, based on measurements of plasma [vitamin A] before and five hours after a large oral dose of vitamin A (50 μmol/kg), have found limited use as a test of intestinal absorptive function.

Vitamin D

The formation and metabolism of vitamin D are described on page 71. Rickets in infancy and childhood, and osteomalacia in adults, are the main forms of vitamin D deficiency (p. 80).

Vitamin E

Eight related tocopherols and tocotrienols possess vitamin E activity; they have antioxidant properties, protect against oxidant (free radical) damage to polyunsaturated fatty acids in cell membranes and help prevent oxidation of low-density lipoprotein (LDL, p. 166). Oxidized LDL may be more atherogenic than native LDL, and there is some evidence that vitamin E may protect against atheromatous coronary heart disease.

Vitamin E deficiency is a rare complication of prolonged and severe steatorrhoea, and of prolonged parenteral nutrition. Altered red cell membrane stability can lead to haemolytic anaemia in children, whilst skeletal muscle breakdown may be responsible for the raised plasma creatine kinase activity observed in both adults and children. Neurological consequences have also been described. Deficiency is investigated by measuring plasma [vitamin E].

Vitamin K

Vitamin K is found in liver and leafy vegetables (as K_1 or phylloquinone) but is also synthesized by colonic bacteria (as K_2 or menaquinone). It is necessary for the post-translational modification in proteins of side-chains of glutamate by gamma-carboxylation. The presence of a second carboxyl group on the glutamate side-chain confers phospholipid-binding properties on the modified protein in the presence of Ca^{2+}. Proteins containing γ-carboxyglutamate include certain clotting factors (II, VII, IX and X) and the bone matrix protein, osteocalcin.

Vitamin K deficiency is most often due to treatment with anticoagulants (e.g. warfarin); it leads to reduced levels of the vitamin K-dependent coagulation factors and, hence, to haemorrhage. Deficiency may also arise in obstructive jaundice, and levels may be low in the new-born (leading to haemorrhagic disease of the new-born). Tests to assess vitamin K status include the prothrombin time – an important test in the investigation and management of jaundiced patients (p. 114) and of those on anticoagulant treatment.

Deficiency of water-soluble vitamins

Thiamin (vitamin B_1)

Dietary thiamin is readily absorbed and phosphorylated to its active form in the liver. Rich sources include wheatgerm, yeast, legumes, nuts and some meats. As its derivative, thiamin pyrophosphate (TPP), thiamine is important as a coenzyme in carbohydrate metabolism, being necessary for oxidative decarboxylation reactions (e.g. conversion of pyruvate to acetyl CoA) and transketolation reactions. Deficiency can lead to mood changes (depression, irritability), defective memory, peripheral neuropathy and, in more extreme cases, to beri-beri with cardiac failure. A clinical diagnosis of thiamin deficiency can be investigated by measuring erythrocyte transketolase activity or urinary thiamin excretion.

Erythrocyte transketolase provides a specific and sensitive index of tissue [thiamin] and is the chemical measurement of choice for investigating possible thiamin deficiency. Enzyme activity is measured in red cell haemolysates before and after addition of TPP.

Urinary thiamin measurements have been extensively used in nutritional surveys; they provide a useful index of deficiency. However, thiamin excretion is considerably influenced by recent dietary intake and by the adequacy of renal function.

Riboflavin (vitamin B_2)

The nucleotides of riboflavin are the prosthetic groups of many enzymes involved in electron transport, and riboflavin is essential for normal oxidative metabolism.

Specific deficiency of riboflavin is characterized by angular stomatitis, cheilosis and skin and eye lesions. Deficiency usually occurs as part of a mixed state involving several vitamins of the B complex, often including thiamin as well. Dietary sources include liver, kidney, milk products.

The activity of glutathione reductase in haemolysed erythrocytes, measured before and after the addition of flavin-adenine dinucleotide (the FAD effect), is a test for riboflavin deficiency.

Niacin

This term includes nicotinic acid and its amide (collectively referred to as niacin). Nicotinamide is a component of nicotinamide adenine dinucleotide (NAD) and its phosphate (NADP); these are coenzymes of many dehydrogenases. The body's requirements for nicotinamide are met partly from dietary niacin, but a substantial part normally comes from metabolism of tryptophan via 3-hydroxykynurenine.

Deficiency can be caused by an inadequate dietary intake. Maize protein is a poor source of tryptophan, and contains a bound form of niacin that is unavailable to the body. It may also be caused by conditions in which large amounts of tryptophan are metabolized along abnormal pathways (e.g. carcinoid syndrome, p. 132), and an acute deficiency can be precipitated by isoniazid treatment. Severe deficiency leads to pellagra, characterized by dermatitis (typically exposed skin parts), diarrhoea and mental changes, including dementia in chronic deficiency. Chemical methods for detecting niacin deficiency measure its excretion in urine or the excretion of its metabolites.

Pyridoxine (vitamin B$_6$)

The term vitamin B$_6$ includes pyridoxine, pyridoxal, pyridoxamine and their 5-phosphate derivatives. Good sources are liver and cereals (whole grain). The active form of the vitamin, pyridoxal phosphate (PP), is the prosthetic group of many enzymes, including the aminotransferases – alanine aminotransferase (ALT) and aspartate aminotransferase (AST) – and amino acid decarboxylases. Deficiency of vitamin B$_6$ nearly always occurs as part of a mixed deficiency of the B vitamins.

As a test for suspected pyridoxine deficiency, the activity of ALT or AST in haemolysed erythrocytes can be determined before and after the addition of pyridoxal phosphate (the PP effect).

Tryptophan load tests provide an alternative way of investigating suspected pyridoxine deficiency. In this test, the 24-hour urinary excretion of xanthurenate or 3-hydroxykynurenine is measured before and after a loading dose of 2 g L-tryptophan. The test stresses pyridoxine-dependent enzymes involved in the further metabolism of kynurenine, normally the main metabolite of tryptophan.

Biotin

This vitamin serves as a coenzyme for carboxylase reactions, including those catalysed by pyruvate carboxylase and acetyl coenzyme A (CoA) carboxylase.

Deficiency in man has been reported during total parenteral nutrition, and very rarely in association with excessive consumption of raw egg whites, which contain the biotin-binding protein avidin. Deficiency symptoms include dermatitis, alopecia, mental depression, nausea and vomiting.

Folic acid

Folic acid functions as a coenzyme in the transport of one-carbon units from one compound to another, and is essential for nucleic acid synthesis. Deficiency leads to impaired cell division, especially manifest as a pancytopenia, with defective red cell maturation (megaloblastic anaemia); folate deficiency is one of the commonest vitamin deficiency states in humans. A large, multicentre Medical Research Council trial demonstrated that folic acid supplementation reduces the occurrence (or recurrence) of neural tube defects (spina bifida, anencephaly and encephalocoele) by about 70 %; the vitamin has to be taken by the mother before conception. Methods of investigation include serum [folate] and erythrocyte [folate]. Good sources are liver, kidney and fresh vegetables.

Cyanocobalamin (vitamin B$_{12}$)

Deficiency of vitamin B$_{12}$ also leads to a megaloblastic anaemia and, additionally, may be associated with demyelination, particularly of the spinal cord, with neurological defects. The vitamin is obtained mainly from animal sources. Deficiency is usually diagnosed by haematological examination of blood and bone marrow specimens, and confirmed by measuring serum [vitamin B$_{12}$] and by investigating vitamin B$_{12}$ absorption from the intestine before and after the administration of intrinsic factor (the Schilling test). These tests are normally all performed by haematology departments.

Examination of gastric secretion for pentagastrin-fast achlorhydria (p. 124), a feature of Addisonian pernicious anaemia, is rarely performed nowadays. Another chemical test of vitamin B_{12} deficiency is measurement of methylmalonic acid (MMA) excretion in urine. Conversion of methylmalonyl-CoA to succinyl-CoA is catalysed by an enzyme that requires vitamin B_{12} as cofactor; urinary excretion of MMA is increased in vitamin B_{12} deficiency.

Ascorbic acid (vitamin C)

Frank scurvy rarely occurs nowadays, but its subclinical form is by no means uncommon, especially among elderly people living alone. Ascorbic acid is involved in the hydroxylation of proline and lysine, during the synthesis of collagen. It is also the most abundant water-soluble reducing agent (anti-oxidant) in man. Rich sources include citrus, blackcurrants and potatoes.

Plasma [ascorbate] measurements provide a poor index of tissue stores, as the concentration falls rapidly when the diet is very deficient in vitamin C. All patients with scurvy have undetectable plasma ascorbate, but not all people with undetectable plasma ascorbate have scurvy. Urinary ascorbate likewise is of no diagnostic value, unless measured as part of a therapeutic trial in an ascorbic acid saturation test.

Buffy layer ascorbate. Leucocyte ascorbate measurements provide a reasonable assessment of tissue stores of ascorbate, but difficulties in obtaining leucocytes uncontaminated by other cellular elements mean that the buffy layer, consisting of leucocytes and platelets (and a few erythrocytes), is normally examined instead. Leucocytes and platelets take up ascorbate against a concentration gradient, and may retain most of their ascorbate even when plasma [ascorbate] has fallen to undetectable levels. Buffy layer [ascorbate] falls at about the same time as clinical evidence of scurvy appears, and seems to give a good indication of the body's stores of the vitamin.

Biochemical assessment of nutritional status

Most types of nutritional assessment determine an individual's fat and protein content and depend on comparison with reference ranges derived from extensive population studies. As well as determining the degree of undernutrition or obesity, this type of assessment allows the response to appropriate treatment (e.g. gain in protein and fat content, loss of fat) to be measured. It may also help to define the potential risk of complications of obesity or undernutrition. Nutritional measures include body weight and height (for determination of BMI), skin-fold thickness as a measure of subcutaneous fat, and mid-arm muscle area (derived from mid-arm muscle circumference and triceps skinfold thickness). Bio-electrical impedance can be measured to determine total body water content, fat and fat-free mass. Estimates of muscle mass can be based on 24-hour urinary creatinine or 3-methylhistidine excretion; both methods depend on the accuracy of urine collections.

Measurements of serum protein concentrations (particularly albumin, transferrin and pre-albumin) are used to determine nutritional status. However, changes in levels of all these proteins are influenced by factors other than nutritional status such as intercurrent illness, or stress, or changes in fluid volume or distribution.

Nutritional support

Nutritional support is required in the presence of severe undernutrition and malnutrition. In addition, patients who are severely ill with sepsis, multiple trauma or extensive burns may develop a marked negative nitrogen balance, demanding nutritional support. Other indications include unconsciousness, clinical cachexia, radiotherapy or chemotherapy, major resection for malignancy, renal failure, the postoperative management of major surgery and complications of surgery, or any circumstances in which the GI tract is not available or is unable to support nutrition (e.g. severe inflammatory bowel disease, gut resection, fistula). Nutritional support may range from the presentation of palatable food, sip or tube feeding, to intravenous feeding.

Intravenous feeding

This is particularly indicated in the short bowel syndrome or in the presence of fistula formation involving the GI tract; it may also be indicated under other circumstances (Table 10.3). Most intravenous feeding is complete, providing all essential nutrients exogenously, and it is then known as total parenteral nutrition (TPN). Because of the irritant effect on the vascular endothelium of the hypertonic solutions that have to be used, potentially leading to thrombosis, delivery is often made into a large central vein to allow rapid dilution of the administered solution. Nutrients can then be given at a pre-defined rate using an appropriate pump and delivery set, usually from a three-litre bag containing all the prescribed ingredients (the 'big bag') for a 24-hour period.

Composition of the feed

Table 10.4 lists the typical composition of the 'big bag' for a 24-hour period. Such a standard regime would suit the majority of patients on first establishing TPN, though the formulation would be unsuitable for some patients (e.g. in the presence of renal disease). Several principles are important:

1 *Energy content.* The complete intravenous feed must provide adequate calories, typically 2000 kcal/24 h; more may be required in some circumstances (e.g. after severe burns). Calories are normally provided as a mixture of carbohydrate (glucose) and fat. In order to provide 1000 kcal as glucose, it is necessary to use *hypertonic* solutions, since about 5 L of 5% dextrose would be needed in order to provide 1000 kcal, whereas the same amount of energy could be provided with 1.25 L of 20% dex-

INDICATIONS FOR TPN
Short bowel syndrome
Radiation enteritis
Acute pancreatitis
Prolonged ileus
Severe inflammatory bowel disease (esp. fistula formation)
Hypermetabolic states (e.g. severe burns, sepsis)

Table 10.3 Principal indications for total parenteral nutrition.

COMPOSITION OF TPN FEED	
Nitrogen	12–14 g (as amino acids)
Fat	900 kcal (as 500 ml of 20% fat emulsion)
Glucose	1000 kcal (as 1.25 L of 20% dextrose)
Sodium	70–100 mmol
Potassium	60–100 mmol
Calcium	5–10 mmol
Magnesium	5 mmol
Phosphate	30 mmol
Trace elements	Present
Vitamins	Present (water-soluble and fat-soluble)
Volume	3 litres

It is emphasized that the above table represents a suitable standard regime only. Individual patients may have requirements that differ considerably from those listed above.

Table 10.4 Total parenteral nutrition: composition of a standard 'big bag'.

trose. Fat, administered as an emulsion, has a higher energy content than glucose, such that 500 mL of a 20% fat emulsion provides about 1000 kcal. The fat emulsion should also provide essential fatty acids.

2 *Nitrogen content.* This is provided in the form of amino acids. The commercially available solutions contain all the essential amino acids. The prescription is normally in the range 12–14 g nitrogen/24 h. Some patients require less nitrogen (e.g. small, elderly patients), while others require more (e.g. hypercatabolic patients with severe burns, multiple trauma).

3 *Electrolyte content.* The requirements for Na^+ and K^+ over the 24-hour period must be stated on each day's 'big bag' prescription. Typically, the Na^+ requirement will be 70–100 mmol/24 h, but more will be needed in the presence of excessive losses of Na^+ (e.g. severe diarrhoea, fistula), and less where there is Na^+ retention (e.g. renal disease, congestive cardiac failure). *Potassium requirements* are more variable. Intracellular repletion, or the administration of glucose and insulin, may increase demands for K^+, whereas requirements will be very small in renal failure or where there is extensive tissue breakdown. A stable patient probably requires 60–100 mmol K^+/24 h.

4 *Vitamins and minerals.* The requirements for calcium and phosphate depend on individual patients' needs, but average requirements are about 5–10 mmol/24 h for calcium and 30 mmol/24 h for phosphate. The magnesium requirement is normally about 5 mmol/24 h. Trace metals and both water-soluble and fat-soluble vitamins are also added to the 'big bag'.

5 *Fluid volume.* This is dictated by clinical circumstances, but 3 L/24 h meets the requirements for most patients (less in the elderly). Depending upon the particular energy prescription, a certain minimum volume will be required to deliver the prescribed number of calories.

Chemical monitoring of patients on total parenteral nutrition

The proper monitoring of patients on TPN requires biochemical, haematological and immunological measurements, together with routine anthropometric tests. An important and potentially serious complication of TPN is sepsis introduced via the catheter, and blood and other cultures may be required. Catheter care and the stipulation that, except in extreme emergencies, the catheter must be used exclusively for the administration of the feed, are important concepts in feeding patients by the parenteral route. This section considers the biochemical measurements that should be made.

Until the patient is stable, it is advisable to measure the plasma urea, creatinine, Na^+, K^+, total CO_2 and glucose concentrations daily, and to keep accurate records of fluid balance. Where there are potentially large electrolyte losses (e.g. via a fistula after surgery on the GI tract, the diuretic phase of acute renal failure), knowledge of (1) the fluid $[K^+]$ and $[Na^+]$ and (2) the volume of the fluid lost assists in the interpretation of abnormal plasma electrolyte values, and is essential in deciding the amount of K^+ and Na^+ to be added to the 'big bag'.

Plasma calcium, phosphate and magnesium should be measured twice weekly, in the absence of severe derangements of these analytes. Mild derangements in 'liver function tests' are sometimes observed during TPN, and these tests (p. 110) should also be carried out twice weekly. Regular measurement of other proteins (i.e. in addition to albumin), used to assay nutritional status, may also be helpful. Measurements of trace metals and vitamins are not often required unless there are specific clinical indications of deficiency.

Twice-weekly 24-hour urine collections should be made so that nitrogen losses can be estimated from the urea excretion; these figures are inevitably underestimates, due to incomplete urine collections and the failure to take account of other routes of nitrogen loss. Moreover, the proportion of urinary N as urea varies with the acid–base status. If proteinuria is significant, these losses must also be determined and taken into account. Despite these drawbacks, the estimated nitrogen losses help to decide whether the nitrogen content of the feed is sufficient to maintain a positive nitrogen balance.

The nutrition team

It cannot be emphasized too strongly that nutritional support is a multidisciplinary affair. The clinical biochemist has an important part to play in advising on the selection of tests, recording the results and advising on the meta-bolic complications that might arise. Ideally, a nutrition team includes representatives from clinical biochemistry, microbiology, pharmacy, dietetics and nursing, in addition to one or more clinicians (often surgeons), all of whom should have special interests in intravenous feeding. As well as advising on policy in this costly area, such a team should be able to offer expert advice and be competent to audit nutritional care.

KEY POINTS

1 Nutritional disorders are common, and are important on a world-wide basis. Broadly speaking, three disorders are recognized: undernutrition, malnutrition and obesity.
2 Clinical biochemical tests may be required for nutritional assessment, particularly measurement of certain vitamins, inorganic ions, trace elements and plasma proteins (e.g. albumin, transferrin).
3 Patients receiving total parenteral nutrition require regular biochemical monitoring. In the uncomplicated patient: daily plasma [urea], [creatinine], [Na+], [K+], [total CO_2], [glucose]; twice-weekly plasma [calcium], [phosphate], [magnesium] and liver function tests; twice-weekly 24-hour urine collections to assess nitrogen requirement.
4 Nutritional status often affects the measurement or interpretation of laboratory tests in clinical biochemistry.

CHAPTER 11

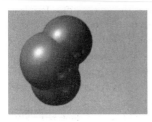

Disorders of Carbohydrate Metabolism

Glucose homeostasis, 149
Diabetes mellitus, 151

Hypoglycaemia, 158

Inherited metabolic
disorders, 159

Diabetes is the most common metabolic disorder, and its incidence is increasing. Biochemical measurements are particularly important in detecting it, monitoring its control, and treating its metabolic complications. Hypoglycaemia occurs in insulin-treated diabetic patients, but is otherwise rare. However, it is an important diagnosis to make, because of its possible consequences. Other disorders of carbohydrate metabolism are uncommon.

In this chapter, we consider diabetes, hypoglycaemia and some of the inherited disorders of carbohydrate metabolism.

Glucose homeostasis

Blood [glucose] is maintained within narrow limits imposed by the undesirable effects of hypoglycaemia, and by the potential for loss in the urine if the renal threshold is exceeded. The liver plays a key role in maintaining blood [glucose]. After a carbohydrate-containing meal, it removes about 70% of the glucose load that is delivered via the portal circulation. Some of the glucose is oxidized, and some is converted to glycogen for use as a fuel under fasting conditions. Glucose in excess of these requirements is partly converted by the liver to fatty acids and triglycerides, which are then incorporated into very low density lipoproteins (VLDL) and transported to adipose tissue stores.

In the fasting state, blood [glucose] is maintained both by glycogen breakdown in the liver and by gluconeogenesis (from glycerol, lactate and pyruvate and from the gluconeogenic amino acids), occurring mostly in the liver, but also in the kidneys. Glucose is spared, under fasting conditions, by the ability of muscle and other tissues to adapt to the oxidation of fatty acids, and by the ability of the brain and some other organs to utilize ketone bodies that are formed under these conditions.

The hormones mainly concerned with regulating glucose metabolism in the fed and fasting states are insulin, glucagon, somatostatin, growth hormone, adrenaline and cortisol. Of these, insulin has the most marked effects in humans (Table 11.1), and is the only hormone that lowers blood [glucose]. Glucagon, growth hormone, adrenaline and cortisol all tend, in general, to antagonize the actions of insulin (Table 11.2).

Insulin secretion

Insulin is synthesized in the β-cells of the islets of Langerhans in the pancreas. It is formed as prepro-insulin, which is rapidly cleaved to pro-insulin. The pro-insulin is packaged into secretory granules in the Golgi apparatus, and cleaved to insulin and C-peptide. Insulin and C-peptide are later released into the circulation in equimolar amounts.

A rise in blood [glucose] is the main stimulus for insulin secretion. Some amino acids (e.g. leucine), fatty acids and ketone bodies also promote insulin secretion. The release of insulin in response to hyperglycaemia is enhanced by the presence of glucose-dependent

EFFECTS OF INSULIN

Tissue	Processes activated by insulin	Processes inhibited by insulin
Liver	Uptake of amino acids and glycerol	Glycogenolysis
	Production of NADPH	Gluconeogenesis
	Synthesis of glycogen, proteins, triglycerides and VLDLs	Ketone body formation
Muscle	Uptake of glucose and amino acids	Triglyceride utilization
	Synthesis of glycogen	
Adipose	Uptake of chylomicrons and VLDLs and of glucose	Lipolysis
	Utilization of glucose	

Table 11.1 The effects of insulin on cellular metabolism.

EFFECTS OF INSULIN ANTAGONISTS

Tissue and hormone	Effects of the various hormones on glucose metabolism			
	Gluconeogenesis	Glycogenolysis	Glycolysis	Glucose uptake
Liver				
Adrenaline	Increased	Increased	Decreased	
Cortisol	Increased			Decreased
Glucagon	Increased	Increased		
Growth hormone	Increased	Increased	Decreased	
Muscle				
Adrenaline		Increased	Increased	
Cortisol				Decreased
Growth hormone				
(a) Short term			Increased	
(b) Long term			Decreased	
Adipose				
Cortisol			Decreased	

Table 11.2 The effects on glucose metabolism of hormones that antagonize the actions of insulin.

insulinotrophic peptide (GIP) or glucagon. GIP is probably the most important factor in the larger release of insulin that occurs in response to an oral glucose load, compared with the same dose of glucose given intravenously. Vagal stimulation also promotes insulin release.

The insulin receptor is located on the cell surface, and is internalized after insulin binding. Within different organs, target enzymes have been identified that serve to explain the known effects of insulin on intermediary metabolism. For instance, activation of glucose transport, induction of hexokinase (or glucokinase) and activation of phosphofructokinase, pyruvate kinase and pyruvate dehydrogenase in the liver are all consistent with insulin's actions of promoting increased glucose uptake and glycolytic breakdown. Stimulation of glycogen synthase accords with the effects of insulin on glycogen formation in the liver.

Diabetes mellitus

Diabetes is common, affecting 1–2% of Western populations, and population screening programmes reveal that many patients are previously unrecognized. It results in chronic hyperglycaemia, usually accompanied by glucosuria and other biochemical abnormalities, expressed as a wide range of clinical presentations ranging from asymptomatic patients with relatively mild biochemical abnormalities to patients admitted to hospital with severe metabolic decompensation of rapid onset that has led to coma. Long-term complications may develop, including retinopathy, neuropathy, nephropathy and vascular disease.

Diabetes may be a secondary consequence of other diseases. For example, in diseases of the pancreas such as pancreatitis or haemochromatosis, there is a reduction in insulin secretion. In some endocrine disorders, such as acromegaly or Cushing's syndrome, there is antagonism of insulin action by abnormal secretion of hormones with opposing activity. Several drugs adversely affect glucose tolerance. Table 11.3 summarizes these different causes. Secondary diabetes is, however, not common.

Most cases of diabetes are not associated with other conditions, but are primary, and fall into two distinct types. In Type I diabetes (insulin-dependent diabetes mellitus, IDDM) there is essentially no insulin secretion, whereas in Type II diabetes (non-insulin-dependent diabetes mellitus, NIDDM) insulin is secreted, but in amounts that are inadequate to prevent hyperglycaemia, or there is resistance to its action.

Type I diabetes usually presents acutely over a period of days or a few weeks in young non-obese subjects, but can occur at any age. In addition to polyuria, thirst and glucosuria, there is often marked weight loss and ketoacidosis. In general, insulin is required for treatment. Islet-cell antibodies that react with the β-cells of the pancreas have been demonstrated in serum from over 90% of patients with newly diagnosed type I diabetes. They have also sometimes been demonstrated in serum several years before the clinical and biochemical features of diabetes develop. Individuals with certain human leucocyte antigens (HLA) have been shown to have a particularly high risk of developing type Ia diabetes.

Type II diabetes generally presents in a less acute manner in older (over 40 years) patients who are obese. Rarely, type II diabetes occurs in young patients. Measurable levels of insulin are present, and the metabolic defect appears to lie either in defective insulin secretion or in insulin resistance. In general, insulin is not required for the prevention of ketosis, as these patients are relatively resistant to its development. However, insulin may be needed to correct abnormalities of blood [glucose]. There appears to be no association between

Table 11.3 Examples of causes of secondary diabetes or of impaired glucose tolerance.

SECONDARY DIABETES AND IMPAIRED GLUCOSE TOLERANCE	
Category of cause	Examples
Drugs	Oestrogen-containing oral contraceptives, salbutamol and some other catecholaminergic drugs, thiazide diuretics
Endocrine disorders	Acromegaly, Cushing's syndrome and Cushing's disease, glucagonoma, phaeochromocytoma, prolactinoma, thyrotoxicosis (occasionally)
Insulin receptor abnormalities	Auto-immune insulin receptor antibodies, congenital lipodystrophy
Pancreatic disease	Chronic pancreatitis, haemochromatosis, pancreatectomy

type II diabetes and either the HLA system or the development of auto-immunity. However, there is a strong genetic element to the disorder.

In established diabetic patients who become pregnant, poor blood glucose control is associated with a higher incidence of intra-uterine death and fetal malformation. Impaired glucose tolerance and hyperglycaemia in pregnancy are associated with an increased incidence of fetal macrosomia and neonatal hypoglycaemia. 'Gestational diabetes mellitus' is the term used to describe the abnormal glucose tolerance or diabetes mellitus that may develop during pregnancy. In the majority of these cases, the response to a glucose tolerance test (GTT) reverts to normal after the pregnancy, but about 50% of patients go on to develop diabetes mellitus within the next seven years.

The diagnosis of gestational diabetes mellitus is made on the basis of an oral GTT. Glucosuria detected at routine antenatal testing may suggest the need for an oral GTT, but may have no significance, since the renal threshold for glucose tends to be lowered in pregnancy. One approach is to select women with appropriate risk factors, such as a family history of diabetes mellitus, or a previous large baby. Also, glucosuria is more significant if detected on the second specimen of urine passed after an overnight fast (i.e. the first specimen passed is discarded). Mild abnormalities should be reassessed not less than six weeks after delivery.

Diagnosis

The diagnosis of diabetes mellitus may be suggested on the basis of the patient's history, or by the results of dipstick tests for glucose on urine specimens. However, urine glucose measurements are inadequate by themselves for diagnosing diabetes. They potentially yield false-positive results in subjects with a low renal threshold for glucose, and in a patient with diabetes may yield false-negative results if the patient is fasting. A provisional diagnosis of diabetes mellitus must always be confirmed by glucose measurements on blood specimens.

The criteria for the diagnosis of diabetes mellitus have been laid down by the World Health Organization (WHO). Separate criteria are described, depending on whether venous or capillary whole blood, or venous or capillary plasma specimens, are used. According to these criteria, a random venous plasma [glucose] of 11.1 mmol/L or more establishes the diagnosis. A single result is sufficient in the presence of typical symptoms, but in their absence a venous plasma [glucose] of 11.1 mmol/L or more should be detected on two separate occasions. Where there is any doubt, an oral glucose tolerance test should be performed (see below), but this is not often necessary.

Blood and plasma glucose

Most laboratory instruments measure plasma [glucose], but some use whole blood. Plasma [glucose] is 10–15% higher than whole blood [glucose], since red cells contain less water per unit volume than plasma. The discrepancy can be greater than this if [glucose] is changing rapidly, because glucose will not have reached equilibration across the red cell membrane. Plasma therefore yields more reliable results. At normal plasma [glucose], there is little difference between results obtained on capillary and venous blood. However, at hyperglycaemic levels, capillary plasma [glucose] may be significantly higher than venous plasma [glucose]. These factors are important in the interpretation of glucose tolerance tests.

If there is likely to be any delay in measuring [glucose] in blood specimens, it is essential either to separate the plasma immediately or to inhibit glycolysis in blood by using a sodium fluoride-containing collection tube. This stabilizes the [glucose] for several hours. Measurements of blood [glucose] that are to be performed using a 'stick' test must be carried out without delay on specimens that do not contain sodium fluoride.

Oral glucose tolerance test (GTT)

Several precautions must be observed in preparing for and in performing the test. It should not be performed on patients who are suffering from an intercurrent infection or the effects of trauma, or who are recovering from a serious illness. Drugs such as corticosteroids and diuretics may impair glucose tolerance, and should be stopped before the test if possible. The patient should have been on an unrestricted diet containing at least 200 g carbohydrate/day for at least three days, and should not have indulged in unaccustomed amounts of exercise. The patient must not smoke before or during the test, nor eat or drink anything other than as specified below.

A GTT is usually performed after an overnight fast, although a fast of 4–5 hours may be enough. The patient is allowed to drink water during the fast. A standard dose of glucose (82.5 g glucose monohydrate or 75 g anhydrous glucose) dissolved in 250–350 mL of water is given by mouth. Smaller amounts of glucose (1.92 g glucose monohydrate or 1.75 g anhydrous glucose/kg body weight) are given to children. During the test, the patient should be

sitting up, or lying over on the right side so as to facilitate rapid emptying of the stomach. Blood specimens are collected before giving the glucose load and after two hours.

Table 11.4 summarizes the criteria for identifying healthy adults, patients with diabetes mellitus and individuals with impaired glucose tolerance for blood and plasma [glucose], and for venous and capillary specimens.

Monitoring the treatment of diabetic patients

There is now excellent evidence that in Type I diabetes, the incidence of long-term complications such as retinopathy can be reduced by achieving tight control, albeit at the expense of an increased frequency of hypoglycaemic episodes. In order to achieve this, insulin doses need to be frequently and carefully adjusted on the basis of multiple daily blood [glucose] measurements. In patients in whom this level of control is unrealistic or is not needed, this requirement can be relaxed. In such patients, and in patients with Type II diabetes, less frequent blood [glucose] measurements can be made, preferably covering different times of the day, although the frequency should be increased at times of illness or when control appears to have deteriorated.

Table 11.4 Diagnostic criteria for diabetes mellitus; their dependence on the nature of the specimens collected for analysis (WHO Expert Committee on Diabetes Mellitus).

DIAGNOSTIC CRITERIA FOR DIABETES MELLITUS		
	Glucose concentration (mmol/L)	
	Fasting	Two hours post-75 g glucose
Normal individuals		
Venous plasma	<7.8	<7.8
Venous blood	<6.7	<6.7
Capillary blood	<6.7	<7.8
Diabetes mellitus		
Venous plasma	≥7.8	and/or ≥11.1
Venous blood	≥6.7	and/or ≥10.0
Capillary blood	≥6.7	and/or ≥11.1
Impaired glucose tolerance		
Venous plasma	<7.8	and 7.8–11.1
Venous blood	<6.7	and 6.7–10.0
Capillary blood	<6.7	and 7.8–11.1

The use of urine testing to monitor diabetes is declining, but it may provide an adequate indication of control in older patients with Type II diabetes, controlled on diet or a small dose of oral hypoglycaemic drug.

Glycated haemoglobin

Blood glucose measurements made at the clinic only indicate the [glucose] at that time, and may be unrepresentative of overall control. The discovery that haemoglobin (Hb) undergoes non-enzymatic glycation has allowed assessment of diabetic control over a longer period.

Glucose reacts spontaneously and non-enzymatically with free amino groups on proteins to form covalent glycated proteins. The extent of glycation depends on the average [glucose] to which the protein is exposed and on the half-life of the protein. Thus, long-lived structural proteins (e.g. lens protein) may be damaged as a result of the abnormal increase in protein glycation found in diabetics. Indeed, it has been suggested that glycation of structural proteins might be responsible for some of the long-term complications of diabetes. Shorter half-life proteins such as Hb also undergo excessive glycation in diabetes.

Several glycated derivatives of Hb exist, derived from the reaction of Hb with glucose, glucose-6-phosphate, etc. These are collectively known as HbA_1. The principal complex is the one formed with glucose itself, HbA_{1c}, which normally forms about 5% of circulating Hb. Methods of measuring both [total HbA_1] and [HbA_{1c}] are available.

Once formed, the glycated Hb stays within the red cell for its lifetime. Since the half-life of the red cell is about 60 days, the glycated Hb value reflects the average level of blood [glucose] over the previous 1–2 months. The extent of the elevation indicates the overall average degree of blood glucose control.

Glycated plasma proteins

Measurement of glycated plasma proteins (the major component of these proteins being albumin), can also be used to monitor diabetic control. The shorter half-life of albumin means that this test reflects control of blood [glucose] over the previous 10–15 days. This has some advantages over glycated haemoglobin measurements, for instance in pregnancy where stringent control is particularly necessary. Plasma fructosamine is a measure of glycated plasma proteins.

Microalbumin

Urinary 'microalbumin' is a term that refers to urinary albumin loss that is greater than normal, but which remains below the threshold of detection by the dipstick tests widely used for detecting the presence of urinary protein. The more sensitive tests required to detect 'microalbuminuria' are performed in the laboratory. There is no analytical difficulty in measuring these low levels of albumin, but there is lack of agreement as to the type of sample to use and how best to express the results. Overnight timed urine collections are increasingly favoured, but random urine samples are often used for convenience. Results are expressed as an albumin excretion rate, or as an albumin : creatinine ratio on a random sample.

Up to 50% of type I diabetics may develop nephropathy, and the detection of microalbuminuria has been shown to signal an eventual progression to diabetic nephropathy. With the benefit of the early warning provided by the detection of microalbuminuria, there is some evidence that meticulous control of diabetes and hypertension, and possibly the use of angiotensin-converting enzyme inhibitors, may delay the progress of the nephropathy.

Metabolic complications of diabetes mellitus

Patients with diabetes can develop severe metabolic derangements potentially leading to coma. The causes can be classified as follows:
• Hyperglycaemia, with or without ketoacidosis.
• Lactic acidosis, with or without hyperglycaemia.

• Hypoglycaemia, due to insulin excess (p. 158).

• Uraemia (p. 61), e.g. due to diabetic nephropathy.

Diabetic ketoacidosis

Diabetic ketoacidosis may be the presenting feature in a patient not previously recognized as having diabetes. In a patient with known diabetes, it may be precipitated by omitting an insulin dose, or by the insulin dose becoming inadequate because of an increase in hormones with opposing action, due to intercurrent infection, trauma, or unusual physical or psychological stress. The clinical features are dehydration, ketosis and hyperventilation ('air hunger').

Ketoacidosis is due to insulin deficiency, accompanied by raised plasma concentrations of the counter-regulatory hormones (adrenaline, cortisol, growth hormone and glucagon). The changes in these circulating hormones result in hyperglycaemia and in mobilization of free fatty acids from adipose tissue, and subsequent increased ketone body production in the liver (Fig. 11.1).

The major metabolic abnormalities result from hyperglycaemia or ketoacidosis, or both. Hyperglycaemia causes extracellular hyperosmolality, which in turn leads to intracellular dehydration as well as to an osmotic diuresis. The osmotic diuresis causes loss of water, Na^+, K^+, calcium and other inorganic constituents, and leads to a fall in circulating blood volume. Ketone bodies stimulate the chemoreceptor trigger zone, so vomiting may exacerbate all these effects. The increased production of ketone bodies causes a metabolic acidosis with associated hyperkalaemia. Lactic acidosis and prerenal uraemia may also be present.

Ketone bodies

Acetoacetate, 3-hydroxybutyrate (β-hydroxybutyrate) and acetone are collectively described as the 'ketone bodies', although 3-hydroxybutyrate is not in fact a ketone. They are most commonly found in the blood in excessive amounts in uncontrolled diabetes.

Levels also increase in starvation, since ketone bodies form an important energy source for many tissues when carbohydrate intake or metabolism is limited. Ketone bodies are synthesized in the liver from acetyl CoA, itself derived from the oxidation of free fatty acids. Some of the acetoacetate may then be reduced to 3-hydroxybutyrate or decarboxylated with the formation of acetone and CO_2.

Acetoacetic acid and 3-hydroxybutyric acid production give rise to a metabolic acidosis, since the liver and other tissues cannot, in general, completely metabolize the increased amounts of these ketone bodies that are being formed. The acidosis is partly compensated by hyperventilation, with reduction in P_{CO_2}. The acidosis causes H^+ to move into cells and K^+ to move out. Increased plasma $[K^+]$ often results from the combined effects of the acidosis and the lack of insulin action that normally promotes K^+ entry into cells.

Laboratory assessment and management of diabetic ketoacidosis

An initial diagnosis is usually made on the basis of the history, clinical examination and dipstick testing of urine for glucose and ketone bodies, and testing of blood [glucose]. Laboratory-based tests on blood are needed to evaluate the severity of the condition more precisely, and to monitor progress during treatment. It is rarely necessary, and indeed may be positively dangerous, to wait for laboratory results before starting emergency treatment. However, further treatment should be based on regular clinical assessment and on chemical measurements in the laboratory.

Plasma glucose, urea, Na^+ and K^+ concentrations are measured on venous blood. Plasma $[Na^+]$ may be normal or low initially. Plasma $[K^+]$ is usually increased, but may be normal. Plasma [urea] is usually increased due to dehydration. Acid–base status is assessed by measurement of venous [total CO_2] or by measurement of arterial 'blood gases' ($[H^+]$, P_{CO_2}, $[HCO_3^-]$ and P_{O_2}). Plasma [total CO_2] is nearly always reduced, often being less than 5 mmol/L in severe cases. Results of blood gas

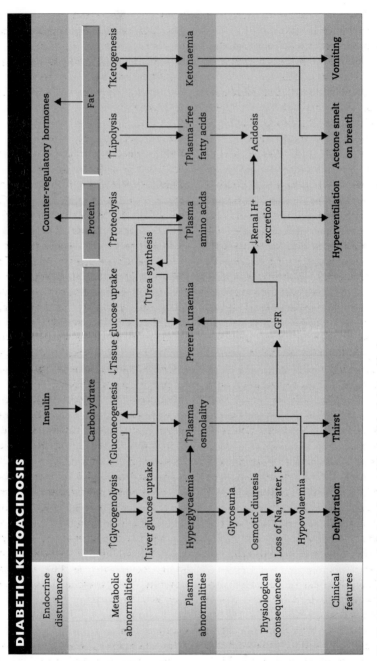

Fig. 11.1 Metabolic and clinical abnormalities in diabetic ketoacidosis.

analysis indicate a metabolic acidosis with compensatory reduction in P_{CO_2}.

Treatment aims to replace fluid and electrolyte deficits, and to correct the metabolic abnormality by infusion of insulin.

Knowledge of the fluid and electrolyte deficits likely to be present helps in planning appropriate therapy. The deficits may be as much as 5–10 L of water, 500 mmol of Na^+, 250–800 mmol of K^+ and 300–500 mmol of base (e.g. HCO_3^-) in patients with severe acidosis. Fluid replacement is usually given initially as isotonic saline. The rate of infusion will depend on the clinical circumstances, but should usually be rapid, at least initially, with careful monitoring of fluid status, often including the use of measurement of central venous pressure. Potassium replacement is usually started early, in the knowledge that the patient has almost certainly developed a large K^+ deficit, and insulin will rapidly cause K^+ to enter the cells from the ECF. Serious hypokalaemia can develop fairly quickly in the absence of early corrective action.

The use of $NaHCO_3$ to correct the acidosis is seldom required except in very severe cases (arterial $[H^+]$ over 100 nmol/L), since restoring normal renal perfusion allows excretion of H^+ and regeneration of HCO_3^-, and the return of metabolism to normal reduces H^+ production. Infusion of $NaHCO_3$ can be hazardous, as rapid correction of the acidosis augments the K^+ influx into cells and can precipitate dangerous hypokalaemia. It may also cause a paradoxical rise in cerebrospinal fluid (CSF) $[H^+]$ rather than a fall, since CO_2 diffuses more rapidly into the CSF than HCO_3^-.

Insulin is usually given as a constant intravenous infusion at 6–10 units/h. Plasma [glucose] is monitored, and once it has fallen to between 10 and 15 mmol/L the intravenous fluid is changed to 5% dextrose. It may be possible to decrease the rate of insulin infusion. This is continued until it is possible to re-establish the patient on oral food and water and a conventional subcutaneous insulin regimen.

The frequency and timing of repeat analyses depends on the severity and nature of the ketoacidosis, and on the method of treatment. For most patients, it is advisable to repeat some of the initial analyses, particularly plasma $[K^+]$, after one hour and thereafter at longer intervals if treatment is progressing satisfactorily.

Nonketotic, hyperglycaemic coma

These patients are usually older than the ketotic group, and typically have Type II diabetes. Insulin deficiency causes effects on carbohydrate metabolism as in diabetic ketoacidosis, but may be less severe, allowing some suppression of ketogenesis. In addition, there may be poorer renal function in older patients, leading to greater losses of water and electrolytes. Severe hyperglycaemia can develop with profound dehydration and a very high plasma osmolality, but no ketosis and minimal acidosis. This condition is often referred to as hyperosmolar nonketotic hyperglycaemia. It should be noted that patients with ketoacidosis may also have a raised osmolality, although this is not so marked.

Treatment of patients with nonketotic hyperglycaemia is similar to the treatment of ketotic hyperglycaemic patients, with administration of fluids and insulin. Because of the hypertonicity, hypotonic saline replacement may be used, although it is important that the osmolality does not fall too quickly. Once the acute illness has resolved, most patients will not require continuing insulin, but will be managed on diet, with or without oral hypoglycaemic agents. There is an increased risk of thrombotic episodes in these patients, and treatment with anticoagulants is generally considered advisable.

Lactic acidosis

If tissue perfusion is affected by extreme dehydration (hyperosmolality), or by the factors that precipitated the original metabolic decompensation (e.g. severe infection, myocardial infarction), tissue anoxia may lead on to lactic acidosis.

Hypoglycaemia

The plasma [glucose] at which hypoglycaemic symptoms appear is very variable, often related more to the rate of fall of blood [glucose] than to the absolute value observed. Arbitrarily, a venous plasma [glucose] below 2.2 mmol/L is the biochemical definition of hypoglycaemia. It is convenient to distinguish between the hypoglycaemia that occurs in response to fasting and the hypoglycaemia that is due to some other stimulus (reactive hypoglycaemia), including the stimulus of a meal. It is often possible to distinguish these two categories on the basis of the patient's history.

Reactive hypoglycaemia

This may be due to drugs (e.g. insulin overdose, accidental or deliberate; sulphonylureas; salicylate overdose in children, but not adults) or poisons (e.g. some toadstools), inborn errors of metabolism (e.g. galactosaemia, hereditary fructose intolerance) or alcohol. It may be brought about by excess alcohol intake, or can be idiopathic in origin. It may occur after meals in patients who have undergone gastric surgery, or in essential reactive hypoglycaemia, which is an idiopathic condition.

Table 11.5 Fasting hypoglycaemia.

Fasting hypoglycaemia

Failure to maintain a normal blood [glucose] in the fasting state is a feature of a number of endocrine conditions, and of some inborn errors of metabolism (pp. 159, 252). Causes of fasting hypoglycaemia are summarized in Table 11.5, subdivided into causes of enhanced glucose utilization and defective glucose production.

Insulinoma

This is usually a small, solitary, benign adenoma of the pancreatic islets that secretes inappropriate amounts of insulin. Occasionally, multiple pancreatic adenomas may be associated with adenomas in other endocrine organs as part of the multiple endocrine neoplasia (MEN I) syndrome (pp. 77, 201). The symptoms may be bizarre, and laboratory investigations play a major part in diagnosis.

Most patients develop symptomatic hypoglycaemia after a fast of 24–36 hours, but in a few the fast may have to last for up to 72 hours before symptomatic hypoglycaemia develops. Blood specimens are collected when hypoglycaemic symptoms develop, or after three overnight fasts. Most patients with an insulinoma will have unequivocal hypoglycaemia in one of these specimens, even if they were asymptomatic. The diagnostic finding in patients suspected of having an insulinoma is a fasting plasma [insulin] that is inappropriately high in relation to the low plasma [glucose].

FASTING HYPOGLYCAEMIA	
Cause	Examples
Enhanced glucose utilization	
Endogenous over-production of insulin	Hyperinsulinism of childhood (nesidioblastosis), insulinoma, pancreatitis, pancreatic tumours (as part of MEN I syndrome)
Defective glucose production	
Endocrine disorders	Adrenocortical insufficiency and hypothyroidism (in both cases, primary and secondary), growth hormone deficiency
Liver disease	Severe portal cirrhosis, acute hepatic necrosis, hepatic tumours
Renal disease	End-stage renal failure
Miscellaneous	Severe malnutrition, starvation, inherited metabolic disorders (e.g. glycogen storage disease type I)

It can be difficult to demonstrate fasting hypoglycaemia satisfactorily in some patients. In these cases, it may still be possible to obtain support for a diagnosis of insulinoma by measuring plasma [C-peptide] during an infusion of exogenous insulin sufficient to induce hypoglycaemia. Exogenous insulin contains little or no C-peptide, and continuous detection of plasma [C-peptide] shows that endogenous insulin release is not suppressed, as it should be in response to hypoglycaemia. This finding is strongly suggestive of insulinoma.

Therapeutic insulin preparations contain little or no C-peptide. Accidental or deliberate overdose of insulin, giving rise to hypoglycaemia, can therefore be distinguished from insulinoma by measuring both plasma [insulin] and plasma [C-peptide].

Other causes of fasting hypoglycaemia

Deficiency of hormones that antagonize insulin activity is an uncommon cause of hypoglycaemia. Some nonpancreatic tumours are associated with hypoglycaemia, mainly in patients with advanced malignant disease. Some of the larger tumours may consume excessive amounts of glucose, but there is also evidence for the production of hormonal insulin-like substances.

Inherited metabolic disorders

Glycogen storage diseases

Glycogen can be synthesized by most tissues, but is stored mainly in liver and muscle. Glycogen metabolism is summarized in Figure 11.2. The glycogen storage diseases are rare inborn errors of carbohydrate metabolism due to deficiency or reduced activity of one or more of the many enzymes involved.

The common feature in this complex group of conditions is an abnormality in the storage of glycogen, usually in increased amounts and sometimes with an abnormal structure. There may also be hypoglycaemia, abnormalities of blood lipids, hyperuricaemia and lactic acidosis. These secondary features are no substitute for tissue enzyme assays, supplemented if required by carbohydrate structural studies.

The commonest glycogen storage disease is Cori type VI (A), due to deficiency of phosphorylase kinase. Glycogen of normal structure accumulates, mainly in liver and muscle. Von Gierke's disease (Cori type I) is due to deficiency of glucose-6-phosphatase, and the glycogen that accumulates (mainly in the liver, kidney and intestine) also has a normal structure. There may be profound fasting hypoglycaemia.

Galactosaemia

The liver is the principal site for the conversion of galactose into glucose. Three defects have been described, due to deficiency of galactose-1-phosphate uridylyltransferase (Gal-1-PUT), galactokinase, or UDPgalactose epimerase (Fig. 11.3). They all interfere with the normal metabolism of galactose, causing a rise in plasma and urine galactose. Galactose gives rise to positive results if urinary side-room tests for reducing substances are performed, unless milk intake is inadequate or vomiting is severe.

Galactosaemia is rare (Table 19.2, p. 248). The commonest and most severe enzymatic defect is due to Gal-1-PUT deficiency. This usually manifests itself in the neonatal period or early in infancy, giving rise to vomiting, accompanied by hypoglycaemia. If galactose-containing foods are given to the child, plasma [galactose] rises, and galactose can be identified in the urine by chromatography. All neonates in some countries (e.g. Scotland) are screened for defective galactose metabolism as an extension of the screening programme for phenylketonuria (p. 250), but the response time is usually too slow for this rapidly fatal condition, and diagnosis is nearly always made following clinical presentation. Treatment is controlled by measurements of blood [galactose-1-phosphate].

Galactokinase deficiency may not present clinically in the neonatal period, and may escape detection until cataracts develop,

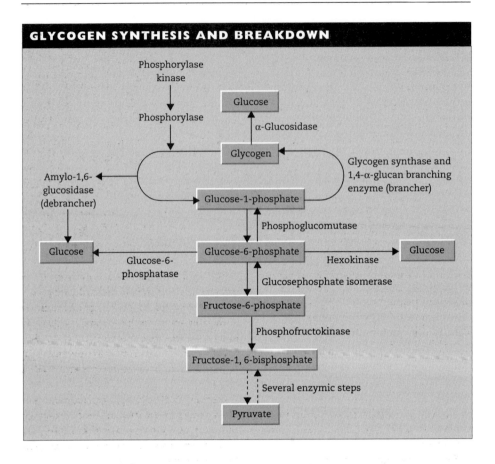

GLYCOGEN SYNTHESIS AND BREAKDOWN

Fig. 11.2 Glycogen synthesis and breakdown. Deficiencies of most of the enzymes named in the figure have been shown to occur in one or more of the many forms of glycogen storage disease. In gluconeogenesis, the hydrolysis of fructose-1,6-bisphosphate by fructose-1,6-bisphosphate is not shown.

unless side-room tests for reducing substances are performed.

Infants who have positive tests for reducing substances in urine should have a urine specimen examined by chromatography. If galactose is identified, blood [galactose] and [galactose-1-phosphate] should be measured. Confirmation of the diagnosis is obtained by measuring erythrocyte enzyme activities.

Miscellaneous causes of glycosuria

Several conditions give rise to glycosuria due to the presence of substances other than glucose in the urine.

Hereditary fructose intolerance. The liver is the principal site for the conversion of fructose into glucose. Deficiency of fructose-1-phosphate aldolase causes intracellular accumulation of fructose-1-phosphate. Vomiting and hypoglycaemia occur after ingestion of fructose-containing foods, usually the disaccharide sucrose. The age of presentation depends on feeding patterns and on the severity of the defect. Most patients develop a strong aversion to sucrose. A fructose tolerance test can be used for the investigation. Patients with the deficiency show marked and prolonged falls in plasma [glucose] and plasma [phosphate] after

CONVERSION OF GALACTOSE TO GLUCOSE

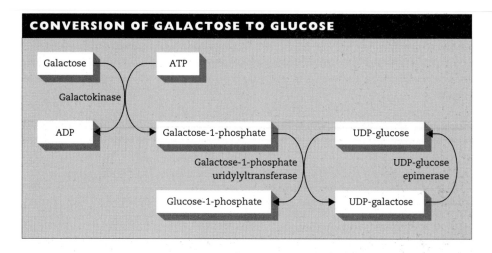

Fig. 11.3 The enzymatic conversion of galactose to glucose. Galactosaemia may be caused by deficiency of any of these three enzymes, but the most common of the three causes is deficiency of galactose-1-phosphate uridylyltransferase. UDP, uridine diphosphate.

fructose administration, as well as fructosuria. Urine chromatography confirms the presence of fructose.

Essential fructosuria is a benign condition caused by fructokinase deficiency. It has to be distinguished from other causes of glycosuria.

Essential pentosuria is a benign inborn error of metabolism in which the sugar L-xylulose is excreted in the urine in excess, due to a defect in NADP-linked xylitol dehydrogenase, one of the enzymes in the glucuronic acid oxidation pathway.

Lactosuria is of no pathological significance. It often occurs in the later stages of pregnancy and while lactation continues after delivery. Its importance stems from the need to distinguish lactosuria from glucosuria.

KEY POINTS

1 In diabetes mellitus, there is chronic hyperglycaemia, usually due to absolute or relative lack of insulin.

2 Both insulin-dependent diabetics (Type I) and non-insulin-dependent diabetics (Type II) are prone to develop long-term vascular and neurological complications. The incidence of these complications can be reduced by strict control of the hyperglycaemia.

3 The diagnosis of diabetes rests on finding plasma [glucose] over 11.1 mmol/L in the presence of symptoms, confirmed by an oral glucose tolerance test if there is any doubt.

4 Ideally, diabetics should use a portable meter to monitor plasma [glucose] and thus adjust insulin dosage. Adequacy of control should also be monitored regularly by measuring HbA_{1c}.

5 Microalbuminuria tends to precede diabetic nephropathy, and should be monitored regularly in Type I diabetics.

6 In the most serious acute complication, diabetic hyperglycaemia with ketoacidosis, insulin and intravenous fluid treatment should be monitored initially by frequent (hourly) plasma [K+] and [glucose] measurements.

7 Hypoglycaemia is a common and potentially dangerous complication of insulin treatment, particularly in tightly controlled diabetics. Insulinomas also cause hypoglycaemia; the diagnosis can be made by demonstrating inappropriately raised plasma [insulin] during fasting.

Case 11.1

A 14-year-old boy was found by his mother in a drowsy and uncooperative state. When the general practitioner arrived, she told her that her son had seemed to be unusually thirsty for the last 1–2 months, and she thought that he had lost weight. Recently, he had been complaining of abdominal pain and discomfort.

He was admitted to hospital as an emergency. On examination he was semiconscious, with deep sighing respiration, a pulse rate of 120/min, a blood pressure of 94/56, and cold extremities. Chemical investigations on blood after admission showed the following:

	Results	Reference range
Plasma analysis		
[Glucose] (mmol/L)	35	3.6–5.8 (fasting)
[K+] (mmol/L)	6.9	3.3–4.7
[Na+] (mmol/L)	128	132–144
[Urea] (mmol/L)	24.5	2.5–6.6
Blood gas analysis		
[H+] (nmol/L)	82	36–44
P_{CO_2} (kPa)	2.9	4.4–6.1
[HCO_3^-] (mmol/L)	7.0	21.0–27.5
P_{O_2} (kPa)	14.0	12–17

What is the probable diagnosis, and how would you confirm this quickly? What principles should guide the treatment of this patient?

Comments on Case 11.1

The patient almost certainly had diabetic ketoacidosis, with typical clinical and biochemical features. The tachycardia, hypotension and cold peripheries suggest marked depletion of extracellular fluid. The arterial sample shows that he has a metabolic acidosis, and the plasma sample contains a high concentration of glucose. The high urea is consistent with renal impairment or dehydration. Ketoacidosis was confirmed by testing a urine specimen for ketone bodies. If he had been too dehydrated to produce urine, a drop of plasma could have been used instead (note that only some people can smell acetone in patients' breath). The mainstays of treatment for patients with diabetic ketoacidosis are:

1 Fluid and electrolyte replacement, starting with saline (150 mmol/L) and containing added potassium chloride (40 mmol/L), usually as a standard regime (e.g. one litre in the first 30 minutes, a second litre in the next hour and a third litre in the following two hours, etc.).

2 Insulin infusion, usually starting at a rate of 6 units/h.

3 Frequent monitoring of the patient's plasma [glucose] and [K+], and monitoring of the central venous pressure. As the treatment takes effect, plasma [K+] is liable to fall rapidly due to the large whole-body K+ deficit, despite the initially raised plasma [K+].

Case 11.2

An elderly man was visited by his son and found to be semiconscious. He had last been seen by neighbours about ten days previously, when he had seemed well. He was admitted to hospital. On examination, he appeared extremely dehydrated. The results of biochemical investigations were as follows:

Plasma analysis	Result	Reference range
[Urea] (mmol/L)	38	2.5–6.6
[Na$^+$] (mmol/L)	151	132–144
[K$^+$] (mmol/L)	4.8	3.3–4.7
[Total CO$_2$] (mmol/L)	18	24–30
[Glucose] (mmol/L)	61	3.6–5.8 (fasting)
Osmolality (mmol/kg)	417	280–290

Comments on Case 11.2

There is severe hyperglycaemia, resulting in a very high osmolality. The hyperglycaemia has driven an osmotic diuresis, resulting in loss of extracellular fluid and consequent reduction in the glomerular filtration rate and retention of urea. The sustained osmotic diuresis causes a loss of water in excess of sodium, explaining the hypernatraemia. The [total CO$_2$] is slightly reduced due to the impaired renal function, but is not as low as would be expected in a case of ketoacidosis with results as abnormal as these. The patients was too dehydrated to produce a urine sample to check for ketones, but a drop of plasma on the ketones square of a urine dipstick gave a negative result.

He had nonketotic hyperglycaemia. This only occurs in patients with Type II diabetes. The insulin concentration required to oppose the ketogenic actions of glucagon is lower than that required to prevent increased glucose production. These patients have sufficient circulating insulin to prevent the ketogenesis, but not enough to prevent the hyperglycaemia. Treatment is by replacement of fluid and electrolyte losses, and by insulin infusion to restore the [glucose]. Once the acute episode is over, insulin is unlikely to be needed.

When the patient recovered, he reported having experienced increasing thirst and polyuria over several weeks. In response to the thirst, he had been drinking several large bottles of lemonade every day.

Case 11.3

A 45-year-old woman who was unable to feed, wash or dress herself because of severe multiple sclerosis was being cared for in a nursing home. About six hours after a visit by relatives, it was found that she could not be roused. On admission to hospital, she was profoundly hypoglycaemic ([glucose] 1.9 mmol/L), and required repeated intravenous infusions of glucose to maintain plasma [glucose] over the next 12–24 h. A sample of blood taken on admission was stored and subsequently analysed for insulin and C-peptide. The results were inappropriately raised, considering the hypoglycaemia. Over the next few days, repeated overnight fasts failed to induce further hypoglycaemia. Eventually, after a prolonged fast of four days, [glucose] dropped to 2.5 mmol/L (not a hypoglycaemic level by strict criteria), at which time insulin and C-peptide were undetectable.

Comments on Case 11.3

The results on admission were suggestive of an insulinoma, with hypoglycaemia and inappropriately elevated insulin and C-peptide levels. However, it proved difficult to induce a further episode of hypoglycaemia. Most patients with an insulinoma will be

Continued on p. 164

Case 11.3 *continued*

hypoglycaemic on one or more occasion after three overnight fasts, even if not symptomatic. Even a prolonged fast failed to induce true hypoglycaemia, and at that time the insulin level was appropriately low. Review of her history revealed no suggestions of previous hypoglycaemic episodes. The clinical staff were accordingly forced to reconsider the initial diagnosis.

The admission sample of blood was sent for toxicological analysis, and was found to contain high concentrations of the oral hypoglycaemic drugs chlorpropamide and glibenclamide. These drugs are sulphonylureas, which act by enhancing pancreatic insulin secretion in response to glucose. Both chlorpropamide and glibenclamide have long half-lives, making hypoglycaemia an occasional problem even when used therapeutically in patients with diabetes.

The patient would have been unable to obtain or take these drugs. It was likely that a relative, distressed by her condition, had administered them. The police were informed, but it was felt that there was insufficient evidence to proceed further

CHAPTER 12

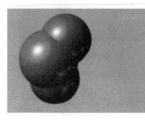

Disorders of Plasma Lipids and Lipoproteins

Lipids, 165
Lipoproteins, 166

Metabolism of plasma
lipoproteins, 167

Investigation of plasma lipid
abnormalities, 169

Lipids

Lipids act as energy stores (triglycerides) and as important structural components of cells (cholesterol and phospholipids). They also have specialized functions (e.g. as adrenal and sex hormones). The main lipids, being insoluble in water, are transported in plasma as particulate complexes with proteins, the *lipoproteins*.

From the clinical viewpoint, it is the strong relationship between plasma lipid levels and the incidence of ischaemic vascular disease, particularly of the coronary arteries, that is of major importance. In this chapter, we outline:
1 The *biochemistry* of the main body lipids.
2 The mechanisms for *lipid transport* in plasma.
3 The importance of lipids, and other factors, in the *pathogenesis of arterial disease*.
4 The role of plasma lipid measurements in *screening for heart disease* and in the *management of hyperlipidaemia*.

Cholesterol

This is a steroid that is present in the diet, but it is mainly synthesized in the liver and small intestine, the rate-limiting step being catalysed by β-*hydroxy-β-methylglutaryl-coenzyme A* (HMG-CoA) *reductase*. Cholesterol is a major component of cell membranes, and acts as the substrate for steroid hormone formation in the adrenals and the gonads. It is present in plasma mainly esterified with fatty acids. The body cannot break down the sterol nucleus, so

cholesterol is either excreted unchanged in bile or converted to bile acids and then excreted. Cholesterol and bile acids both undergo an enterohepatic circulation.

Triglycerides

These are fatty acid esters of glycerol, and are the main lipids in the diet. They are broken down in the small intestine to a mixture of monoglycerides, fatty acids and glycerol. These products are absorbed, and triglycerides are resynthesized from them in the mucosal cell. Most of these *exogenous* triglycerides pass into plasma as *chylomicrons* (see below).

Endogenous triglyceride synthesis occurs in the liver, from fatty acids and glycerol. The triglycerides synthesized in this way are transported as *very low density lipoproteins* (VLDL) (see below).

Fatty acids

These are mostly straight-chain monocarboxylic acids. They are mainly derived from dietary or tissue triglyceride, but the body can also synthesize most of them, apart from certain polyunsaturated (essential) fatty acids. Fatty acids act as an alternative or additional energy source to glucose.

Phospholipids

These have a structure similar to triglycerides, but a polar group (e.g. phosphorylcholine) replaces one of the three fatty acid components. The presence of both polar and nonpolar (fatty acid) groups gives the phospholipids their characteristic detergent properties. Phospholipids are mainly synthesized in the liver and small intestine; they are important constituents of cells, and are often present in cell membranes.

Lipoproteins (Table 12.1)

Cholesterol and its esters, triglycerides and phospholipids are all transported in plasma as lipoprotein particles. Fatty acids are transported bound to albumin.

Lipoprotein particles comprise a peripheral envelope, consisting mainly of phospholipids and free cholesterol (which have both water-soluble polar and lipid-soluble nonpolar groups) with some *apolipoproteins*, and a central nonpolar core (mostly triglyceride and esterified cholesterol). The molecules in the envelope are distributed in a single layer in such a way that the polar groups face out towards the surrounding plasma, while the nonpolar

groups face inwards towards the lipid core in which the insoluble lipids are carried. *Most lipoproteins are assembled in the liver or small intestine.* Five main types of lipoprotein particle can be recognized:

1 *Chylomicrons* are the principal form in which dietary triglycerides are carried to the tissues.

2 *Very low density lipoproteins (VLDL)* are triglyceride-rich particles that form the major route whereby endogenous triglycerides are carried to the tissues from the liver and, to a lesser extent, from the small intestine.

3 *Intermediate-density lipoproteins (IDL or 'VLDL remnants')* are particles formed by the removal of triglycerides from VLDL during the transition from VLDL to LDL.

4 *Low-density lipoproteins (LDL)* are cholesterol-rich particles, formed from IDL by the removal of more triglyceride and apolipoprotein.

5 *High-density lipoproteins* are of two main types, HDL_2 and HDL_3. They probably act as a means whereby cholesterol can be transported from peripheral cells to the liver, prior to excretion.

A sixth type of lipoprotein particle, *Lp(a),* is synthesized in the liver and has about the same

Table 12.1 Properties of the five main classes of lipoproteins.

LIPOPROTEINS

Property	Chylomicrons	VLDL	IDL	LDL	HDL
Physical properties					
Diameter (nm)	100–500	30–80	25–30	20–35	5–10
Density (kg/L)	<0.95	<1.006	1.006–1.019	1.019–1.063	>1.063
Electrophoresis	Stay at origin	Pre-β	β	β	α_1
Lipoprotein composition (approximate percentages)					
Triglyceride	90	65	35	10	5
Cholesterol	5	20	40	50	35
Phospholipid	5	10	15	20	35
Protein	1	5	10	20	25
*Apolipoprotein composition**	C, B, E, (A)	C, B, E, (A)	B, (C, E, A)	B	A, C, E, (B)

*The main apolipoprotein components are listed in descending order of amount (trace components in parentheses).

lipid composition as LDL *(see below)*. The physiological role of Lp(a) is not known, but it has been shown to compete with plasminogen for tissue plasminogen receptors.

The apolipoproteins

The protein components of the lipoproteins, the apolipoproteins, are a complex family of polypeptides that promote and control the lipid transport in plasma and uptake into tissues. They are separable into four main groups (apoA, B, C and E), some of which may be subdivided, and apo(a).

ApoA. These are synthesized in the liver and intestine. They are initially present in chylomicrons in lymph, but they rapidly transfer to HDL.

ApoB is present in plasma in two forms, $apoB_{100}$ and $apoB_{48}$. $ApoB_{100}$ is the protein component of LDL, and is also present in chylomicrons, VLDL and IDL. $ApoB_{48}$ (the N-terminal half of $apoB_{100}$) is only found in chylomicrons. $ApoB_{100}$ is recognized by specific receptors in peripheral tissues (see below).

ApoC. This family of three proteins (apoC-I, apoC-II and apoC-III) is synthesized in the liver and incorporated into HDL.

ApoE is synthesized in the liver, incorporated into HDL, and transferred in the circulation to chylomicrons and VLDL. There are three major isoforms (apoE2, apoE3 and apoE4) at a single genetic locus, giving rise to several genotypes (E3/3, E2/3, E2/4, etc.). ApoE is probably mainly involved in the hepatic uptake of chylomicron remnants and IDL; it binds to apoB receptors in the tissues.

Apo(a) is present in equimolar amounts to $apoB_{100}$ in Lp(a). It has a high carbohydrate content and has a similar amino acid sequence to plasminogen.

Enzymes involved in lipid transport

Four enzymes of relevance to clinical disorders need to be described:

1 *Lecithin cholesterol acyltransferase (LCAT)* transfers an acyl group (fatty acid residue) from lecithin to cholesterol, forming a cholesterol ester. In plasma, this reaction probably takes place exclusively on HDL, and may be stimulated by apoA-I.

2 *Lipoprotein lipase* is attached to tissue capillary endothelium and splits triglycerides, present in chylomicrons and VLDL, to glycerol and free fatty acids. Its activity increases after a meal, partly as a result of activation by apoC-II, present on the surface of triglyceride-bearing lipoproteins.

3 *Hepatic lipase* has an action similar to that of lipoprotein lipase.

4 *Mobilizing lipase*, present in adipose tissue cells, controls the release of fatty acids from adipose tissue into plasma. It is activated by catecholamines, growth hormone and glucocorticoids (e.g. cortisol), and inhibited by glucose and by insulin.

Metabolism of plasma lipoproteins

The above description of the lipoproteins and apolipoproteins is an oversimplification, and the following points should be emphasized:

1 Plasma lipids and apolipoproteins exist in a dynamic state. There is interchange of lipids both (a) between different lipoprotein particles and (b) with tissues.

2 There is considerable variation in the size and composition of individual lipoprotein particles within each lipoprotein class.

Chylomicron metabolism (Fig. 12.1)

Chylomicrons are formed in the intestinal mucosa after a fat-containing meal, and reach the systemic circulation via the thoracic duct. They then transfer apoA to HDL and acquire apoC and apoE from HDL. The apoC-II then activates lipoprotein lipase in the tissues, and triglycerides are progressively removed from the hydrophobic core of the chylomicrons. As the size of the particles decreases, the more hydrophilic surface components (apoC, unesterified cholesterol and phospholipid) transfer to HDL. The triglyceride-poor *chylomicron remnants* are taken up by the liver, where they are catabolized.

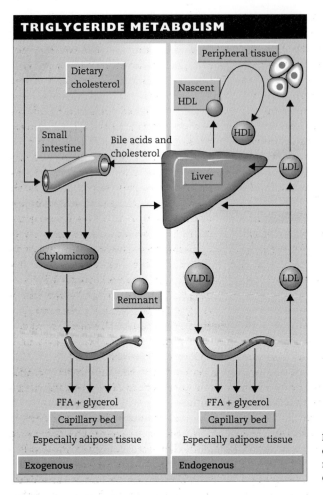

TRIGLYCERIDE METABOLISM

Fig. 12.1 Endogenous and exogenous triglyceride metabolism (see text for details).

VLDL and IDL metabolism (Fig. 12.1)

Most VLDL is secreted into plasma by the hepatocytes ('endogenous' VLDL), but some originates from the intestinal mucosa ('exogenous' VLDL). Hepatic synthesis is increased whenever there is increased hepatic triglyceride synthesis, e.g. when there is increased transport of fatty acids to the liver, or after a large carbohydrate-containing meal.

When first produced, VLDL consists mainly of triglycerides and some unesterified cholesterol, with apoB$_{100}$ and lesser amounts of apoE. ApoC-II is then acquired, mainly from HDL, and triglycerides are removed from the VLDL 'core' in a manner analogous to that for chy-

lomicrons. The residual particles are known as 'VLDL remnants', or IDL, which are either rapidly converted to LDL or removed from the circulation to the liver.

LDL metabolism

Probably all LDL arises from VLDL metabolism in man. The LDL particles are rich in cholesterol esters, probably derived from HDL; apoB$_{100}$ is the only apolipoprotein. LDL is removed from the circulation by two processes; one *regulated*, the other *unregulated*.

The *regulated mechanism* involves the binding of LDL to *specific apoB$_{100}$ receptors* present on the 'surface pits' of hepatocytes and other peripheral tissue cells. The entire LDL particle is incorporated into the cell by invagination of the cell membrane. Inside the cell, the particle fuses with lysosomes; apoB is then broken down and the cholesterol esters are hydrolysed, thereby making unesterified cholesterol available to the cell. The size of the intracellular cholesterol pool regulates:

1 The rate of cholesterol synthesis in the cell, through the effect of cholesterol on HMG-CoA reductase.

2 The number of LDL-apoB receptors on the cell surface.

The unregulated mechanism involves receptor-independent mechanisms of cholesterol uptake by cells; these are present particularly in macrophages. These mechanisms are brought into operation especially when plasma [cholesterol] is increased.

HDL metabolism

This heterogeneous group of particles (HDL_2, HDL_3, etc.) is formed in the liver and intestinal mucosa. The HDL particles then undergo fairly complex exchanges of lipid and protein with other plasma lipoproteins. However, the main point to note is that free cholesterol in tissues transfers to HDL in plasma. The cholesterol is then esterified by LCAT and transferred to LDL, which, in turn, is mainly taken up by the liver (see above). Thus, HDL forms the principal route whereby cholesterol can return from peripheral tissues to the liver.

Investigation of plasma lipid abnormalities

Most laboratories measure plasma [total cholesterol], [HDL cholesterol] and [triglycerides]. Further tests to characterize the lipoprotein abnormalities may be indicated in a few patients. The investigations are mainly of value in the investigation and management of ischaemic vascular disease.

Plasma total cholesterol

Plasma [cholesterol] is affected by both within-individual and between-individual factors. However, these tend to be long-term effects. Diet, for example recent meals, does not affect plasma [cholesterol] much in the short term. This means that random [cholesterol] can be measured to assess risk:

Diet. The amount and composition of dietary fat affect plasma [cholesterol]. In particular, those fats containing mainly polyunsaturated fatty acids, such as those in fish and vegetable oils, tend to lower plasma [cholesterol], whereas those fats containing mainly saturated fatty acids, such as animal fat and butter, tend to raise plasma [cholesterol]. Dietary fibre may have a small effect in lowering plasma [cholesterol]. The consumption of one to three units of alcohol per day causes a significant rise in plasma [HDL cholesterol]. Dietary cholesterol intake has relatively little effect on plasma [cholesterol].

Exercise. When regular, this tends to cause a rise in plasma [HDL cholesterol] and a small fall in plasma [total cholesterol].

Age. In developed countries, plasma [cholesterol] rises with age. This is probably related to diet.

Sex. In women, plasma [total cholesterol] is lower before the menopause, and plasma [HDL cholesterol] is higher. These differences disappear after the menopause.

Race. It is likely that the marked racial differences, with particularly high plasma [cholesterol] in north Europeans, are mainly due to dietary and environmental factors rather than genetic differences.

Numerous studies have shown that the incidence of ischaemic heart disease is directly correlated with plasma [cholesterol] (Fig. 12.2), even within the 'reference range'. There is no clear cut-off between values for normal risk and increased risk, although risk rises particularly rapidly above about 6.5 mmol/L. Because of this association, it is inappropriate to employ reference ranges for plasma [cholesterol] in the usual way, as these imply health without increased risk of disease. Instead, it seems more appropriate to define a desirable concentration (e.g. below 5 mmol/L).

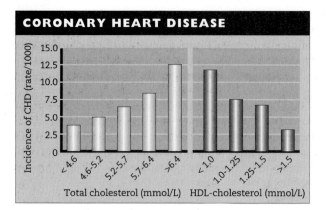

Fig. 12.2 The variation in incidence of coronary heart disease (CHD) with the plasma concentrations of cholesterol (histograms drawn from data in Martin *et al*, (1986) Serum cholesterol, blood pressure and mortality: implications from a cohort of 361, 662 men. *Lancet* ii, 933–6.) and HDL-cholesterol (histograms drawn from data in Castelli *et al*. (1986) Incidence of coronary heart disease and lipoprotein cholesterol levels. *Journal of the American Medical Association* **256**, 2835–8.).

Plasma [total cholesterol] is a rather unsatisfactory measurement, since it represents the sum of the various ways in which cholesterol is transported in plasma. In fact, whereas raised plasma [LDL-cholesterol] is associated with an *increased* risk of ischaemic heart disease, raised plasma [HDL-cholesterol] is associated with a *decreased* risk of ischaemic heart disease and seems to have a protective effect.

Plasma triglycerides
Plasma [triglycerides] also show variations with age and sex, but more especially with diet. There is, in addition, a very considerable within-individual variation, which makes interpretation of a single result difficult.

Specimen collection
It is very important to collect specimens for plasma lipid and lipoprotein studies under the appropriate, standardized conditions:

1 The patient should have been leading a normal life in terms of diet (including alcohol consumption) and exercise for at least the previous fortnight.

2 Blood specimens should be collected after an overnight fast of 10–14 hours, if triglyceride measurements are to be performed.

3 Venous stasis should be minimal.

Routine investigations
The following investigations should be requested initially in a patient suspected to be at risk of ischaemic heart disease or lipid disorder:

1 Plasma [cholesterol].

2 Plasma [fasting triglycerides].

3 Plasma [HDL-cholesterol], if plasma [cholesterol] is raised or if additional risk factors are present.

Measurement of plasma [HDL-cholesterol] helps to define the risk of ischaemic heart disease in patients with raised [total cholesterol]. It is also needed for the diagnosis of hyper-α-lipoproteinaemia.

Specialized investigations
A large number of specialized investigations, including ultracentrifugation, apolipoprotein and enzyme studies, lipoprotein electrophoresis, and molecular genetic studies may occasionally be helpful.

Cautionary note
Results of plasma lipid and lipoprotein investigations can be misleading, often showing hypertriglyceridaemia and sometimes reduced plasma [cholesterol], in specimens collected during or within a few weeks after a serious

illness (e.g. a myocardial infarction or a major operation). However, specimens collected within 24 h of a myocardial infarction may be used to determine the need for subsequent cholesterol-lowering treatment.

The primary hyperlipoproteinaemias
(Table 12.2)

The causes of hyperlipoproteinaemia are complex, and different disease mechanisms can give rise to similar lipid patterns. The approach adopted here will be primarily descriptive, based on the observed lipid abnormalities.

Increased plasma lipid concentrations may be due to:

1 Genetic factors.
2 Environmental factors.
3 A combination of the above.
4 Other diseases (secondary).

Primary hypercholesterolaemia

In about 95% of patients with primary hypercholesterolaemia, the abnormality is due to a combination of dietary factors and a number of so far unidentified genetic abnormalities in handling cholesterol.

In the minority of patients who have *familial hypercholesterolaemia*, there is a specific genetic defect in the production or nature of high-affinity tissue $apoB_{100}$ receptors (or in the

Table 12.2 The primary hyperlipoproteinaemias (genetic classification).

structure of the $apoB_{100}$ itself, so that it is not recognized by the normal receptor). Heterozygotes have about 50% of normal receptor activity, and homozygotes have no receptor activity. Many heterozygotes have *tendon xanthomas,* and over 50% will have symptoms of coronary artery disease by the fourth or fifth decade. In homozygotes, heart disease often presents in the second decade. Plasma [cholesterol] is usually raised to 8–15 mmol/L in heterozygotes, and is even higher in homozygotes.

Familial hypertriglyceridaemia

This group of conditions is associated with defects either in the production or in the catabolism of VLDL. Plasma [triglycerides] and [VLDL] are increased but, whereas plasma [cholesterol] is often also moderately increased, plasma [HDL] is often reduced. Patients have an increased risk of ischaemic heart disease.

In some patients, there is chylomicronaemia in addition to increased plasma [VLDL]. This pattern may be brought on by alcohol excess, and is also seen in diabetics. These patients may have eruptive xanthomas and attacks of acute pancreatitis.

Familial combined hyperlipidaemia

This disorder is difficult to classify, and the method of inheritance is unclear. Even in the same family, the gene does not always express

PRIMARY HYPERLIPOPROTEINAEMIAS			
	Concentrations in plasma		
Hyperlipoproteinaemia	Cholesterol	Triglycerides (fasting)	Lipoproteins mainly affected
Familial hypercholesterolaemia	↑↑	N (or ↑)	LDL
Familial hypertriglyceridaemia	↑ or N	↑↑	VLDL (and chylomicrons)
Familial combined hyperlipidaemia	↑ or N	↑ or N	LDL and/or VLDL
Remnant hyperlipoproteinaemia	↑	↑	IDL and chylomicron remnants
Lipoprotein lipase deficiency (or apoC-II deficiency)	↑ or N	↑↑	Chylomicrons and VLDL

itself in the same way, as there may be increased plasma [LDL] only, increased plasma [VLDL] only, or increases in both. The incidence of ischaemic heart disease is three to four times greater than in the general population.

Remnant hyperlipoproteinaemia
This is an uncommon disorder characterized clinically by cutaneous xanthomas and a high risk of premature ischaemic heart disease. In the plasma, there is an increase in cholesterol-rich but otherwise VLDL-like particles; these are probably IDL (i.e. 'VLDL remnants'). On electrophoresis, they give rise to a characteristic broad β-band. Both plasma [cholesterol] and [triglycerides] are increased; plasma [LDL] is decreased.

This disorder is probably due to a combination of factors. There is abnormal conversion of VLDL to LDL. This is usually associated with the apoE2/2 genotype. However, since as many as 1% of normal individuals have this genotype, whereas the incidence of remnant hyperlipoproteinaemia is only about 1 in 5000, an additional factor must be present.

Remnant hyperlipoproteinaemia responds well to treatment with fibric acid derivatives (e.g. gemfibrozil), so its recognition is important. Ultracentrifuge studies provide the definitive means of confirming the diagnosis.

Lipoprotein lipase deficiency
This is a rare autosomal recessive disorder causing hypertriglyceridaemia and chylomicronaemia. The incidence of ischaemic heart disease and acute pancreatitis is increased; eruptive xanthomas often occur. The primary defect is deficiency of either lipoprotein lipase or its activator, apoC-II.

Treatment involves restriction of normal dietary fat and replacement by means of triglycerides containing fatty acids of medium chain-length (C_8–C_{11}); these are less prone to lead to chylomicron formation.

Other inherited defects
Hyper-α-lipoproteinaemia is an inherited abnor-mality, giving rise to increased plasma [HDL] and mildly increased plasma [cholesterol]. Patients have a reduced incidence of ischaemic heart disease. The only importance of hyper-α-lipoproteinaemia is that treatment for the raised plasma [cholesterol] should not be given.

Secondary hyperlipidaemia
Probably less than 20% of cases of hyperlipidaemia are secondary to other disease. Patterns of abnormality tend to vary, even within a single disease; plasma [cholesterol] or [triglycerides], or both, may be affected.

Hypercholesterolaemia is often a marked feature of hypothyroidism and of the nephrotic syndrome; in these two disorders, there is increased plasma [LDL]. It also occurs in cholestatic jaundice, but in this condition there is an accumulation of abnormal discoid particles rich in phospholipid and unesterified cholesterol, and an additional abnormal lipoprotein – lipoprotein X – is detectable. Coronary artery disease tends to develop in those patients with long-standing secondary hyperlipidaemia

Hypertriglyceridaemia, secondary to other disease, is most commonly due to diabetes mellitus or to alcoholism. It may also occur in chronic renal disease and in patients on oestrogen therapy, including women taking oestrogen-containing oral contraceptives.

The effects of alcohol on plasma lipids are complex. Regular drinking of small amounts increases plasma [HDL] without affecting other lipoprotein particles. Some heavy drinkers develop hypertriglyceridaemia due to increased plasma [VLDL], possibly as a result of increased direction of fatty acid metabolism into triglyceride synthesis in the liver.

The hyperlipidaemia secondary to diabetes mellitus is also complex. Increased plasma [VLDL] is the usual finding, but plasma [LDL] is often increased also, whereas plasma [HDL] is reduced.

The primary hypolipoproteinaemias
Three rare familial diseases require brief mention. Their recognition has helped with

the understanding of normal lipoprotein metabolism.

Tangier disease is due to an increased rate of apoA-I catabolism. Only traces of HDL are detectable in plasma, and plasma [LDL cholesterol] is also reduced. Cholesterol esters accumulate in the lymphoreticular system, probably due to excessive phagocytosis of the abnormal chylomicrons and VLDL remnants that result from the apoA-I deficiency.

Abetalipoproteinaemia is associated with a complete absence of apoB. The lipoproteins that normally contain apoB in significant amounts (i.e. chylomicrons, VLDL, IDL and LDL) are *absent* from plasma. Plasma [cholesterol] and [triglycerides] are very low.

Hypobetalipoproteinaemia is due to decreased synthesis of apoB. Plasma [VLDL] and [LDL], although reduced, are not absent.

Secondary hypolipidaemia
Greatly reduced plasma [cholesterol] occurs whenever hepatic protein synthesis is depressed, as in protein-energy malnutrition (e.g. kwashiorkor in children), severe malabsorption, or some forms of chronic liver disease.

Hyperlipidaemia and arterial disease
The following associations are now clearly established:

1 Increased plasma [LDL cholesterol], and hence plasma [total cholesterol], is *positively* correlated with the incidence of ischaemic heart disease (Fig. 12.1).

2 Increased plasma [HDL cholesterol] is *negatively* correlated with the incidence of ischaemic heart disease. This is presumably explained by the role of HDL in transporting cholesterol from the peripheral tissues to the liver (Fig. 12.1).

3 Increased plasma [triglyceride] is *positively* correlated with the incidence of ischaemic heart disease, but the association is weaker than that with plasma [cholesterol].

4 Plasma [Lp(a)] is *positively* associated with the incidence of ischaemic heart disease, independently of other lipoprotein fractions. The

effect *may* be due to competition between Lp(a) and plasminogen for endothelial cell receptors, thereby inhibiting thrombolysis.

Plasma [cholesterol], hypertension and cigarette smoking are the major risk factors for ischaemic heart disease. It is essential to recognize that the separate effects of each risk factor are *multiplicative* rather than additive, so it is especially important to treat patients who have more than one risk factor.

Screening for hypercholesterolaemia
In populations with a high incidence of hypercholesterolaemia, the simplest and most cost-effective strategy for reducing the incidence of ischaemic heart disease is a widely based publicity campaign to reduce plasma [cholesterol] in the population at large, by encouraging an appropriate diet. An additional approach would be to *target* treatment to those at highest risk, identified by *screening* for raised plasma [cholesterol].

At present, the optimal screening strategy applied by the general practitioner might be to screen patients with a family history of hyperlipidaemia or early cardiovascular mortality, or with diabetes mellitus, ischaemic heart disease, or raised blood pressure — particularly if present in a smoker.

Screening strategies whereby members of the general public are encouraged, sometimes by commercial interests, to arrange for their own plasma cholesterol measurements to be performed (e.g. in supermarkets or other retail outlets) may be less satisfactory unless there are stringent safeguards (p. 2). These require the quality of the results to be monitored regularly and appropriate counselling about diet, the implications of the result, etc., to accompany every cholesterol result. Without this advice, the screening process is largely valueless, and may lead to inappropriate action or unwarranted anxiety on the part of the patient.

Treatment of hyperlipidaemia
It is possible to lower plasma [LDL cholesterol] by dietary or other means, but the most effective therapy, usually leading to reductions of

between 20% and 30%, is achieved by HMG-CoA reductase inhibitors ('statins'). It is this class of drug that has been used mainly in the clinical trials mentioned below.

Primary prevention. Large-scale clinical trials have now shown that cholesterol lowering (by an average 20%) in hyperlipidaemic men with [total cholesterol] over 6.5 mmol/L, *but with no clinical or ECG evidence of cardiovascular disease*, can reduce cardiovascular death and nonfatal myocardial infarction by about 30%.

Secondary prevention. In patients with previous myocardial infarction or with angina, trial results are even more conclusive. Cholesterol reduction by about 25% reduced all-cause mortality by 30% and cardiac events by over 40%.

Choice of therapy in individuals with raised [cholesterol] or with ischaemic heart disease is often not straightforward, and other risk factors, such as hypertension, smoking and lack of exercise, must be considered. In general, changes in lifestyle and diet should be tried first. However, those with ischaemic heart disease or those who have raised lipid levels and do not respond to these simpler measures should be considered for drug therapy, usually with statins.

KEY POINTS

1 The main lipids of clinical importance in plasma are cholesterol and triglyceride. These are insoluble in water and are transported in plasma as protein/lipid complexes known as lipoproteins.

2 The principal lipoproteins in plasma are chylomicrons, very low density lipoproteins (VLDL), low-density lipoproteins (LDL), and high-density lipoproteins (HDL).

3 Increased plasma [cholesterol] and [triglyceride], whether primary or secondary to other diseases such as diabetes, are associated with an increased risk of arterial disease,

particularly coronary atheroma leading to myocardial infarction.

4 It has recently been shown, both in asymptomatic individuals and those with a previous history of ischaemic heart disease, that reduction of raised plasma [cholesterol] leads to a reduced incidence of heart disease in those treated.

5 Effective, but rather expensive, treatments for the above groups of patients are now available. Appropriate strategies for screening have been developed to balance health benefit against cost.

CHAPTER 13

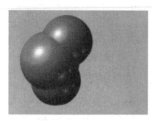

Disorders of Iron and Porphyrin Metabolism

Iron metabolism, 175
  Dietary iron and iron
    absorption, 175
  Iron transport, storage and
    utilization, 177
  Iron excretion and sources of
    loss, 177

Laboratory assessment of
  iron status, 177
Iron deficiency, 179
Iron overload, 179
Iron poisoning, 180

Porphyrin metabolism, 180
  Chemical investigation of
    the porphyrias, 181
  Abnormal derivatives of
    haemoglobin, 183

Iron is an essential element present mainly in the porphyrin complex, haem, and in iron storage proteins, ferritin and haemosiderin. *Iron-deficiency anaemia* is a serious global problem. There are also clinical problems with *acute iron overdose*, since free iron is toxic, and with *chronic iron overload*, which is associated with organ damage, particularly to the liver.

Haem, which is present in haemoglobin, myoglobin and cytochromes, is formed by insertion of ferrous iron, Fe^{2+}, into protoporphyrin (Fig. 13.1). The porphyrins are synthesized in the body by a fairly complex chain of reactions. Clinical disorders of porphyrin metabolism — the porphyrias — are relatively rare, but can arise from inherited or acquired abnormalities of this pathway.

In this chapter, we discuss iron metabolism and its disorders and, separately, the porphyrias and lead poisoning.

Iron metabolism

The adult human possesses about 70 mmol (4 g) of iron. Iron balance is regulated by alterations in the intestinal absorption of iron. There is only a limited capacity to increase or decrease the rate of loss of iron.

Dietary iron and iron absorption
(Fig. 13.2)

The normal intake of iron is about 0.2–0.4 mmol/day (10–20 mg/day). Good sources are liver, fish and meat. Normally, about 5–10% of dietary iron is absorbed by an active transport process. Most absorption occurs in the duodenum. The rate of absorption is controlled by physiological factors:

State of iron stores in the body. Absorption is increased in iron deficiency, and decreased when there is iron overload. The mechanism is unclear.

Rate of erythropoiesis. When this rate is increased, absorption may be increased even though the iron stores are adequate or overloaded.

The rate of absorption is also influenced by the contents of the diet and by the nature of gastrointestinal secretions, as follows:

Contents of diet. Substances that form soluble complexes with iron (e.g. ascorbic acid) facilitate absorption. Substances that form insoluble complexes (e.g. phytate) inhibit absorption.

The chemical state of the iron. Iron in the diet does not usually become available for absorption unless released during digestion. This depends, at least partly, on gastric acid

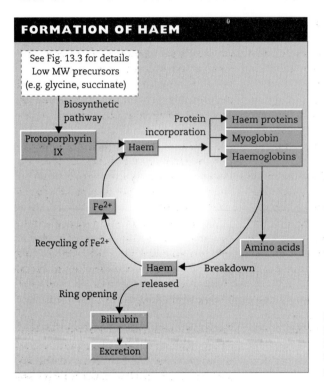

Fig. 13.1 Schematic diagram illustrating the formation of haem, its incorporation into haem proteins and subsequent metabolism to bilirubin.

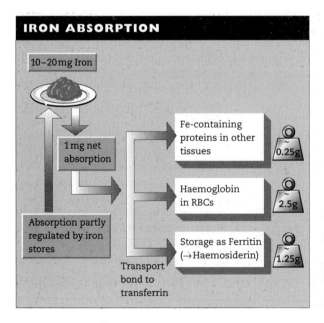

Fig. 13.2 Summary of the absorption, transport and utilization of iron. Total body iron stores (g) for the main iron-containing proteins are shown on the right side of the figure.

production; Fe^{2+} is more readily absorbed than Fe^{3+}, and the presence of H^+ helps to keep iron in the Fe^{2+} form. Iron in haem (in meat products) can be absorbed while still contained in the haem molecule.

Iron transport, storage and utilization

After being taken up by the intestinal mucosa, iron is either (i) incorporated into ferritin and retained by the mucosal cells, or (ii) transported across the mucosal cells directly to the plasma, where it is carried mainly combined with *transferrin*. Iron retained by mucosal cells is lost from the body when the cells are sloughed. Mucosal cell retention is influenced by the body's iron status, being reduced in iron depletion and increased in states of iron overload.

Binding sites on transferrin are normally about 30–50% saturated; the total iron circulating bound to transferrin is normally about 50–70 μmol (3–4 mg).

Table 13.1 Reference ranges for iron status.

Iron in plasma is taken up by cells and either incorporated into haem or stored as ferritin (or haemosiderin, probably formed by condensation of several molecules of ferritin).

Iron released by the breakdown of Hb, at the end of the erythrocyte's life, is normally efficiently conserved and later reused.

Iron excretion and sources of loss

Iron excreted in the faeces is principally *exogenous*, i.e. dietary iron that has not been absorbed by the mucosal cells and transported into the circulation.

In males, there is an average loss of *endogenous* iron of about 20 μmol/day (1 mg/day) in cells desquamated from the skin and the intestinal mucosa. Females may have additional losses due to menstruation or pregnancy. Urine contains negligible amounts of iron.

Laboratory assessment of iron status

This is necessary in the investigation of iron deficiency states and iron overload. The following tests are used (for reference ranges, see Table 13.1).

IRON STATUS

	Iron (μmol/L)	Ferritin (μg/L)	TIBC (μmol/L)	TIBC saturation (%)
Reference ranges				
Males	14–32	15–350*	45–72	30–50
Females	10–28	8–300*	45–72	30–50
Physiological changes				
Premenstrual	↓	N	N	↓
Steroid contraceptives	↑	N	↑	N
Pregnancy	Variable†	↓	↑	↓
Disease states				
Iron deficiency	↓	↓	↑	<30
Iron overload	↑	↑	N or ↓	up to 100
Infections, neoplasms	↓	↑ or N	↓	N
Hypoplastic anaemia	↑	↑ or N	N or ↓	>40

N, Normal; ↑, increased; ↓, decreased
*A plasma [ferritin] below 20 μg/L suggests that the body's iron stores are depleted.
† See p. 178.

Plasma iron

This is of limited diagnostic value, since levels fluctuate widely in health. Much of this variation appears to be random, but some specific causes can be recognized:
- *Diurnal variation*, with higher values in the morning.
- *Menstrual cycle*, with low values just before and during the menstrual period.
- *Oral contraceptives*, which cause increased plasma [iron].
- *Pregnancy*, which tends to cause increased plasma [iron]. However, it is often accompanied by iron deficiency so that plasma [iron] falls.

Measurements of plasma [iron] do *not* provide an adequate index of iron status. Although plasma [iron] is low in iron deficiency and is raised in iron overload, these changes occur relatively late when iron stores have already become either completely depleted or seriously overloaded. In addition, plasma [iron] also alters in conditions not associated with changes in iron stores. Acute infections or trauma precipitate a rapid fall in plasma [iron]. Chronic inflammatory disorders (e.g. rheumatoid arthritis) and malignant diseases are also associated with low levels.

Plasma [iron] determination is only required for diagnostic purposes for a few conditions, e.g. in suspected cases of acute iron poisoning and in the assessment of individuals with an increased risk of haemochromatosis.

Plasma ferritin

Plasma [ferritin] is closely related to body iron stores, whether these are decreased, normal or increased, whereas plasma [iron] only becomes abnormal in the presence of gross abnormalities of iron storage. A low, or low normal, plasma [ferritin] indicates the presence of depleted iron stores. Ferritin is one of the acute-phase reactants (p. 88) and, as such, may increase in infections or other acute disorders; in these patients, ferritin measurements should be repeated after recovery from the acute stress.

Increased plasma [ferritin] is found in iron overload, irrespective of the cause, and in many patients with liver disease or cancer. A normal plasma [ferritin] virtually excludes untreated iron overload.

Determination of plasma [ferritin] currently provides the most useful measure of iron status widely available on a routine basis.

Plasma transferrin, total iron-binding capacity (TIBC) and iron saturation

Normally, nearly all the iron-binding capacity is due to transferrin, and about 40 % of its binding sites are occupied by iron. Transferrin has a much longer half-life in plasma than iron, and plasma [transferrin] shows fewer short-term fluctuations. Transferrin levels fall in protein-energy malnutrition, during the acute-phase response, with infections, neoplastic disease and chronic liver disease. Synthesis increases in iron deficiency.

[Transferrin] can be measured directly, but can also be measured indirectly as the ability of plasma protein (largely transferrin) to bind iron, the so-called *total iron-binding capacity* of plasma (TIBC). The ratio of plasma [iron] to [transferrin] (or TIBC) then determines the transferrin (or TIBC) saturation.

In iron-deficiency anaemia, the low serum [iron] is typically associated with an increase in transferrin concentration (and TIBC). This leads to a low saturation of transferrin (and TIBC) with iron. Conversely, in iron overload, serum [iron] is high and transferrin is normal or low, i.e. high percentage saturation of TIBC (Table 13.1). This effect is particularly marked in haemochromatosis, in which saturation of the TIBC usually rises above 60 % fairly early in the disorder.

As with plasma [iron], there is little place for determining plasma [transferrin] or TIBC as a routine measure of iron status. However, in the detection of early or latent haemochromatosis, plasma TIBC saturation should be measured. Also, in patients being treated with erythropoietin for the anaemia of chronic renal failure, the percentage saturation of TIBC is a better index of available iron than plasma [ferritin], and it is also a better guide to the need to give iron treatment.

The plasma transferrin (or TIBC) is also helpful in determining the significance of very high plasma [ferritin] in patients with disordered liver function of unknown cause, in whom the differential diagnosis may be between haemochromatosis and malignancy. A high plasma [ferritin] in the absence of an increased percentage saturation of TIBC indicates that cancer is more likely to be the diagnosis.

Iron deficiency (Table 13.2)

Worldwide, this is the commonest single nutrient deficiency. The main causes are deficient intake (including reduced bioavailability from dietary fibre, phytates, etc.), impaired absorption (e.g. intestinal malabsorptive disease, abdominal surgery) and excessive loss (e.g. menstrual, gastrointestinal bleeding). Tests for the presence of occult blood in faeces (p. 299) should be performed if no source of blood loss is apparent.

In patients who develop iron deficiency,
1 plasma [ferritin] falls, then
2 plasma [transferrin] and TIBC increase, after which:

3 plasma [iron] falls, and finally
4 anaemia becomes evident.

A microcytic, hypochromic anaemia is characteristic, and storage iron is absent from macrophages in the bone-marrow aspirate. In general, plasma [ferritin] is the best diagnostic test for iron deficiency (renal failure is one of the few exceptions, see above).

Iron overload (Table 13.2)

This is much less common than iron deficiency. Diagnosis is not usually difficult once the possibility has been considered. Increased plasma [iron] with normal [transferrin] (or TIBC) often lead to 100% saturation of transferrin (or TIBC). Plasma [ferritin] is increased, often to more than 1000 µg/L. More common causes are:

1 Increased intake and absorption.

(a) Acute overdose, mainly occurring in children, may cause severe or even fatal symptoms, due to the toxic effects of free iron in plasma (see below).

(b) Chronic overload occurs when the diet contains excess absorbable iron (e.g. acid-containing food cooked in iron pots). Iron deposits form, e.g. in liver causing hepatic fibrosis, and in myocardium causing myocardial damage.

Table 13.2 Causes of iron deficiency and excess.

IRON DEFICIENCY AND OVERLOAD	
Iron deficiency	**Iron overload**
Decreased intake	Excessive intake
Poor diet	Over-supplementation with iron tablets
Prolonged weaning (milk: poor iron source)	Repeated blood transfusions
Malabsorption	Iron utensils (esp. with acid foodstuffs)
Increased requirements (in the presence of inadequate intake)	
Adolescence	
Pregnancy	
Menstruating females	
Excessive iron losses	Excessive absorption
Menorrhagia	Haemochromatosis
Gastrointestinal losses	
Genito-urinary losses	
Excessive blood donations	

2 Parenteral administration of iron, including repeated blood transfusions.
3 Idiopathic (genetic) haemochromatosis.

Genetic (primary) haemochromatosis

This autosomal recessive disorder, evident in homozygotes, is probably due to an unregulated increase in the intestinal absorption of dietary iron. At least 90% of affected individuals are male, suggesting that iron losses in menstruation and pregnancy may protect females. Excessive iron deposits build up as haemosiderin in the liver, leading to a macronodular cirrhosis in untreated individuals. Fibrotic damage to the pancreas (with diabetes mellitus) and heart involvement are also described. Other clinical features include skin pigmentation ('bronzed diabetes'), endocrine organ involvement (testicular atrophy) and arthritis with chondrocalcinosis.

Genetic haemochromatosis can be detected at the preclinical stage in affected members of a family in which an index case has occurred. The haemochromatosis gene is closely linked to the genes that determine human leucocyte antigens (HLA). In families at risk, apparently unaffected members with a susceptible HLA genotype should have regular (e.g. twice-yearly) measurements of plasma [iron], [ferritin] and TIBC. The first abnormalities to appear in plasma are increased [ferritin] and percentage saturation of TIBC; if either of these becomes abnormal, liver biopsy is indicated. Case-finding for affected relatives is important, since treatment by phlebotomy can prevent the disease from progressing.

Iron poisoning

This is potentially life-threatening, particularly in children. Early clinical symptoms, which include epigastric pain, nausea and vomiting, often with haematemesis, may settle but be followed later by acute encephalopathy and circulatory failure. Acute liver and renal failure may also develop. Treatment involves giving desferrioxamine, an iron-chelating agent, which binds the iron in plasma, and the resulting complex is excreted in urine.

Serum iron values >90 μmol/L require treatment. An immediate intramuscular injection of desferrioxamine is followed by gastric lavage, leaving desferrioxamine in the stomach.

Porphyrin metabolism

Porphyrins are tetrapyrroles, some of which are intermediates in the formation of haem. Haem itself is formed when Fe^{2+} combines with protoporphyrin IX. Most cells can synthesize haem, but bone marrow and liver cells are the most active. Inherited or acquired defects in the enzymes that are involved in protoporphyrin IX formation can lead to overproduction of pathway intermediates, with different clinical consequences. These conditions, which are relatively rare, are collectively known as the porphyrias. The biosynthetic pathway for haem synthesis is summarized in Figure 13.3.

Most of the porphyrias are at least partly genetically determined. Different stages in haem synthesis are affected in each disease, and many different symptoms may be present. Excessive porphyrin production occurs either in bone marrow (erythropoietic porphyrias) or liver (hepatic porphyrias).

Erythropoietic porphyrias (Table 13.3)

The erythropoietic porphyrias are very rare disorders characterized by an increase in red-cell porphyrins. As well as the congenital diseases, there are some acquired disorders in which erythrocyte [porphyrins] are increased, such as lead poisoning (p. 182) and iron deficiency. Over 90% of red-cell porphyrin is normally present as zinc protoporphyrin.

Accumulation of porphyrins in the skin leads to photosensitivity. The symptom is explained by the strong absorption of light of 400 nm wavelength by porphyrins present in the upper epidermis, which causes the porphyrin molecule to become activated. It is speculated that the consequent release of free radicals may cause local lysosomal damage and release of lysosomal enzymes. Unlike the hepatic por-

SYNTHESIS OF HAEM

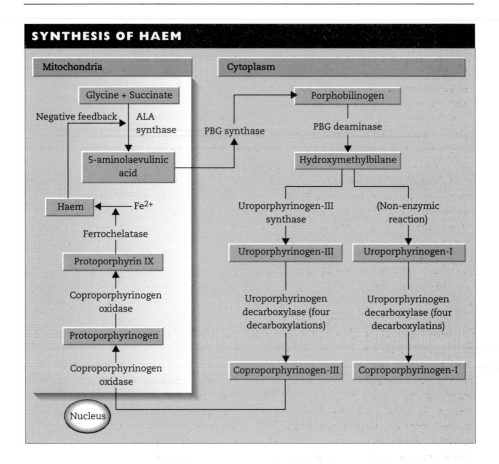

Fig. 13.3 The intracellular distribution of the enzymatic steps in the synthesis of haem. In the presence of uroporphyrinogen-III synthase, the formation of porphyrins from PBG (via hydroxymethylbilane, an unstable intermediate) is mainly directed along the series III pathway and thence onwards towards haem.

phyrias, acute abdominal symptoms do not occur.

Hepatic porphyrias (Table 13.3)

Most of the hepatic porphyrias present as acute disorders, with symptoms that include acute abdominal pain and vomiting, peripheral neuropathy and mental disturbance. Red-cell porphyrins are not increased, but skin sensitivity to sunlight may be present in some types. In acute intermittent porphyria, drugs such as barbiturates, oral contraceptives and alcohol may precipitate an acute attack. Acute abdominal and neurological symptoms tend to occur in those porphyrias in which there is overproduction of aminolaevulinic acid (ALA) and porphobilinogen (PBG), both of which probably have direct neurotoxic effects (Fig. 13.3).

Chemical investigation of the porphyrias

Only about 10–20% of patients with the enzyme defects of the hereditary porphyrias ever develop symptoms. Because of the protean manifestations of the porphyrias, the diagnosis is likely to be suspected much more often than it is present. The presence or absence of porphyria can be diagnosed by relatively simple screening tests in most laboratories. The complex tests necessary to fully

THE PORPHYRIAS

Type of porphyria	ALA in urine	PBG in urine	Porphyrins in urine	Porphyrins in faeces	Porphyrins in red cells
Hepatic porphyrias (erythrocyte porphyrins normal)					
Acute intermittent porphyria	↑ or N	↑↑↑	Polymers of PBG	No	No
Variegate porphyria	↑ or N	↑↑	Copro III, PBG polymers	Copro III, Proto IX, and others	No
Hereditary copro-porphyria	(↑) or N	↑↑	Copro III, PBG polymers	Copro III	No
Porphyria cutanea tarda	No	No	Uro I & III and others	Yes	No
Erythrocyte porphyrins increased					
Congenital erythrocytic porphyria			Uro I & copro I		Copro I, Proto IX, Zn proto
Protoporphyria			Variable	Proto IX	Proto IX
Lead poisoning	↑↑	↑ or N	Copro III		Zn proto

ALA: 5-aminolaevulinic acid; copro: coproporphyrin; uro: uroporphyrin; PBG: porphobilinogen.

Table 13.3 Chemical investigations in the porphyrias.

investigate established cases should be performed in specialist laboratories.

The screening tests available require fresh samples (some porphyrins are unstable), and include qualitative and quantitative tests for ALA and PBG (which are increased in the acute porphyrias), total urinary and faecal porphyrins and whole blood [total porphyrins].

Lead poisoning

After absorption from the lungs or intestine, lead is carried in the blood mainly on the surface of red cells, and is usually stored in bone. Its main toxic effects are peripheral neuropathy, abdominal pain, anaemia and encephalopathy. Three types of diagnostic and public health problems need to be considered:

Patients with symptoms or signs that may be explained by a diagnosis of lead poisoning. If lead poisoning is present, blood [lead] will be markedly raised.

Occupational hazard, where healthy workers may be exposed to increased risk of poisoning. Screening those at risk by sensitive tests is required.

Exposure to lead in the general population, e.g. lead in water, food, petrol, etc.

Lead inhibits many enzyme systems, but most of its effects can be attributed to inhibition of several stages of porphyrin synthesis, including PBG synthase activity (Fig. 13.3). The latter effect leads to accumulation and increased urinary excretion of precursor metabolite, ALA. Erythrocyte [zinc protoporphyrin] is also increased.

The following tests may be useful when investigating the possibility of lead poisoning:

1 Tests demonstrating the presence of excess lead:

(a) Blood [lead].

(b) Chelatable lead excretion in urine after giving ethylenediamine tetraacetic acid (EDTA), calcium salt.

2 Tests demonstrating the toxic effects of lead (Table 13.4).

Blood [lead] has several drawbacks as the sole measure of either lead poisoning or over-exposure. Although it correlates significantly with other biological indices of lead poisoning, there are variations in individual susceptibility to a given blood [lead]. Partly for this reason, it has proved difficult to establish 'acceptable' blood lead levels in a healthy population. Also, the measurement of blood [lead] is technically demanding.

Chelatable lead excretion is a measure of the amount of lead excreted in the 24-hour period after a 60-minute intravenous infusion of 1 g calcium EDTA. The test is an excellent index of lead overexposure, but is rather tedious and is unsuitable for screening purposes.

Table 13.4 Chemical investigation of suspected lead poisoning.

Abnormal derivatives of haemoglobin (Table 13.5)

These all reduce the oxygen-carrying capacity of the blood. The abnormal derivatives of Hb can all be identified by means of their characteristic absorption spectra, and it is possible to measure the various derivatives quantitatively if they are present in sufficient amounts.

Methaemoglobin

This is oxidized haemoglobin (Hb), the Fe^{2+} normally present in haem being replaced by Fe^{3+}; the ability to act as an O_2 carrier is lost. The normal erythrocyte contains small amounts of methaemoglobin, formed by spontaneous oxidation of Hb.

Methaemoglobin is normally reconverted to Hb by reducing systems in the red cells, the most important of which is NADH-methaemoglobin reductase.

Excess methaemoglobin may be present in

LEAD POISONING

Test	Finding	Comment
Blood lead	Increased	Screening. Raised levels require follow-up tests.
Erythrocyte PBG synthase activity	Decreased	Sensitive, but interpretation complicated by genetic differences in activity
Urinary ALA excretion	Increased	Sensitive, but requires timed urine.
Erythrocyte [Zn protoporphyrin]	Increased	Avoids timed urine, so preferred in young children.

ABNORMAL HAEMOGLOBINS

Haemoglobin derivative	Description
Methaemoglobin	Fe^{3+} replaces Fe^{2+}. Genetic or acquired causes.
Haematin	Protoporphyrin containing Fe^{3+}, released from methaemoglobin. May combine with albumin to form methaemalbumin.
Sulphaemoglobin	Produced by oxidation of Hb in presence of SH-containing compounds. Often present with methaemoglobin.
Carboxyhaemoglobin	Very stable compound where CO replaces O_2 in oxyhaemoglobin. Unable to transport O_2.

Table 13.5 Abnormal forms of haemoglobin.

the blood because of increased production or diminished ability to convert it back to Hb. If there is more than 20 g/L of methaemoglobin, cyanosis develops.

Both genetically determined and acquired conditions can cause methaemoglobinaemia; the acquired group is much the commoner. Haemolysis sometimes occurs in cases of methaemoglobinaemia, and methaemoglobin then appears in the urine, giving it a brownish colour.

Genetic causes of methaemoglobinaemia include, firstly, a group of haemoglobinopathies, collectively termed haemoglobin M, where an amino acid substitution stabilizes haemoglobin in the Fe^{3+} form. A second group has a deficiency in the enzyme system that reduces methaemoglobin. Reducing agents (such as ascorbic acid or methylene blue) work effectively in the second group, but are ineffective in the first group.

Acquired methaemoglobinaemia usually arises following the ingestion of large amounts of drugs, e.g. phenacetin, the sulphonamides, excess of nitrites, or certain oxidizing agents present in the diet. Treatment with reducing agents is also effective in reversing acquired methaemoglobinaemia.

Sulphaemoglobin

This is formed when Hb is acted on by the same substances as those that cause acquired methaemoglobinaemia, if they act in the presence of sulphur-containing compounds such as hydrogen sulphide that may arise from bacterial action in the intestine. Sulphaemoglobin and methaemoglobin are often present at the same time in these patients.

Sulphaemoglobin cannot act as an O_2 carrier, nor can it be converted back to Hb.

Because of its spectroscopic characteristics, patients with even a mild degree of sulphaemoglobinaemia are cyanosed.

Carboxyhaemoglobin (COHb)

Carbon monoxide is a colourless, odourless gas that avidly combines with the haem moiety in haemoglobin and cytochrome enzymes. It combines at the same position in the Hb molecule as O_2, but with an affinity about 200 times greater than oxygen. As a result, even small quantities of CO in the inspired air cause the formation of relatively large amounts of COHb, with a corresponding reduction in the O_2-carrying capacity of the blood. This is due not only to the blocking effect of CO on O_2-binding sites, but also to a shift to the left of the oxygen dissociation curve (Fig. 3.4) that occurs even when only one of the four O_2-binding sites on Hb is occupied by CO. As little as 1% CO in the inspired air can be fatal in minutes.

In general, non-smokers have COHb values of less than 1%, except in some city dwellers. However, values of as much as 10% occur in heavy smokers. Acute poisoning (smoke inhalation, faulty heaters or flues, car exhaust fumes, attempted suicides) gives rise to nonspecific symptoms of lethargy, headache, nausea that may proceed to confusion, agitation and deep coma. When poisoning is suspected, COHb levels can be measured in the laboratory. Urgent treatment with 100% oxygen and, where necessary, cardiorespiratory resuscitation and treatment of cerebral oedema should be instituted. Hyperbaric oxygen is particularly helpful in the more serious cases, especially when COHb levels are 30% or more (concentrations above 40% usually result in unconsciousness, and may be fatal).

KEY POINTS

1 About 1 mg of dietary iron is absorbed daily. This is transported in blood in transferrin, and stored mainly as ferritin and haemosiderin.

2 Most of the body iron is present in haem.

3 The best routine measure of iron stores is plasma [ferritin].

4 Plasma [iron] is of limited diagnostic value on its own, except in acute poisoning.

5 Iron-deficiency anaemia is common and may be due to inadequate dietary iron, malabsorption or excessive blood losses.

6 Iron overload is rarer. It may be due to excessive iron intake or administration, or a genetically determined increase in iron absorption (haemochromatosis).

7 Hepatic porphyrias are associated with an acute presentation and the appearance of the porphyrin precursors aminolaevulinic acid (ALA) and porphobilinogen (PBG) in the urine. Specific diagnosis depends on analysis of the types of porphyrin excreted to excess in urine and faeces.

8 Lead inhibits several stages in porphyrin synthesis. In suspected lead poisoning, blood lead and other specialist tests may be of value.

9 Abnormal forms of the major haem protein, haemoglobin, may interfere with blood O_2 transport.

CHAPTER 14

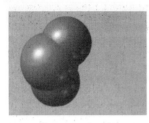

Disorders of Purine Metabolism

Purine metabolism, 186
Plasma urate, 186
   Hyperuricaemia, 186
Primary gout, 189

Diagnosis of primary gout, 189
Treatment of primary gout, 189

HGPRT deficiency, 190
Secondary gout, 190

The clinical importance of purines rests largely on the disorders characterized by increased plasma [urate]. Urate accumulation may arise either from increased intake of urate or its precursors, from increased production in the body, or from defects in renal elimination. The main manifestations are due either to formation of urate crystals in joints, causing *gout*, or deposition of urate crystals in the renal tract, causing *renal calculi*.

Purine metabolism

The purine bases, adenine and guanine, and corresponding nucleosides (purine base – ribose, e.g. adenosine) and nucleotides (nucleoside – phosphate, e.g. adenosine 5'-monophosphate, AMP) are present in nucleic acids and in other metabolically important compounds (e.g. adenosine triphosphate, ATP). Partly obtained from the diet, purines are also synthesized *in vivo* (Fig. 14.1), regulation probably occurring through the reaction catalysed by 5-phosphoribosyl-1-pyrophosphate (PRPP)-amidotransferase.

Nucleic acids are broken down to nucleotides, nucleosides and bases (mainly hypoxanthine and guanine), which in turn are partly converted to uric acid and excreted as urate. However, a 'salvage pathway' whereby purine bases are partly reused for nucleotide synthesis, by reactions catalysed by hypoxan-

thine phosphoribosyltransferase (HGPRT) and adenine phosphoribosyltransferase (APRT), is also important (Fig. 14.1). These 'salvaged' nucleotides can be used for nucleic acid synthesis.

About 70% of urate excretion normally occurs through the kidney, and the rest through the intestine; output via the intestine is increased in renal disease.

Plasma urate

Plasma [urate] varies with the following physiological factors:

1 *Sex*. Plasma [urate] reference range is higher in males (0.12–0.42 mmol/L) than females (0.12–0.36 mmol/L).

2 *Obesity*. Plasma [urate] tends to be higher in the obese.

3 *Social class*. The more affluent social classes tend to have a higher plasma [urate].

4 *Diet*. Plasma [urate] rises in individuals taking a high-protein diet, i.e. a diet that is also rich in nucleic acids, and in those with a high alcohol consumption.

5 *Genetic factors* are important.

Hyperuricaemia (Table 14.1)

Solutions of monosodium urate become supersaturated when the concentration exceeds 0.42 mmol/L. However, the relationship between the presence and severity of

SYNTHESIS OF IMP, AMP AND GMP

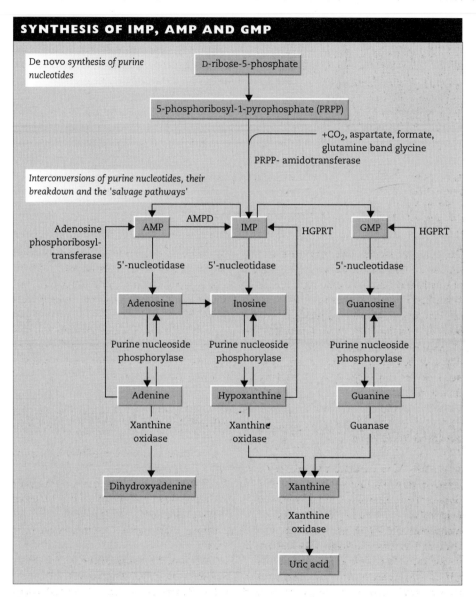

Fig. 14.1 The upper part of this figure is a simplified representation of the synthetic pathway leading to the *de novo* synthesis of inosinic acid (IMP), a purine nucleotide that can then be converted to adenylic acid (AMP) and guanylic acid (GMP) by complex reactions, indicated by the upper pair of curved arrows.

The lower part of the figure shows the breakdown of AMP, IMP and GMP to the corresponding purines, and their further metabolism to uric acid (the main end-product of purine metabolism) and dihydroxyadenine. It also shows, with another set of curved arrows, the salvage pathways for re-forming AMP, IMP and GMP from their corresponding purine bases, by reactions catalysed by hypoxanthine-guanine phosphoribosyltransferase (HGPRT) and by adenine phosphoribosyltransferase.

HYPERURICAEMIA

Category	Primary	Secondary
Overproduction of urate Increased de novo purine synthesis	Specific enzymic defects (e.g. PRPP-synthase or PRPP-amidotransferase overactivity) Idiopathic	Specific enzymic defects (e.g. complete HGPRT deficiency in the Lesch–Nyhan syndrome, glucose-6-phosphatase deficiency in von Gierke's disease
Increased turnover of pre-formed purines Myeloproliferative disorders		Polycythaemia rubra vera
Lymphoproliferative disorders		Lymphoma, lymphocytic leukaemia, paraproteinaemias (e.g. myeloma)
Miscellaneous		Carcinomatosis, secondary polycythaemia, exfoliative dermatoses
Defective elimination of urate	Idiopathic	Volume depletion Renal: chronic renal failure, lead nephropathy Drugs: diuretics, low-dose salicylates Metabolic acidosis: lactic acidosis, ketoacidosis

Table 14.1 Examples of causes of hyperuricaemia.

hyperuricaemia and the development or arthritis or renal calculi is more complex than simple considerations of solubility might suggest.

Increased plasma [urate] may be due to either overproduction or defective elimination of urate.

Overproduction of urate

The following metabolic causes may occur:

1 Increased activity of the rate-limiting enzyme in de novo nucleotide synthesis, PRPP-amidotransferase, or increased concentration of its substrate, PRPP.

2 Increased activity of those pathways of nucleotide metabolism that lead to urate formation, as compared to those that lead to the formation of nucleic acids.

3 Increased rate of nucleic acid breakdown, as occurs whenever there is an increased rate of cell turnover or destruction.

4 Decreased activity of the 'salvage pathway' due to absence or deficiency of HGPRT.

5 Increased activity of xanthine oxidase. When this occurs, it is probably a secondary rather than a primary effect.

Defective elimination of urate

Renal excretion of urate is a complex process. Except for a small fraction bound to plasma proteins, urate is completely filtered at the glomerulus; this is then mostly reabsorbed in the proximal tubule. In the distal tubule, there is both active secretion and postsecretory reabsorption at a more distal site. These processes can all be affected by disease or drugs:

1 Glomerular filtration rate. When the GFR becomes reduced for any reason (p. 51), urate retention occurs.

2 Distal tubular secretion. Lactic acid, 3-

hydroxybutyric acid and some drugs (e.g. thiazide diuretics) compete with urate for this excretory pathway. Any condition giving rise to lactic acidosis or ketosis tends to be associated with hyperuricaemia.

3 *Distal tubular reabsorption.* Most uricosuric drugs (e.g. probenecid) act by decreasing tubular reabsorption of urate.

Salicylates and many other uricosuric agents have paradoxical and dose-dependent effects on the renal tubular handling of urate. With *low* doses, salicylates mainly reduce distal tubular secretion, tending to cause hyperuricaemia. With *high* doses of salicylates, however, reduction of tubular reabsorption is the dominant effect, and there is increased urate excretion.

Primary gout

This is characterized by recurrent attacks of mono-articular arthritis, usually in men. In patients with hyperuricaemia, it is likely that supersaturation of urate (above 0.42 mmol/L) causes crystals to accumulate in connective tissues (e.g. joints) over a long period prior to symptoms developing.

The acute symptoms of gout are probably due to trauma or local metabolic changes causing crystals of monosodium urate to shed into the joint cavity. The crystals are phagocytosed by leucocytes and macrophages and cause damage to membranes within the leucocytes. Lysosomal contents and other mediators of the acute inflammatory response (cytokines, prostaglandins, free radicals, etc.) are then released, causing both the systemic and the local acute manifestations of gout.

Most patients with primary gout have an impaired renal fractional excretion of urate, i.e. an inappropriately low urinary urate output if the raised plasma [urate] is taken into consideration. A minority of patients show clear evidence of overproduction of urate and markedly increased urinary urate output. In a few cases, partial deficiency of HGPRT has been demonstrated.

The risk that a previously asymptomatic individual will develop gout varies with the plasma [urate]. The annual incidence is very low when plasma [urate] is below 0.42 mmol/L, but rises progressively with higher concentrations.

Patients with primary gout often show deposition of urate as tophi in soft tissues. Some also develop renal stones, mainly composed of uric acid, but the incidence varies widely, largely depending on the presence of other contributory factors such as dehydration or a low urinary pH.

Diagnosis of primary gout

The diagnosis is often made clinically on the basis of the distribution of the joint involvement, a past history of similar episodes (especially if responsive to colchicine) and the presence of a raised plasma [urate]. However, not all cases are typical clinically, and it should be remembered that:

1 A high plasma [urate] makes the diagnosis of gout probable, but not certain.

2 A small minority of patients with gout have a normal plasma [urate] at the time of an attack.

For the definitive diagnosis of gout, it may be necessary to aspirate joint fluid during an acute attack. This is then examined microscopically, and the finding of needle-shaped urate crystals that show negative birefringence establishes the diagnosis.

Treatment of primary gout

In an acute attack, anti-inflammatory drugs (e.g. indomethacin) are usually prescribed. Uricosuric drugs and allopurinol should be avoided at this stage.

Long-term treatment aims to reduce plasma [urate]. Factors known to increase plasma [urate], such as a high-protein diet, alcohol and certain drugs, should be avoided. Weight reduction, uricosuric drugs (e.g. probenecid) and inhibitors of urate synthesis (e.g. allopurinol) may be required. In patients in whom urate stones seem likely to form, a high fluid intake and alkalinization of the urine reduce the likelihood of stone formation.

Allopurinol (an isomer of hypoxanthine)

inhibits xanthine oxidase, thereby causing a fall in plasma [urate] and in urinary [urate].

HGPRT deficiency

The Lesch–Nyhan syndrome is a very rare inherited condition that usually presents in early childhood with choreo-athetosis, mental retardation and self-mutilation. The activity of HGPRT is greatly diminished or undetectable. In the absence of HGPRT, the salvage pathway is inoperative, and purines cannot be reconverted to nucleotides (Fig. 14.1); instead, they are converted to urate. Urinary [urate] is greatly increased, and uric acid calculi may form in the urinary tract. Plasma [urate] is usually increased.

Partial HGPRT deficiency is another rare inherited condition that causes a severe form of primary gout. Patients usually present with this condition in early adult life. Both plasma [urate] and urinary excretion of urate are increased.

Secondary gout

Hyperuricaemia may occur as a complication of several disorders, all of which affect either urate production or excretion, or both. These conditions, although commonly causing hyperuricaemia, are only rarely associated with the joint manifestations of gout. They include overproduction and defective elimination of urate.

Overproduction of urate

Myeloproliferative disorders. Polycythaemia rubra vera is probably the most common of these disorders, which are associated with signs of gout; this is due to increased turnover of red cell precursors causing hyperuricaemia.

Cytotoxic drug therapy. Increased rates of cell turnover cause hyperuricaemia. Renal failure may occur due to deposition of urate crystals in the collecting ducts and ureters. Maintenance of a high fluid intake and prophylaxis with allopurinol usually prevent this.

Psoriasis. The hyperuricaemia is thought to be due to an increased rate of cell turnover in the skin.

Hypercatabolic states and starvation. There may be both an increased rate of cell destruction and impaired urate excretion due to an associated lactic acidosis.

Defective elimination of urate

Chronic renal disease. Plasma [urate] rises in uraemia due to the reduced glomerular filtration rate, but clinical gout is very unusual.

Diuretic therapy. Most effective diuretics (e.g. chlorothiazide, frusemide) cause hyperuricaemia by reducing distal tubular secretion of urate.

Inherited metabolic disorders. Those that are associated with lactic acidosis, such as type I glycogen storage disease (von Gierke's disease), often cause hyperuricaemia.

Hypertension and ischaemic heart disease are commonly associated with hyperuricaemia for a variety of reasons, such as obesity and drug treatment.

KEY POINTS

1 In humans, urate is the main end-product of nucleic acid and purine metabolism.
2 Urate in plasma and tissue fluids is close to the limit of its solubility.
3 Urate is mainly excreted in the urine.
4 Plasma urate may rise either due to increased production, e.g. increased cell turnover, or decreased excretion.
5 Primary gout is characterized by arthritis due to an inflammatory reaction to the deposition of urate crystals in joints. Urate may be deposited in connective tissue elsewhere, and urate renal stones may also form.

CHAPTER 15

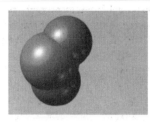

Abnormalities of Thyroid Function

Thyroid hormone synthesis, action and metabolism, 191
Regulation of thyroid function, 192
Investigations to determine thyroid status, 192
Selective use of thyroid function tests, 194
Interpreting results of thyroid function tests, 195
Situations in which TSH usually provides the correct estimate of thyroid status, 195
Common situations in which TSH results may be misleading, 197
Causes of abnormal results for thyroid hormone measurements, 198
Monitoring the treatment of thyroid disease, 199
Miscellaneous chemical tests and thyroid diseases, 200
Medullary carcinoma of the thyroid (MCT), 201

Thyroid hormones are essential for normal growth, development and metabolism. Hormone production by the thyroid gland is tightly regulated through the hypothalamic–pituitary–thyroid axis.

Thyroid disease is common, particularly in women, with a prevalence in the community of 3–5%. Although primary diseases of the thyroid gland are the most common, pituitary disease and the use of certain drugs that alter thyroid hormone synthesis or metabolism can also give rise to thyroid dysfunction. Once diagnosed, thyroid disease is easily treated, with an excellent long-term outcome for most patients.

This chapter outlines the pathways of thyroid hormone synthesis and metabolism. The tests used in diagnosis and management of thyroid disease are described, together with guidance on their interpretation.

Thyroid hormone synthesis, action and metabolism

Synthesis

Thyroxine (T4) and small amounts of tri-iodothyronine (T3) and reverse T3 (rT3) are all synthesized in the thyroid gland (Fig. 15.1) by a process involving:
• *Trapping of iodide* from the plasma by the thyroid gland.
• *Oxidation of iodide to iodine by thyroid peroxidase.*
• *Incorporation of iodine* into tyrosyl residues on thyroglobulin in the colloid. Mono-iodotyrosine and di-iodotyrosine (MIT and DIT) are formed.
• *Production of T3 and T4* by coupling iodotyrosyl residues in the thyroglobulin molecule.
• *Splitting off of T4 and T3* from thyroglobulin following its reabsorption from the colloid.
• Release of T4 and T3 into the circulation.
These stages are shown diagrammatically in Figure 15.2.

Thyroxine, a pro-hormone, is produced exclusively by the thyroid. *The biologically active hormone is T3*, and about 85% of plasma T3 is formed by outer-ring (5′) mono-deiodination of T4 in liver, kidneys and muscle (Fig. 15.3). Thyroxine also undergoes inner-ring (5) mono-deiodination in nonthyroidal tissues, with the production of metabolically inactive rT3.

Plasma transport and cellular action

Thyroid hormones are transported in plasma

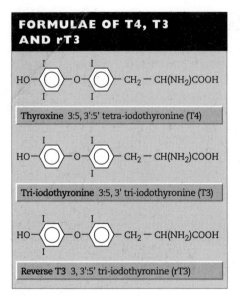

FORMULAE OF T4, T3 AND rT3

Thyroxine 3:5, 3':5' tetra-iodothyronine (T4)

Tri-iodothyronine 3:5, 3' tri-iodothyronine (T3)

Reverse T3 3, 3':5' tri-iodothyronine (rT3)

Fig. 15.1 The formulae of the thyroid hormones, T4 and T3, and of rT3.

almost entirely bound, reversibly, to plasma proteins. Thyroxine-binding globulin (TBG) binds about 70% of plasma T4 and 80% of plasma T3. Thyroxine-binding pre-albumin and albumin also bind thyroid hormone.

Approximately 0.05% of plasma T4 and 0.2% of plasma T3 are free (i.e. unbound to protein). Only the free fractions can cross the cell membrane and affect intracellular metabolism. After binding to high affinity binding sites on the plasma membrane, the hormones are actively transported into cells by an adenosine triphosphate (ATP)-dependent mechanism. In the cell, T3 acts mainly at the nucleus, where it binds to specific receptors that in turn activate T3-responsive genes. These genes appear to exert a number of effects on cell metabolism, which include a stimulation of basal metabolic rate and the metabolism of lipids, carbohydrates and proteins.

Regulation of thyroid function
(Fig. 15.3)
The most important regulator of thyroid homeostasis is thyroid-stimulating hormone (TSH, or thyrotrophin). This peptide hormone

comprises a specific beta subunit, which is required for binding to the TSH receptor, and an alpha subunit, which is common to the gonadotrophins; both subunits are required for bioactivity. The subunits contain carbohydrate chains that are essential for the biological activity of the molecule. Modifications to these carbohydrate residues occur in different thyroid states, which alter both the bioactivity of the molecule and its plasma half-life. For example, in primary hypothyroidism, TSH has increased bioactivity and an increased plasma retention time, whilst in secondary hypothyroidism the bioactivity of the molecule is diminished. Most immunoassays are unable to recognize modifications to the carbohydrate chains.

The production of TSH is controlled by a stimulatory effect of the hypothalamic tripeptide, thyrotrophin-releasing hormone (TRH, or thyroliberin), mediated by a negative feedback from circulating free T3 and free T4. It is thought that the hypothalamus, via TRH, sets the level of thyroid hormone production required physiologically, and that the pituitary acts as a 'thyroid-stat' to maintain the level of thyroid hormone production that has been determined by the hypothalamus.

Dopamine, somatostatin and glucocorticoids appear also to be involved in inhibiting the release of TSH, and these agents together with the interleukins may be important modifiers of TSH release in nonthyroidal illness (NTI).

Investigations to determine thyroid status
The tests used to investigate thyroid dysfunction can be grouped into:
• Tests that establish whether there is thyroid dysfunction, i.e. plasma TSH and thyroid hormone (T4 and T3) measurements.
• Tests to elucidate the cause of thyroid dysfunction, i.e. thyroid auto-antibody and serum thyroglobulin measurements, thyroid enzyme activities, biopsy of the thyroid, ultrasound and isotopic thyroid scanning.

Measurement of plasma TSH and thyroid

SYNTHESIS OF T4 AND T3

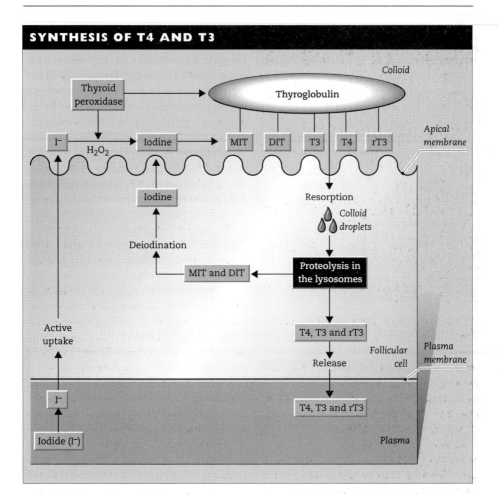

Fig. 15.2 The synthesis of T4 and T3 in the thyroid gland. The metabolism of T4 is described in Fig. 15.3. Di-iodotyrosine (DIT) and mono-iodotyrosine (MIT) are hormonally inactive; their iodine content is conserved.

hormones should be performed to determine the patient's thyroid status before requesting the more demanding tests that seek to determine the cause of the thyroid dysfunction.

Plasma thyrotrophin (reference range 0.3–5.0 mU/L)
The measurement of plasma [TSH] in a basal blood sample by immunometric assay provides the single most sensitive, specific and reliable test of thyroid status in both overt and subclini-

cal thyroid disease. In primary hypothyroidism, plasma [TSH] is increased, whilst in primary hyperthyroidism plasma [TSH] is below 0.1 mU/L. There are exceptions to this, and both raised and undetectable plasma [TSH] may be found in some euthyroid patients (Table 15.1).

Plasma free T4 (reference range 10–27 pmol/L)

Plasma free T3 (reference range 3–9 pmol/L)
Free thyroid hormone concentrations are independent of changes in the concentration and affinity of thyroid-hormone binding proteins and theoretically provide a more reliable means

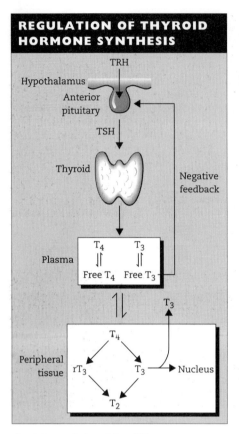

REGULATION OF THYROID HORMONE SYNTHESIS

Fig. 15.3 Regulation of thyroid hormone synthesis and metabolism.

of diagnosing thyroid dysfunction than measurement of total hormone concentrations. Several assay techniques have been developed to measure free hormone concentrations. These methods produce results that show good agreement in most ambulant patients, however, in patients with nonthyroidal illnesses, results may not always correlate well with one another due to various assay artefacts.

Plasma total T4 (reference range 70–150 nmol/L)

Plasma total T3 (reference range 1.2–2.8 nmol/L)

More than 99% of T4 and T3 circulate in plasma bound to protein. The concentrations

of plasma total T4 and total T3 are therefore greatly influenced by the plasma concentrations of thyroid hormone-binding proteins, particularly TBG. Both plasma [total T4] and [total T3] change in parallel in euthyroid patients if plasma [TBG] alters, e.g. in women taking oestrogen-containing oral contraceptives or in pregnancy; their concentrations may rise into the hyperthyroid range. However, plasma [free T4] and [free T3] remain normal if pituitary–thyroid homeostasis is maintained. Table 15.2 lists the common causes of abnormal plasma [total T4] and [total T3] in euthyroid patients.

Plasma [total T4] discriminates well between euthyroid, hyperthyroid and hypothyroid states if there are no abnormalities in plasma [TBG]. Plasma [total T3] also provides a useful test for hyperthyroidism, as values are often raised proportionately more than plasma [total T4] in these patients. However, measurement of plasma [total T3] is of *no value* in investigating patients with suspected hypothyroidism, as normal results are often found.

Selective use of thyroid function tests

Many laboratories measure basal plasma [TSH] as the initial test of thyroid function. This test is not infallible, but is least likely to produce an abnormal result in nonthyroidal illness and in patients on various forms of drug treatment. It can detect both overt and subclinical disease. A normal plasma [TSH] virtually excludes primary thyroid dysfunction. If an abnormal result is obtained, plasma thyroid hormone measurements are made to confirm that thyroid dysfunction is present, and to determine the severity of the disease.

Initial measurement of both TSH and free T4 together can provide a more satisfactory method of assessing thyroid status, since in some situations a single TSH result may be misleading. If this strategy is followed, a significant number of cases will arise in which one test will be abnormal whilst the complementary test will be normal. It is thus essential to understand and appreciate the factors that can affect the results of thyroid function tests.

ABNORMAL PLASMA [TSH] IN EUTHYROID PATIENTS

Undetectable plasma [TSH]	Increased plasma [TSH]
Pregnancy, during the first 20 weeks Treated hyperthyroid patients within 6 months of becoming euthyroid Ophthalmic Graves' disease Various kinds of nonthyroidal illness* Nontoxic multinodular goitre Treatment with dopaminergic drugs or with high doses of glucocorticoids	Subclinical hypothyroidism Amiodarone During the recovery stage following various nonthyroidal illnesses*

*Nonthyroidal illness is discussed on p. 197.

Table 15.1 Causes of an abnormal plasma [TSH] in some euthyroid patients.

ABNORMAL PLASMA [THYROID HORMONES] IN EUTHYROID PATIENTS

Increased plasma [total T4]	Increased plasma [total T3]	Decreased plasma [total T4] and [total T3]
Nonthyroidal illness T4 auto-antibodies Variant albumins, TBG excess	TBG excess T3 auto-antibodies	Non-thyroidal illness TBG deficiency

Table 15.2 Causes of abnormal plasma [thyroid hormones] in euthyroid patients.

Interpreting results of thyroid function tests

Figure 15.4 provides a guide to the interpretation of thyroid function tests.

Situations in which TSH usually provides the correct estimate of thyroid status

Overt primary hyperthyroidism

Plasma [TSH] is nearly always below 0.1 mU/L, due to feedback inhibition on the pituitary. Plasma free and total T4 and T3 concentrations are nearly always increased in patients with overt hyperthyroidism. In a very small percentage of hyperthyroid patients, plasma [total T4] and [free T4] are both normal, whereas both plasma [total T3] and [free T3] are increased; this condition is known as T3 hyperthyroidism or T3 thyrotoxicosis.

Overt primary hypothyroidism

Plasma [TSH] is invariably increased, often to more than 20 mU/L, as feedback inhibition of the pituitary (Fig. 15.3) is diminished, and plasma [free T4] and [total T4] are usually low. Plasma free T3 and total T3 measurements are of no value here, since normal concentrations are often observed.

Subclinical primary thyroid disease

Thyroid disease presents as a spectrum of clinical and biochemical features of varying severity. The clinical diagnosis of mild thyroid disorders is often difficult, and the only bio-

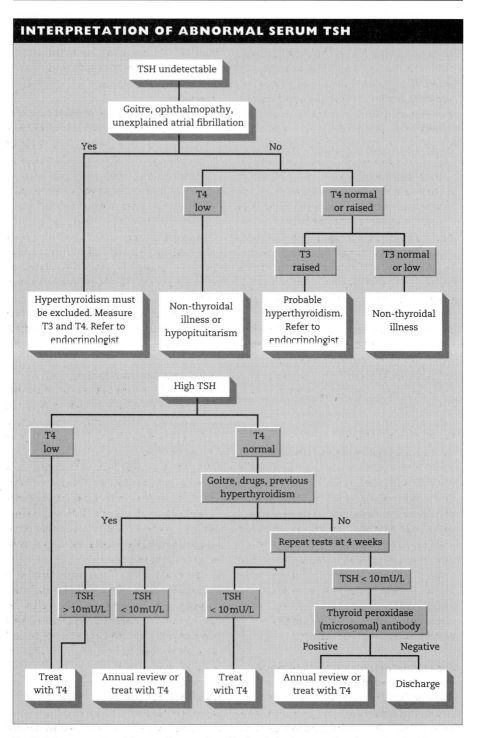

Fig. 15.4 Interpretation of abnormal serum thyroid-stimulating hormone (TSH). Reprinted with permission from Rae P., Farrar J., Beckett G.J. & Tort A.D. (1993) Assessment of thyroid status in elderly people. *Br Med J* **307**, 177–180.

chemical abnormality may be an abnormal plasma [TSH]. For example, many clinically euthyroid patients with multinodular goitre or with exophthalmic Graves' disease may have a plasma [TSH] below 0.1 mU/L but have plasma [total T4] and [free T4] in the upper part of their respective reference ranges. In all these patients, production of TSH has been suppressed despite the fact that their plasma [free T4] is not abnormally high. Some of the patients may remain euthyroid, but others progress to overt hyperthyroidism. This combination of chemical findings is sometimes termed 'subclinical hyperthyroidism', but this description is unsatisfactory, since it rests solely on the results of chemical investigations. Similarly, there are patients with 'subclinical hypothyroidism' in whom plasma [TSH] is elevated, but plasma [free T4] and [free T3] are normal.

Before the diagnosis of subclinical thyroid disease can be made, causes of an abnormal plasma [TSH] other than thyroid disease must be excluded. These include pregnancy, nonthyroidal illnesses, drug treatment, and assay interference.

Paediatrics and the neonate

Plasma TSH is widely used to screen for congenital hypothyroidism in the neonate (p. 252). Marked changes in thyroid function occur in the early days of life, with an initial surge in TSH and thyroid hormone after delivery, followed by a marked decline in hormone levels over the next few days. Hormone levels then show a slow decline until adult values are reached at about the age of ten. It is essential to apply appropriate age-related reference ranges.

Common situations in which TSH results may be misleading

Assay interference from endogenous heterophilic antibodies

Some individuals have antibodies in their plasma that react with a range of animal immunoglobulins (heterophilic antibodies). These antibodies interfere with a wide range of immunoassays, and can produce a spurious increase in TSH. For example, a normal or elevated TSH result may be found in some thyrotoxic patients due to this interference.

Pregnancy

TSH is a reliable indicator of thyroid status in the second and third trimester of pregnancy, but in the first trimester a plasma [TSH] of <0.1 mU/L may be found in up to 3% of patients. This is due to the weak thyrotrophic effect of placental human chorionic gonadotrophin (hCG), which is present in high concentrations particularly in the first trimester.

Free thyroid hormone levels decline in pregnancy, and trimester-related reference ranges must be applied. Plasma [TBG] increases during pregnancy, resulting in elevated plasma [total T4] and [total T3].

Transient postpartum thyroid dysfunction may occur in up to 15% of women, but this is usually subclinical.

Secondary thyroid disorders

Plasma [TSH] is normal in about half of patients with central (pituitary) hypothyroidism, but the circulating TSH has been shown to have reduced bioactivity. Plasma [total T4] or [free T4] are usually low.

Very rarely, hyperthyroidism is due to a TSH-secreting tumour. Persistent hyperthyroid symptoms, with elevated [thyroid hormones] and raised or normal TSH, is consistent with this diagnosis, once the common problems of assay interference or nonthyroidal illness have been eliminated.

Abnormal pituitary T3 receptor function is another rare cause of hyperthyroidism. In this disorder, the thyrotroph is resistant to the normal negative feedback regulation, so that plasma thyroid hormone levels are raised, and there are hyperthyroid symptoms and a normal or raised plasma [TSH].

Nonthyroidal illness and the sick euthyroid syndrome

In patients attending or admitted to hospital suffering from any of a wide range of chronic or acute nonthyroidal illnesses (NTIs), abnormalities in thyroid function tests, in particular a low plasma [T3], may often be found even though the patients are clinically euthyroid; this has been termed the *sick euthyroid syndrome*.

Several mechanisms are involved, including:
• Alterations in the hypothalamic–pituitary–thyroid axis, e.g. resulting from increased release of dopamine, cytokines, cortisol and somatostatin, which inhibit TSH release.
• Changes in the affinity characteristics and in the plasma concentrations of the thyroid hormone-binding proteins. These changes give rise to alterations in the plasma concentrations of both the free and total thyroid hormones.
• Impaired uptake of thyroid hormones by the tissues.
• Decreased production of T3 in the peripheral tissues.
• Changes in the T3 occupancy and function of the T3 receptors.

The contribution of each of the above mechanisms may vary with the severity and stage of the illness, and thus the pattern of thyroid function tests may be extremely variable and may mimic the profile seen in primary or secondary thyroid disease. Interpretation of thyroid function tests is complicated further by the effects

Table 15.3 Examples of drugs that alter thyroid hormone synthesis, secretion and metabolism.

of drugs and methodological problems associated with free hormone measurements.

Although TSH is the most reliable of the thyroid function tests in hospitalized patients, a TSH of <0.1 mU/L is twice as likely to be due to NTI as to hyperthyroidism, and an increased TSH is as likely to be due to recovery from illness as to hypothyroidism. Because of the poor predictive value of thyroid function tests in hospitalized patients, these tests should only be requested if the reason for hospital admission is considered on clinical grounds to be related to a thyroid problem.

Drug treatment
Several drugs can, by themselves, affect the results of thyroid function tests; examples are given in Table 15.3. The combination of nonthyroidal illness and certain forms of drug treatment can have marked effects on thyroid function test results.

Causes of abnormal results for thyroid hormone measurements

Abnormalities in binding proteins
Alterations in the concentrations or affinities of plasma thyroxine-binding proteins can produce the following misleading results for thyroid hormone measurements:
• *Abnormal plasma TBG concentrations* occur frequently (Table 15.4), leading to parallel

DRUGS AFFECTING THYROID FUNCTION

Mechanism	Example of drug
Decrease in TSH Secretion	Dopamine, glucocorticoids
Decrease in thyroid hormone secretion	Lithium, amiodarone*
Increase in thyroid hormone secretion	Iodide, amiodarone*
Decrease in thyroidal synthesis	Carbimazole, propylthiouracil, lithium
Increase in TBG	Oestrogens, tamoxifen
Decrease in TBG	Androgens, glucocorticoids
Displacement of thyroid hormones from plasma proteins	Furosemide, fenclofenac, salicylates
Increased hepatic metabolism	Phenytoin, carbamazepine
Impaired T4 and T3 conversion	Beta antagonists, amiodarone*
Impaired absorption of thyroxine	Cholestyramine, aluminium hydroxide

*Amiodarone has a number of effects on thyroid hormone metabolism.

changes in total thyroid hormone concentrations. The affinity and binding capacity of TBG for thyroid hormones may be diminished by NTI and by drugs (e.g. salicylates), leading in turn to decreases in [total T3] and [total T4].

• *Abnormal plasma albumin and pre-albumin concentrations* may influence the results for plasma [total T4] and [total T3] to a small extent. Free hormone concentrations are unrelated to changes in the concentration of these proteins, but in practice some methods for free hormone measurement are unreliable and produce results that are influenced by changes in the concentration and binding capacity of albumin.

• *Genetic variants of both albumin and pre-albumin* have been described in which the affinity of these binding proteins for T4 is increased. These variants give rise to increased plasma [total T4]. Plasma TSH, total T3 and free T3 measurements are usually all normal if the patient is euthyroid, as also is plasma [free T4] if measured by a reliable method.

• *Endogenous antibodies to thyroid hormone* may occur in patients with auto-immune thyroid disease. These antibodies interfere with many of the assay methods for both free and total thyroid hormones and produce apparently elevated results. Plasma TSH measurements provide the most reliable indications of thyroid status in these patients, as they are not affected by these auto-antibodies.

Monitoring the treatment of thyroid disease

Management of hypothyroidism

Replacement therapy in patients with *primary hypothyroidism* aims to restore the euthyroid state both clinically and, if possible, biochemically. It is desirable to normalize both plasma [free T4] and TSH concentrations, but in a few patients normal plasma [TSH] can only be achieved in the presence of a modest elevation in plasma [free T4].

Following a change in the prescribed dose of thyroxine, it may be six to eight weeks before the thyroid function tests again stabilize, and TSH results must be interpreted with caution during this stabilization period.

Some hypothyroid patients may not take their replacement thyroxine regularly, but may take some shortly before attending the follow-up clinic. Such poor compliance is indicated by finding that the plasma [free T4] and plasma [TSH] are both abnormally high.

Excessive thyroxine replacement may be recognized from the patient's symptoms and on clinical examination. It may also be suspected or confirmed by finding that plasma [TSH] is less than 0.1 mU/L.

In *pregnancy*, T4 requirements increase, and hypothyroid patients should be monitored regularly.

In patients with *secondary hypothyroidism*, the objective of replacement therapy is to maintain

Table 15.4 Causes of an abnormal plasma [thyroxine-binding globulin].

ABNORMAL PLASMA [TBG]	
Increased plasma [TBG]	**Decreased plasma [TBG]**
Oral contraceptives	Nonthyroidal illness
Pregnancy	Genetic causes
Oestrogen therapy	Protein-losing states
Genetic causes	Drugs (see Table 15.3)
Drugs (see Table 15.3)	
Note that many drugs may bind to thyroxine-binding globulins (TBGs) and thereby decrease the binding capacity of these proteins for thyroid hormones, but without affecting plasma [TBG].	

plasma [free T4] or [total T4] in the upper half of the reference range.

In patients with papillary and follicular *carcinoma of the thyroid*, the aim of treatment is to give sufficient thyroxine to suppress plasma [TSH] to undetectable levels.

Management of hyperthyroidism

Plasma free or total thyroid hormone concentrations can be used to provide a satisfactory index of the progress of the untreated disease. These tests also provide the best indications of the adequacy or otherwise of antithyroid drug treatment. The therapeutic objective is to maintain plasma [total T4] or [free T4] in the upper half of the reference range. Measurement of plasma [TSH] is not a reliable guide of thyroid status during the first four to six months of treatment for hyperthyroidism, since TSH levels may still be suppressed even when plasma thyroid hormone concentrations have become abnormally low. Plasma [TSH] can be used to determine the adequacy of treatment after normal thyrotroph responsiveness has returned.

After radioactive iodine treatment, the likelihood that patients will eventually develop hypothyroidism is high. Long-term follow-up of these patients with periodic measurements of both plasma [TSH] and either [total T4] or [free T4] is essential.

Patients treated by subtotal thyroidectomy are more likely to remain euthyroid than are patients treated with radioactive iodine or with antithyroid drugs. However, they may have temporary disturbances of thyroid function tests in the early postoperative period, and it is advisable to monitor these patients for six months before deciding whether thyroid replacement treatment is needed. The decision should then be based on clinical assessment supplemented by measurements of both plasma [TSH] and either [total T4] or [free T4].

Miscellaneous chemical tests and thyroid disease
Thyroid auto-antibodies

Several types of antibody to thyroid tissue have been detected in serum, usually from patients with thyroid disease. Measuring these antibodies helps to demonstrate the presence of auto-immune disorders.

• *Thyroid peroxidase (microsomal antigen) and thyroglobulin antibodies* are present in the serum of patients with immunologically mediated thyroid disease (e.g. Hashimoto's thyroiditis, Graves' disease). They may also be found in a small proportion of healthy individuals, the incidence being higher in relations of patients with hyperthyroidism. The highest titres of these antibodies are found in the serum of patients with Hashimoto's thyroiditis, one or both antibodies being present in 90% of patients. The main indications for measuring antithyroglobulin and antithyroid peroxidase antibodies are to confirm a diagnosis of Hashimoto's thyroiditis and to distinguish ophthalmic Graves' disease from other possible diagnoses. In patients with subclinical hypothyroidism the presence of antithyroid peroxidase antibodies is a strong indicator for the need for replacement therapy, as such patients are at high risk of developing overt disease.

• *Thyrotrophin-receptor antibodies* (TRAbs) are IgG antibodies directed against TSH receptors in the thyroid, and are involved in the pathogenesis of Graves' disease by promoting hormone synthesis and thyroid hypertrophy. Thyrotrophin-receptor antibody measurements can be readily measured, and the results may be of value in:

• Predicting neonatal hyperthyroidism in babies born to mothers with high TRAbs in the last weeks of pregnancy (TRAbs cross the placenta).

• Distinguishing between postpartum thyroiditis and Graves' disease. Undetectable TRAbs are found in thyroiditis, whilst TRAbs are positive in 90% of patients with Graves' disease.

Thyroglobulin

Many differentiated papillary and follicular carcinomas of the thyroid synthesize and secrete thyroglobulin. In patients with these diseases, measurement of serum [thyroglobulin] is of value in monitoring progression of the disease, and in assessing response to treatment; plasma [thyroglobulin] above 5 μg/L suggests that residual tumour is present.

Thyroid enzymes

Inherited metabolic disorders of thyroid hormone synthesis are all rare. For their specific recognition, measurements of iodinated tyrosines or of the activities of the enzymes involved in thyroxine synthesis may be required.

Tests affected by thyroid dysfunction

Several other chemical tests may be affected by changes in thyroid status. For example, in hyperthyroidism:
- *Glucose tolerance tests* may show a diabetic type of response.
- *Plasma calcium* and alkaline phosphatase may be increased.
- *Plasma cholesterol may be low.*
- *Liver function tests* may be abnormal.

Medullary carcinoma of the thyroid (MCT)

This tumour of the parafollicular, calcitonin-

Table 15.5 Characteristic tumours in the multiple endocrine neoplasia (MEN) syndromes.

producing cells (C-cells) of the thyroid gland accounts for about 10% of thyroid cancers. Nonfamilial cases account for 80% of all cases of MCT. The familial form of the disease may occur in conjunction with neoplasia of other endocrine tissues, a syndrome known as multiple endocrine neoplasia (MEN). A description of MEN is given in Table 15.5.

Plasma [calcitonin] is often greatly increased in patients with MCT, but plasma [calcium] is usually normal. A raised plasma [calcitonin] may occur in other conditions, including Hashimoto's thyroiditis, chronic renal failure and diseases associated with transformed neuroendocrine cells (e.g. carcinoid tumours and phaeochromocytoma).

In patients with MCT, plasma [calcitonin] increases by two to five times above the basal level following combined calcium and pentagastrin administration, whereas normal subjects show little or no response. The test is usually performed by taking a blood sample for basal plasma [calcitonin], after which the patient is given an intravenous infusion of calcium gluconate (2 mg/kg body weight over 1 min). Pentagastrin is then given intravenously (0.5 μg/kg body weight over 50 seconds), after which the plasma [calcitonin] response is monitored over the next two minutes. DNA mutational analysis should also be performed in patients with suspected MCT.

TUMOURS ASSOCIATED WITH MEN SYNDROMES		
MEN I	MEN IIa	MEN IIb
Hyperparathyroidism	Medullary carcinoma of the thyroid (97%)	Medullary carcinoma of the thyroid (90%)
Tumours secreting:	Phaeochromocytoma (30%)	Phaeochromocytoma (45%)
Gastrin	Hyperparathyroidism (50%)	Associated abnormalities:
Insulin		Mucosal neuroma (100%)
Glucagon		Marfan habitus (65%)
Vasoactive intestinal		Megacolon
polypeptide (VIP)		
Pancreatic polypeptide		
Pituitary tumours		

Values in brackets show the percentage of patients having the condition.

KEY POINTS

1 Plasma [TSH] is usually the single best test for assessing thyroid status. Plasma [TSH] is elevated in primary hypothyroidism and suppressed to <0.1 mU/L in primary hyperthyroidism. A normal plasma [TSH] usually excludes a primary thyroid disorder.

2 Plasma [free T4] or [total T4] can help assess the severity of thyroid disease and distinguish subclinical from overt disease.

3 Plasma [free T3] or [total T3] can help determine the severity of hyperthyroidism and to identify patients with T3 hyperthyroidism.

4 Free thyroid hormone measurements correlate more closely with thyroid status than total hormone measurements, which are heavily influenced by changes in the concentration of thyroid hormone-binding proteins.

5 Thyroid function tests are often abnormal in patients with nonthyroidal illness, and should not be requested in hospitalized patients unless the presenting complaint might be due to thyroid disease.

6 In certain situations (nonthyroidal illness, secondary thyroid disease, early treatment of hyperthyroidism and early pregnancy), TSH results alone may be misleading.

Case 15.1

A 30-year-old housewife attended her general practitioner. She had lost weight (6 kg in the previous three months), was irritable and felt uncomfortable in the recent hot spell of weather. She was taking an oestrogen-containing oral contraceptive. On clinical examination, her palms were sweaty, and she had a fine tremor of the fingers when her arms were outstretched. There was no thyroid enlargement or bruit, and no eye signs. The following results were reported for thyroid function tests:

Plasma analysis	Result	Reference range
[TSH] (mU/L)	<0.1	0.3–5.0
[Free T4] (pmol/L)	20	10–27
[Total T4] (nmol/L)	160	70–150
[Free T3] (pmol/L)	20	3.0–9.0
[Total T3] (nmol/L)	6	1.2–2.8

What is the diagnosis in this patient, and on which results was this diagnosis based?

Comments on Case 15.1

The patient had T3 thyrotoxicosis, and the diagnosis was based on the increased plasma [free T3] and undetectable [TSH], in the presence of a normal plasma [free T4]. The fact that the patient was taking an oestrogen-containing oral contraceptive would account for the increased plasma [total T4] and some of the increase in [total T3], since the oestrogen content would cause an increase in plasma [TBG].

In patients with thyrotoxicosis but no goitre, it is important to perform a thyroid scan to help determine the cause of the hyperthyroidism. This patient's thyroid showed a diffuse and increased uptake of ^{131}I, and TSH-receptor antibodies were detected in her serum. This patient had Graves' disease but no goitre; this is thought to arise when thyroid-stimulating immunoglobulins are present but thyroid-growth immunoglobulins are absent.

Case 15.2

A 65-year-old widow had been receiving treatment for primary hypothyroidism with thyroxine (150 mg/day) for the previous 12 months. She felt well and was clinically euthyroid; her weight had been steady. Results of thyroid function tests performed at a routine follow-up out-patient attendance were:

Plasma analysis	Result	Reference range
[TSH] (mU/L)	0.2	0.3–5.0
[Free T4] (pmol/L)	28	10–27
[Free T3] (pmol/L)	6.0	3.0–9.0

Are these results indicative of satisfactory therapeutic control, or would you want to adjust the patient's dosage of thyroxine?

Comments on Case 15.2

The aim of thyroxine replacement treatment for primary hypothyroidism is to keep the patient clinically euthyroid and to render plasma [TSH] normal (it would have been much increased before thyroxine treatment was started). In many of these patients, it is necessary to give sufficient thyroxine to increase the plasma [free T4] to above the upper reference value in order to normalize plasma [TSH].

In this patient, although she was clinically euthyroid, the plasma [free T4] was above normal and [TSH] was below normal, but not so suppressed as to be undetectable (i.e. it was not <0.1 mU/L). It was decided not to reduce the thyroxine dosage, and to reassess the patient three months later.

Case 15.3

A 35-year-old secretary attended for follow-up review of her treatment for Graves' disease. Carbimazole administration (15 mg three times/day) had been started one month before. The results for thyroid function tests were as follows:

Plasma analysis	Result	Reference range
[TSH] (mU/L)	<0.1	0.3–5.0
[Free T4] (pmol/L)	<5	10–27
[Free T3] (pmol/L)	2.5	3.0–9.0

Comment on the acceptability of these results. If they are not acceptable, what would you do?

Comments on Case 15.3

Plasma TSH measurements are not a reliable indicator of thyroid status in the early months of treating hyperthyroid patients, as the responsiveness of the thyrotrophs lags behind the fall in plasma [free T4] and [free T3] for several weeks. During these early months, plasma free thyroid hormone measurements provide the most reliable indication of thyroid status. In this patient, the results for plasma [free T4] and [free T3] clearly indicated the need to reduce the dosage of carbimazole immediately.

Case 15.4

A 38-year-old factory worker attended her general practitioner because she was always tired and had a feeling of discomfort in her neck. She had been gaining weight. On clinical examination, she was found to have a goitre. The following results were reported for thyroid function tests:

Plasma analysis	Result	Reference range
[TSH] (mU/L)	45	0.3–5.0
[Free T4] (pmol/L)	10	10–27
[Free T3] (pmol/L)	4.2	3.0–9.0

Antimicrosomal and antithyroglobulin antibodies were present in the patient's serum in very high titre.

What is the diagnosis? Comment on whether all these tests needed to be requested in this patient.

Comments on Case 15.4

The patient has hypothyroidism. However, she still had sufficient functioning thyroid tissue, when stimulated by the very high plasma [TSH], to be able to maintain plasma [free T4] and [free T3] within their reference ranges. It should be noted that it was not appropriate to have requested the free T3 measurement, since about 50 % of patients with hypothyroidism have a normal plasma [free T3].

The very high titres of antimicrosomal and antithyroglobulin antibodies in this patient's serum indicate that she had hypothyroidism due to Hashimoto's thyroiditis.

CHAPTER 16

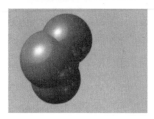

Disorders of the Adrenal Cortex and Medulla

Regulation of adrenal steroid hormone synthesis and secretion, 205
Investigation of suspected

adrenocortical hyperfunction, 208
Investigation of suspected adrenocortical hypofunction, 212

Hyperaldosteronism, 215
Inherited adrenocortical enzyme defects, 217
Phaeochromocytoma, 218

The adrenal gland consists of two distinct tissues of different embryological origin, the outer cortex and inner medulla. The cortex secretes glucocorticoid, mineralocorticoid and sex steroid hormones, whilst the medulla secretes catecholamines, principally adrenaline. Although there are important interactions between the cortex and medulla (e.g. cortisol is required for adrenaline synthesis), it is convenient to study their pathology separately. Disorders of the adrenals are uncommon, but they often have to be considered in an individual patient's differential diagnosis. The need for specific and sensitive screening tests is therefore important; additional tests can then be used to confirm or refute the results of screening tests.

After a brief review of the control of steroid hormone secretion from the adrenal cortex and the action of the different steroid hormones, the investigation of adrenocortical hyperfunction and hypofunction will be discussed. Hypersecretion of aldosterone is then discussed, followed by a brief review of congenital enzyme defects in the adrenal cortex. Finally, the investigation of catecholamine hypersecretion from an adrenomedullary tumour (phaeochromocytoma) is discussed.

Regulation of adrenal steroid hormone synthesis and secretion

Three zones can be recognized in the adrenal cortex (Fig. 16.1). The outermost zona glomerulosa is the site of synthesis of aldosterone, the principal mineralocorticoid. The deeper layers of the cortex, the zona fasciculata and zona reticularis, synthesize glucocorticoids, of which cortisol is the most important in man. Sex steroid production also occurs in the adrenal cortex, mainly in the zona reticularis.

Glucocorticoid secretion

Glucocorticoids have widespread metabolic effects on carbohydrate, fat and protein metabolism. In the liver, cortisol stimulates gluconeogenesis, amino acid uptake and degradation, and ketogenesis. Lipolysis is increased in adipose tissue, and proteolysis and amino acid release promoted in muscle.

Adrenocorticotrophic hormone (ACTH) is the main stimulus to cortisol secretion. Three factors regulate ACTH (and therefore cortisol) secretion:

1 *Negative feedback control.* ACTH release from the anterior pituitary is stimulated by hypothalamic secretion of corticotrophin-releasing hormone (CRH). Increased plasma

THE ADRENAL CORTEX

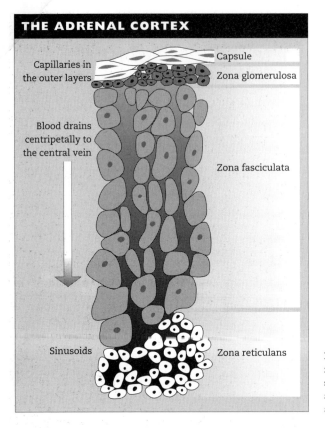

Capillaries in the outer layers

Capsule

Zona glomerulosa

Blood drains centripetally to the central vein

Zona fasciculata

Sinusoids

Zona reticulans

Fig. 16.1 The morphological zonation of the adrenal cortex, showing the three types of cells and their particular structural arrangement.

[cortisol] or synthetic glucocorticoids suppress secretion of CRH (Fig. 16.2).

2 *Stress* (e.g. major surgery, emotional stress) leads to a sudden large increase in CRH (and ACTH) secretion; the negative feedback control mechanism is temporarily overridden.

3 *The diurnal rhythm of plasma [cortisol].* This control mechanism is related to the rhythm of an individual's sleeping–waking cycle (Fig. 16.3). Cortisol levels are highest at the start of the working day, falling to lowest levels at the onset of sleep.

In the circulation, glucocorticoids are mainly protein-bound (about 90%), chiefly to cortisol-binding globulin (CBG or transcortin). Plasma [CBG] is increased in pregnancy and with oestrogen treatment (e.g. oral contraceptives). It is decreased in hypoproteinaemic states (e.g. nephrotic syndrome). Parallel changes occur in plasma [cortisol].

The biologically active fraction of cortisol in plasma is the free (unbound) component, though most assays measure the total (i.e. bound plus free) concentration.

Aldosterone secretion

The principal physiological function of aldosterone is to conserve Na^+, mainly by facilitating Na^+ reabsorption and reciprocal K^+ or H^+ secretion in the distal renal tubule and in other epithelial cells. Although its rate of production is less than 1% of the rate of cortisol production, aldosterone is a major regulator of water and electrolyte balance, as well as blood pressure.

The renin–angiotensin system is the most important system controlling aldosterone secretion. Potassium ions and ACTH are also stimulatory.

1 *Renin* is a proteolytic enzyme produced by

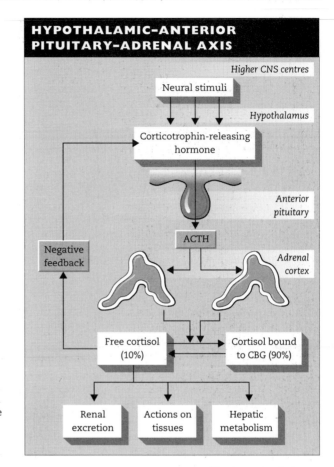

HYPOTHALAMIC–ANTERIOR PITUITARY–ADRENAL AXIS

Higher CNS centres

Neural stimuli

Hypothalamus

Corticotrophin-releasing hormone

Anterior pituitary

ACTH

Adrenal cortex

Negative feedback

Free cortisol (10%)

Cortisol bound to CBG (90%)

Renal excretion

Actions on tissues

Hepatic metabolism

Fig. 16.2 The hypothalamic–anterior pituitary–adrenal axis and the fate of cortisol following its release. CBG, cortisol-binding globulin.

the juxtaglomerular apparatus of the kidney and released into the circulation in response to a fall in circulating blood volume or renal perfusion pressure, and by loss of Na+. Its action on renin substrate is described on p. 18.

2 *Potassium.* Aldosterone is released in response to increases in plasma [K+], and exerts its effects on the distal renal tubule, causing an increased output of K+ in the urine.

3 *ACTH.* This control mechanism is relatively unimportant, except possibly in stress conditions and in congenital adrenal hyperplasia due to 21-hydroxylase deficiency.

No specific aldosterone-binding protein has been demonstrated.

Cortisol and ACTH measurements

Serum [cortisol] and plasma [ACTH]

Serum measurements are preferred for cortisol and plasma for ACTH (the latter is also unstable). Specimens must be collected without venous stasis between 8 a.m. and 9 a.m. and between 10 p.m. and 12 p.m. because of the diurnal rhythm (Fig. 16.2). Temporary, often large, increases in these hormones may be observed as a response to emotional stress.

Urinary cortisol excretion

Cortisol is removed from plasma by the liver and mostly converted to a number of metabol-

DIURNAL RHYTHM OF CORTISOL SECRETION

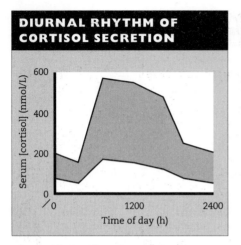

Fig. 16.3 The diurnal rhythm of cortisol secretion; the shaded area represents values that lie within the reference range. There is a similar rhythm for the secretion of adrenocorticotrophic hormone (ACTH) by the anterior pituitary.

ADRENOCORTICAL HYPERFUNCTION

ACTH-dependent
1 Pituitary (Cushing's disease)
2 Ectopic
3 Ectopic CRH or related peptides
4 ACTH therapy

ACTH-independent
1 Adrenal adenoma
2 Adrenal carcinoma
3 Glucocorticoid therapy
4 Micronodular hyperplasia (partially ACTH-dependent)

From P.J. Trainer and A. Grossman (1991) The diagnosis and differential diagnosis of Cushing's syndrome. *Clinical Endocrinology* **34**, 317–30.

Table 16.1 Causes of adrenocortical hyperfunction.

ically inactive compounds, excreted in the urine mainly as conjugated metabolites (e.g. glucuronides).

A small amount of cortisol is excreted unchanged in the urine. Urinary cortisol excretion is related to the biologically active plasma [free cortisol] during the period of urine collection. In normal individuals, urinary cortisol excretion is less than 250 nmol/24 h, and the cortisol : creatinine ratio in an early morning specimen of urine is less than 25 μmol cortisol : mol creatinine.

Investigation of suspected adrenocortical hyperfunction

Adrenocortical hyperfunction leads to the clinical condition known as Cushing's syndrome (Table 16.1); the condition may also arise from administration of ACTH or glucocorticoids therapeutically (iatrogenic Cushing's syndrome). Most ACTH-dependent forms of Cushing's syndrome lead to diffuse adrenocortical hyperplasia, but about 10–15% of patients demonstrate a macronodular hyperplasia.

Patients with suspected adrenocortical hyperfunction should be investigated according to a logical scheme:
1 *Screening tests (out-patient):* to assess whether a clinical diagnosis of adrenocortical hyperfunction is likely to be correct.
2 *Confirmatory tests (in-patient):* to confirm or exclude the provisional diagnosis of adrenocortical hyperfunction.
3 *Tests to determine the cause:* to ascertain (a) the *site* of the pathological lesion (adrenal cortex, pituitary or elsewhere?); and (b) the *nature* of the pathological lesion.
A suggested plan of investigation is shown in Figure 16.4. Table 16.2 gives a summary of the commonly observed (but not invariable) findings in these hormonal tests.

Screening tests
The clinical suspicion of Cushing's syndrome arises quite commonly, whereas the incidence is very low, if iatrogenic causes are discounted. Effective screening tests need to be sensitive (p. 8) but do not have to be specific (p. 8), since further tests will confirm the provisional diagnosis.

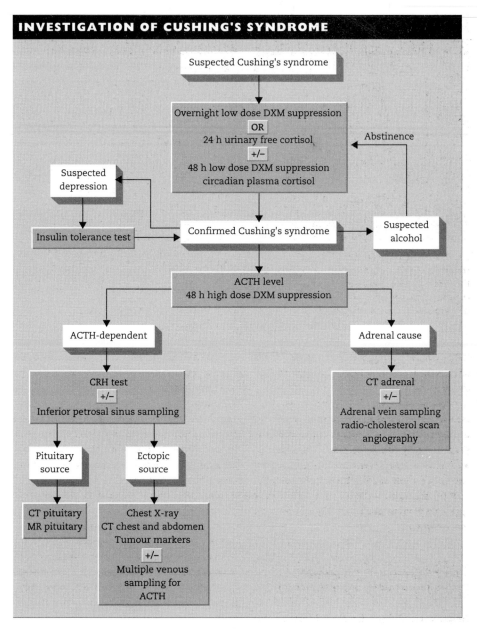

Fig. 16.4 Algorithm for the investigation of suspected Cushing's syndrome and elucidation of its cause. CRH, corticotrophin-releasing hormone; CT, computed tomography; DXM, dexamethasone; MR, magnetic resonance.

ADRENAL HYPERFUNCTION: BIOCHEMICAL TESTS

Test	Cushing's disease	Adrenal tumour	Ectopic ACTH-secreting tumour
Tests to confirm the diagnosis			
Serum [cortisol]	Increased	Increased	Increased
Dexamethasone, low-dose test	Not suppressed	Not suppressed	Not suppressed
Urinary cortisol*	Increased	Increased	Increased
Diurnal rhythm	Lost	Lost	Lost
Insulin-induced hypoglycaemia	No response	No response	No response
Tests to differentiate the cause			
Plasma [ACTH]	Normal or increased	Not detectable	Increased or much increased
Dexamethasone, high-dose test	Suppressed	Not suppressed	Not suppressed
CRH test (p. 212)	Increased response	No response	No response

*This test may be performed on a 24-hour collection of urine or on an early morning specimen when the results are expressed as the urinary cortisol : creatinine ratio.

Table 16.2 Results of hormonal tests in patients with adrenal hyperfunction.

The initial screening test for adrenocortical hyperfunction is a low-dose dexamethasone suppression test that can be performed on an out-patient basis. Measurement of urinary free cortisol is a less satisfactory alternative.

Low-dose dexamethasone suppression test

Dexamethasone suppresses the secretion of CRH (negative feedback – Fig. 16.2); ACTH and cortisol levels fall. In the *overnight suppression test*, the patient takes dexamethasone (1 mg) at 11–12 p.m. the night before attending the out-patient clinic. Serum [cortisol] is measured on a blood specimen the following morning at 8–9 a.m. A cortisol value of less than 50 nmol/L in this sample effectively excludes Cushing's syndrome. The *48-hour suppression test* is superior, but less convenient. Dexamethasone (0.5 mg) is taken every six hours, beginning at 9 a.m. on the first day, and serum [cortisol] is measured 48 hours later (interpretation as for overnight

test). The true-positive rate is reported to be better than 97%, with a false-negative rate of less than 1% for the 48-hour test.

Drugs that induce hepatic microsomal enzymes (e.g. phenytoin, phenobarbitone) may increase dexamethasone metabolism, with premature lowering of its blood level below that required to achieve suppression of CRH secretion (false-negative result).

Urinary free cortisol

This is an acceptable screening test, but it suffers from the disadvantage that an incomplete collection of urine may lead to a false-negative result. Cushing's syndrome is excluded if the excretion is <250 nmol/24 h. An alternative is to determine the urinary cortisol : creatinine ratio on an early morning specimen.

Interpretation of screening tests

The screening tests usually serve to distinguish simple non-endocrine obesity from obesity due to Cushing's syndrome. Abnormal results may, however, be obtained in depressed or extremely anxious patients, in the presence of severe intercurrent illness, or in alcoholism (pseudo-Cushing's syndrome). Further tests (on an in-patient basis) rule out pseudo-Cushing's syndrome and help determine the specific cause of the adrenocortical hyperfunction.

Confirmatory tests

In-patient tests that assist in the diagnosis of Cushing's syndrome include assessment of diurnal rhythm, which is lost early in the disease. Patients need to be hospitalized for at least 48 hours prior to stress-free venepuncture (e.g. in-dwelling catheter) to obtain meaningful results. It is also convenient to collect a series of 24-hour urine samples for urine free cortisol measurement.

Patients with pseudo-Cushing's syndrome may also show abnormal results in these further tests. However, in response to a hypoglycaemic stimulus, the pseudo-Cushing's patient will increase secretion of CRH, ACTH and cortisol; in true Cushing's syndrome, there is little or no response (see next section).

In alcoholism, other clues (e.g. raised mean cell volume, abnormal liver function tests) may be helpful; abstinence will lead to normalization of the hypothalamic–pituitary–adrenal axis.

Insulin hypoglycaemia test

This tests the integrity of the hypothalamic–pituitary–adrenal (HPA) axis, and is sometimes necessary to allow true Cushing's syndrome to be distinguished from depressive illness. The test is contraindicated in patients with epilepsy or heart disease.

Insulin is administered intravenously (typically 0.15 U/kg) to lower blood glucose to 2.2 mmol/L or less while monitoring serum cortisol. Samples for simultaneous measurement of glucose and cortisol are taken basally (before insulin) and at 30, 45, 60 and 90 min after intravenous insulin injection. The test requires close supervision, with glucose available for immediate injection if symptoms of severe hypoglycaemia develop. Failure to achieve a glucose level of 2.2 mmol/L invalidates the test, and

repetition, with insulin incremented in steps of 0.05 U/kg, may be necessary.

Interpretation of results. Serum [cortisol] normally reaches its maximum at 60 or 90 minutes, the level reached being at least 425 nmol/L with an increment above the basal (pre-insulin) level of at least 145 nmol/L. Patients with Cushing's syndrome, whatever the cause, do not respond normally to insulin-induced hypoglycaemia. There is often a high basal serum [cortisol] and usually little or no increase in serum [cortisol], despite the production of an adequate degree of hypoglycaemia.

Determining the cause of Cushing's syndrome

Once the diagnosis is established, other investigations may help to determine the cause (Table 16.2); difficulties sometimes arise in distinguishing between ectopic ACTH production and Cushing's disease. Biochemical results need to be considered together with the findings from other methods of investigation, particularly radiological – e.g. computed tomography (CT) scanning.

Plasma [ACTH]

Plasma [ACTH] should be measured on blood specimens collected both in the morning and the evening (e.g. at 8 a.m. and 10 p.m.).

If ACTH is undetectable, this is diagnostic of a functional adrenal tumour, and should be confirmed by an abdominal CT scan to detect an adrenal mass. Rare types of nodular adrenocortical disease (also ACTH-independent) are also described.

If the patient has Cushing's disease (pituitary-dependent Cushing's syndrome), ACTH will be present in plasma in normal or increased amounts, particularly in the evening specimen. Results for plasma [ACTH] overlap considerably for patients with Cushing's disease and ectopic ACTH secretion. However, a very high plasma [ACTH] points to an ectopic ('non-endocrine') origin.

The following additional tests are used to distinguish Cushing's disease from ectopic ACTH secretion.

High-dose dexamethasone suppression test

This uses 2 mg dexamethasone six-hourly for 48 hours in an attempt to suppress cortisol secretion. Basal (pre-dexamethasone) serum cortisol or 24-hour urine free cortisol is compared with the same at the end of the 48-hour period. Suppression is defined as a fall to less than 50% of basal value. An overnight suppression test using a single dose of 8 mg dexamethasone is reported to achieve similar diagnostic accuracy to the standard 48-hour high-dose test.

About 90% of patients with Cushing's disease show suppression of cortisol output. In contrast, only 10% of patients with ectopic ACTH production (or with adrenal tumours) show suppression.

CRH stimulation test

This test measures the ACTH and cortisol levels basally and 60 minutes after injection of 100 µg CRH. Most patients with Cushing's disease show normal or exaggerated ACTH and cortisol responses to human CRH, whereas patients with ectopic ACTH-secreting or adrenocortical tumours show no response. However, about 10% of patients with Cushing's disease fail to respond. False-positive responses in patients with ectopic ACTH production are unusual. Together, the high-dose dexamethasone suppression test and the CRH test provide almost 100% specificity and sensitivity in the diagnosis of Cushing's disease.

Finally, as many as 70% of patients with ectopic ACTH secretion also secrete one or more marker peptides (e.g. carcinoembryonic antigen, gastrin, somatostatin and calcitonin), so a peptide marker screen may assist in difficult cases.

Other chemical tests

Potassium. Hypokalaemic alkalosis may be a prominent feature of ectopic ACTH production, possibly due to the increased output of mineralocorticoids or high cortisol levels (with renal loss of K^+ and H^+ in the urine). Patients with Cushing's syndrome are often treated with diuretics (for hypertension and oedema), and this treatment may itself lower the plasma $[K^+]$.

Selective venous sampling. Blood specimens can be collected from selected sites for measurement of plasma [ACTH], to help identify the source of the ACTH (e.g. the inferior petrosal sinus : peripheral vein [ACTH] ratio, which increases on CRH injection, would support a pituitary source for the ACTH).

Pituitary function tests (Chapter 17) may be abnormal in Cushing's syndrome due to the suppressive effect of cortisol on the hypothalamus and pituitary. Luteinizing hormone (LH) and thyroid-stimulating hormone (TSH) responses to luteinizing hormone-releasing hormone (LH-RH) and to thyrotrophin-releasing hormone (TRH) are often impaired, and the increase in plasma [growth hormone] in response to hypoglycaemia is reduced.

Glucose tolerance test. Patients with adrenocortical hyperfunction may develop steroid-induced diabetes and have a diabetic type of response to an oral glucose tolerance test (p. 152).

Investigation of suspected adrenocortical hypofunction

Adrenocortical insufficiency may be primary (e.g. destruction of the gland itself by tuberculosis or autoimmune disease) or secondary (e.g. hypothalamic or pituitary disease leading to ACTH deficiency or after long-term steroid therapy). The causes are listed in Table 16.3.

In primary adrenal failure, patients present with lethargy, weakness, nausea and weight loss. They are typically hypotensive, with characteristic hyperpigmentation affecting the buccal mucosa, scars and skin creases. The condition may present itself when a patient suffers trauma, infection or undergoes surgery. Often there is hypoglycaemia with hyponatraemia, hyperkalaemia, raised serum urea levels and acid–base disturbance. The condi-

ADRENOCORTICAL HYPOFUNCTION

Primary adrenocortical insufficiency (Addison's disease)
1 Autoimmune adrenalitis
2 Infective (e.g. TB, CMV, histoplasmosis, meningococcal)
3 Secondary tumour deposits
4 Infiltrative lesions (e.g. amyloidosis, haemochromatosis)
5 Congenital adrenal hyperplasia or hypoplasia
6 Drugs (e.g. etomidate)

Secondary to pituitary disease
1 Congenital deficiency (isolated or with GH deficiency)
2 Pituitary tumours (functional or nonfunctional)
3 Infections (e.g. TB, syphilis)
4 Secondary tumour deposits
5 Vascular lesions (e.g. postpartum haemorrhage)
6 Trauma
7 Iatrogenic (e.g. surgery or radiotherapy)
8 Secondary to hypothalamic disease
9 Others

Table 16.3 Causes of adrenocortical hypofunction.

tion is life-threatening, and requires urgent investigation if suspected.

The hypotension and electrolyte abnormalities are generally less severe in secondary adrenal insufficiency with preservation of aldosterone secretion; the patient is typically pale. Where hypothalamic or pituitary disease is the cause, associated deficiency of other pituitary hormones may be found. An enlarging pituitary tumour often first affects gonadotrophin secretion (with loss of libido and secondary sexual characteristics), followed by loss of growth hormone, thyrotrophin and ACTH.

The diagnosis of adrenocortical hypofunction is relatively straightforward, once the suspicion of the condition arises. Patients should be immediately referred to hospital, and blood

should be collected for basal measurements of plasma urea, electrolytes, glucose, serum cortisol and plasma ACTH concentrations *before* the patient is given cortisol. Definitive tests for the diagnosis of this condition should be carried out later, after the crisis. A suggested plan of investigation is shown in Figure 16.5.

Diagnosis of primary adrenal hypofunction (Addison's disease)

Cortisol and ACTH measurements

A normal serum [cortisol] at 8 a.m. (or normal 24-hour urinary free cortisol) does *not* exclude Addison's disease; patients may be able to maintain a normal basal output but be unable to secrete adequate amounts of cortisol in response to stress. Nevertheless, a serum [cortisol] below 50 nmol/L at 8 a.m. is strong presumptive evidence for Addison's disease, whilst a value (at 8 a.m.) of 550 nmol/L or more (in the absence of steroid therapy) makes the diagnosis extremely unlikely. Simultaneous measurement of cortisol and ACTH improves diagnostic accuracy such that a low serum cortisol (< 200 nmol/L) and a raised ACTH (> 200 ng/L) is diagnostic of adrenal failure.

Short tetracosactrin (Synacthen) test

Stimulation of the adrenal cortex with synthetic ACTH (tetracosactrin, Synacthen) allows confirmation of the diagnosis of Addison's disease and an assessment of adrenocortical reserve. For patients with equivocal results, it allows a firm diagnosis to be made or dismissed. Basal cortisol is measured and a further measurement is taken 30 minutes after an intramuscular injection of 0.25 mg tetracosactrin.

A normal response is defined as a rise in serum [cortisol] to at least 500 nmol/L. A normal response excludes primary adrenocortical insufficiency. Conversely, failure of cortisol to respond to Synacthen, together with an elevated plasma ACTH, confirms primary adrenocortical insufficiency. Adrenocortical hypofunction secondary to hypothalamic or pituitary disease is also extremely unlikely if

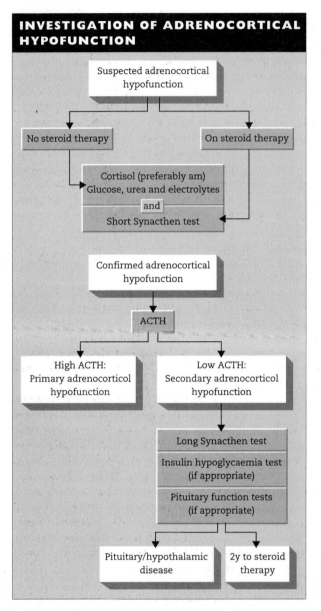

INVESTIGATION OF ADRENOCORTICAL HYPOFUNCTION

Suspected adrenocortical hypofunction

No steroid therapy

On steroid therapy

Cortisol (preferably am)
Glucose, urea and electrolytes
and
Short Synacthen test

Confirmed adrenocortical hypofunction

ACTH

High ACTH:
Primary adrenocorticol hypofunction

Low ACTH:
Secondary adrenocorticol hypofunction

Long Synacthen test

Insulin hypoglycaemia test (if appropriate)

Pituitary function tests (if appropriate)

Pituitary/hypothalamic disease

2y to steroid therapy

Fig. 16.5 Suggested plan of investigation of adrenocortical hypofunction.

the response is normal, since, in the prolonged absence of ACTH, the cells of the adrenal cortex would have atrophied.

Severe emotional stress, treatment with glucocorticoids within 12 hours prior to the tetracosactrin injection, and the taking of oestrogen-containing oral contraceptives may invalidate the test. Where a patient with suspected Addison's disease is receiving steroid therapy, a steroid that does not cross-react in the cortisol assay should be prescribed (e.g. dexamethasone). With this proviso, adrenal reserve in patients on steroid therapy can also be assessed using this test.

Diagnosis of secondary adrenocortical insufficiency

The finding of a low serum cortisol accompanied by a low plasma ACTH would support a diagnosis of adrenocortical insufficiency secondary to hypothalamic or pituitary disease. Whilst the atrophied adrenocortical cells fail to respond in the short Synacthen test, the gland can become responsive over a longer period of stimulation using the so-called depot (long) Synacthen test.

Depot (long) Synacthen test

Serum cortisol is measured on a basal sample and on further samples taken between five and eight hours after intramuscular injection of 1 mg depot Synacthen on each of three successive days. In Addison's disease, the cortisol fails to rise above 600 nmol/L at 5–8 hours after the third injection. In secondary adrenocortical insufficiency, a stepwise increase in the cortisol response after successive injections is observed. Poor responses to prolonged tetracosactrin tests may occur in patients with hypothyroidism (primary or secondary). In patients with hypothyroidism, adrenal function cannot be satisfactorily assessed until the thyroid deficiency has been corrected.

Patients who receive prolonged steroid therapy are at risk of secondary adrenal hypofunction on withdrawal of steroid treatment, and the same test can be used to assess their reserve. Occasionally, it may be necessary to test the full integrity of the hypothalamic–pituitary–adrenal axis using the insulin hypoglycaemia test (reducing insulin dose to 0.1 U/kg).

Other pituitary function tests

Other pituitary functions will almost certainly be abnormal by the time hypopituitarism is severe enough to produce adrenocortical hypofunction. It is usual in these patients, therefore, to measure basal concentrations of free T4 and TSH, LH and follicle-stimulating hormone (FSH) in plasma or serum and to investigate dynamic growth hormone responses in addition to the cortisol response.

Adrenal antibodies. A diagnosis of autoimmune Addison's disease can be made in patients who have idiopathic Addison's disease if they have adrenal antibodies in their serum.

Electrolytes. Electrolyte abnormalities are common. There is loss of Na^+ in urine, extracellular fluid volume depletion and there may be hyponatraemia, all of which can become severe in untreated patients, especially in Addisonian crisis. There is retention of K^+, with diminished urinary excretion and a tendency to hyperkalaemia. Acid–base disturbances are not usually observed unless complications develop (e.g. due to vomiting).

Hyperaldosteronism

Primary hyperaldosteronism (Conn's syndrome or low-renin hyperaldosteronism)

This is due to an adrenal adenoma (65% cases) or bilateral nodular hyperplasia (most remaining cases). Adrenal carcinoma is a very rare cause.

Conn's syndrome is a rare cause of hypertension. It may be suspected in a hypertensive patient with low plasma $[K^+]$, found in about 80–90% of such patients. $[K^+]$ depletion arises from renal losses, and may lead to muscle weakness and renal tubular defects; more severe hypokalaemia can lead to life-threatening cardiac arrhythmias. Other causes of hypertension with a reduced plasma $[K^+]$ need to be considered in the differential diagnosis (e.g. essential hypertension with *diuretic* therapy).

Secondary hyperaldosteronism

This is much more common, and is only sometimes associated with hypertension. It is due to conditions that stimulate the secretion of renin, often as a result of reduced renal Na^+ filtration (e.g. congestive heart failure, cirrhosis, Na^+ deprivation). These conditions are usually clearly diagnosed so further investigation of the renin–angiotensin–aldosterone system is not necessary. Probably the commonest cause of secondary hyperaldosteronism is diuretic therapy.

Investigation of primary hyperaldosteronism

Preliminary screening studies depend on the fact that aldosterone causes retention of Na^+ by the kidney, associated with loss of K^+ and H^+ in the urine. The changes in plasma $[K^+]$ are potentially of greatest diagnostic value.

Plasma potassium

This is the principal screening investigation. The patient should not be undergoing treatment with diuretics (which may lower plasma $[K^+]$). Liquorice or carbenoxolone preparations stimulate mineralocorticoid receptors directly, and must also be avoided. Ideally, plasma $[K^+]$ should be measured either before the patient starts treatment with hypotensive drugs or diuretics, or after the patient has been taken off such treatment (and off liquorice, etc.) for at least one month. Spuriously high plasma $[K^+]$ must be avoided by minimizing both venous stasis and forearm exercise during venepuncture. It is also important to measure *plasma* $[K^+]$, not serum $[K^+]$, in these patients.

In affected patients, plasma $[K^+]$ may be lower than 3.0 mmol/L, but values of 3.3 mmol/L and below should be regarded as suspicious. Plasma $[Na^+]$ may be slightly increased with a mild metabolic alkalosis, and urinary K^+ excretion may be inappropriately high for the degree of hypokalaemia.

Primary aldosteronism is occasionally associated with an intermittently reduced plasma $[K^+]$. If the first result is normal, but clinical suspicion is strong, plasma $[K^+]$ should be measured again after a few weeks. Such patients can also be placed on a high Na^+ intake (150–200 mmol/day) for two weeks, after which plasma $[K^+]$ is measured again.

Special investigations

Patients found to have hypokalaemia, or to develop hypokalaemia in the presence of an Na^+ load, require further investigation; other causes of hypokalaemia (e.g. diuretics, laxa-tives, liquorice) and secondary causes of hypertension should have been excluded.

Plasma renin activity (PRA). Primary hyperaldosteronism can be distinguished from secondary hyperaldosteronism by measuring either PRA or angiotensin II. PRA measurement is technically more straightforward, and has the theoretical advantage that its activity is rate-limiting in the formation of angiotensin II. Simultaneous measurement of aldosterone adds to the diagnostic value:

1 If PRA is *low*, the patient may have primary hyperaldosteronism. A high plasma [aldosterone] or 24-hour urinary excretion of aldosterone, or both, confirms the diagnosis. A high plasma [aldosterone] : PRA ratio in the supine position after an overnight fast has been reported to be more specific and sensitive for Conn's syndrome than other tests that were assessed.

2 If PRA is *high*, the patient has secondary hyperaldosteronism, and steps should be taken to identify its cause, if not already apparent.

Distinction between adenoma and hyperplasia

This is important, since adenomas are curable by surgery, whereas this is of no value in the treatment of adrenal hyperplasia. In general, hypokalaemia is more severe and aldosterone levels are higher with adenomas, which also tend to affect younger individuals. Imaging techniques may allow identification of an adenoma. The following biochemical investigations are relevant:

Adrenal vein sampling with measurement of the aldosterone : cortisol ratio can be used to localize an adenoma. If the patient has an adenoma, the aldosterone : cortisol ratio is higher in the adrenal vein draining this gland than in the inferior vena cava; the reverse is true for the suppressed, contralateral gland. The aldosterone : cortisol ratio is higher in *both* adrenal veins than in the inferior vena cava in patients with idiopathic adrenal hyperplasia.

A further test depends on the fact that the hyperplastic gland is still under some degree of renin-angiotensin control, whilst the adenoma is predominantly under ACTH control. Since ACTH levels are falling over the period 8 a.m. to 11.30 a.m., plasma [aldosterone] tends to fall over this period in the patient with an adenoma. In contrast, plasma [aldosterone] tends to rise when hyperplasia is the cause. For the test to be effective, the patient needs to be supine at 8 a.m., up and about before the 11.30 a.m. sample, and also 'volume-expanded'.

Inherited adrenocortical enzyme defects

Striking anatomical changes take place in the adrenal cortex immediately after birth; these

Fig. 16.6 Steroid biosynthetic pathway in the adrenal cortex. Enzymes are shown in italic, and major steroid products are shown in bold. The conversion of corticosterone to aldosterone is restricted to the zona glomerulosa.

are associated with marked alterations in the pattern of steroid output. There is a period of transition during the first six months of an infant's life, during which the pattern of fetal steroid metabolism changes to the normal childhood pattern, which closely resembles the adult pattern.

A number of enzyme deficiencies have been identified that are associated with abnormal steroid secretion or action. Figure 16.6 shows a simplified steroid biosynthetic pathway and some of the known sites of enzyme defect.

Congenital adrenal hyperplasia (CAH)

21-Hydroxylase deficiency (Fig. 16.6)
This is an autosomal recessive condition (about one in 10 000 live births in Caucasians) that may impair synthesis of cortisol and aldosterone. The low cortisol promotes ACTH secretion, so that the adrenal gland becomes hyperplastic. Severe cases show evidence of mineralocorticoid deficiency, with salt and

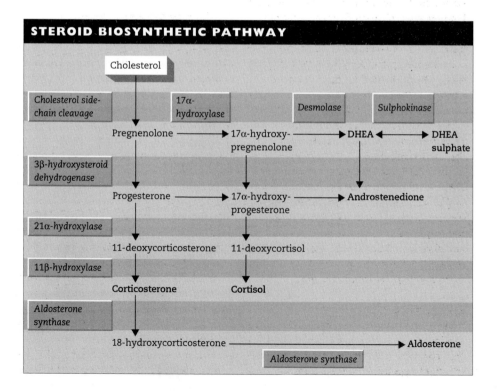

STEROID BIOSYNTHETIC PATHWAY

water loss and possible adrenal crisis. Steroids accumulate before the enzyme block, and are diverted to moderately strong androgens (e.g. androstenedione, which is metabolized to testosterone in peripheral tissues) with the possibility of virilization of the female fetus and precocious sexual development in the male. Late presentation (adult life) is also possible in less severe cases (p. 238).

The diagnosis can be established by measurement in plasma of 17-hydroxyprogesterone, or other steroids that accumulate before the block, and by gene probing for 21-hydroxylase. Treatment with glucocorticoids (e.g. cortisol) suppresses the excessive output of ACTH and limits the excessive androgen production. It may also be necessary to administer a mineralocorticoid.

Other enzyme defects in steroid metabolism

Deficiencies of other steroid pathway enzymes are described, but are rare. Inherited or acquired deficiencies in the enzyme that converts cortisol to cortisone (11β-hydroxysteroid dehydrogenase or 11β-HSD) lead to an interesting form of hypertension, the syndrome of apparent mineralocorticoid excess. Two forms of 11β-HSD are described, the liver or L form and the kidney or K form; the condition specifically affects the K form. The conversion of cortisol to cortisone is thought to be important in protecting the mineralocorticoid receptor from excess occupancy by cortisol (cortisone is a poor agonist for this receptor). Cortisol accumulates in the cell, and acts like a mineralocorticoid with accompanying hypertension and associated hypokalaemia. A similar picture can be produced by inhibiting the R enzyme by liquorice extracts.

Phaeochromocytoma

These tumours arise from chromaffin cells (90% are in the adrenal medulla; the rest can occur anywhere from the base of the brain to the testes). About 5% of tumours are bilateral and about 10% are malignant. They secrete excessive amounts of either noradrenaline or adrenaline (usually both) with increased excretion of catecholamines and their metabolites in the urine.

Phaeochromocytoma is a rare cause of hypertension (less than 0.1% of cases). Characteristically, this is episodic. Even when the hypertension is present all the time, episodic attacks of symptoms (e.g. headache, pallor, palpitations, sweating, panic attacks, abdominal pain) tend to occur. Such features are important when selecting the time for collecting specimens for laboratory investigation.

Phaeochromocytoma sometimes occurs as a familial condition, in association with the multiple endocrine neoplasia (MEN) IIa and IIb syndromes (p. 201).

Diagnosis

Urine tests

Chemical tests usually involve measurement of 24-hour urinary excretion of catecholamine metabolites: (i) metadrenaline and normetadrenaline or (ii) 4-hydroxy-3-methoxymandelic acid (HMMA), the metabolite normally excreted in the largest amount.

Measurement of 24-hour urinary metadrenaline and normetadrenaline (added together) has a sensitivity and specificity of about 90% and is preferred to measurement of HMMA, which is less accurate. Measurement of urinary free catecholamines by high-performance liquid chromatography (HPLC) is probably the most sensitive and specific method, but one that is not widely available.

Several points concerning the collection and timing of urine specimens for catecholamine investigations should be noted:

1 *Drugs* can increase (e.g. vasodilators) or decrease (e.g. reserpine) the release of catecholamines. Others affect their metabolism (e.g. monoamine oxidase inhibitors), or interfere with certain analytical methods (e.g. labetalol). Investigations for phaeochromocytoma should preferably be started *before* initiation of drug treatment.

2 *Diet.* Interference from dietary constituents is possible (e.g. HMMA measurement requires

the patient to be on a vanilla-free diet). Local laboratory requirements for any dietary restrictions should be consulted.

3 *Timing of urine collections* is important in order to minimize false-negative results. When the clinical index of suspicion is high:

Patients who have 'attacks'. If the patient is normotensive between attacks, a single baseline set of measurements should be made, and the patient should be instructed to start a second 24-hour urine collection when the next 'attack' occurs.

Patients with persistent hypertension. Determination of 24-hour urinary excretion of catecholamines or metabolites need only be performed once.

When the clinical index of suspicion is low (e.g. a middle-aged or elderly patient who is hypertensive, but without paroxysmal symptoms), there is little justification for requesting these investigations, which should be restricted to those with appropriate symptoms or young patients with hypertension.

Plasma catecholamines

In some studies, this assay has been found to be a more sensitive test for phaeochromocytoma than the urinary metabolite determinations just described, but this has not been a universal experience. The measurement is not widely available. Plasma and urinary measurements provide different information.

Urinary excretion of catecholamines and their metabolites relate to total catecholamine production during the collection period. Plasma measurements only reflect catecholamine output in the previous few minutes; plasma free noradrenaline has a half-life of about two minutes in plasma. Thus, if a tumour is secreting catecholamines intermittently, plasma measurements may fail to detect any abnormality, whereas results for urinary measurements may be abnormally high.

Plasma catecholamine measurements can be used to help localize an extra-adrenal phaeochromocytoma, by determining concentrations in blood specimens obtained from veins draining possible tumour sites. However, this is rarely needed, as CT scanning and magnetic resonance (MR) scanning are effective. Tumours may also be detected by radionuclide imaging.

KEY POINTS

1 Patients with suspected adrenocortical hyperfunction should be screened by the low-dose overnight or 48-hour dexamethasone suppression test, or measurement of urine free cortisol. A positive result requires confirmation (diurnal rhythm, serial 24-hour urine free cortisol measurements). Pseudo-Cushing's syndrome (severe depression, alcoholism, severe intercurrent illness) may need to be distinguished by the insulin hypoglycaemia test. Plasma adrenocorticotrophic hormone (ACTH) measurement, the high-dose dexamethasone suppression test and the corticotrophin-releasing hormone (CRH) test help establish the cause.

2 The diagnosis of primary adrenal hypofunction is best made by simultaneous measurement of cortisol and ACTH (early morning) followed by the short tetracosactrin (Synacthen) test. Secondary hypofunction is assessed by the long Synacthen test and tests of pituitary hormone reserve. Patients on long-term steroid therapy may require the whole axis tested with the insulin hypoglycaemia test.

3 Hyperaldosteronism is most commonly secondary (e.g. liver disease, congestive heart failure, kidney disease). Primary hyperaldosteronism (Conn's syndrome) is rare. Diagnosis is suspected in hypertensive patients with hypokalaemia (with no other explanation for low plasma K[+]). Confirmation is by measurement of plasma renin activity (PRA) and aldosterone.

4 Phaeochromocytoma is a catecholamine-secreting tumour of the adrenal medulla or extra-chromaffin tissue. It is a rare cause of hypertension. Biochemical diagnosis depends on measurement of certain urinary metabolites of catecholamines (e.g. the total metadrenaline and normetadrenaline) or urinary free catecholamines.

Case 16.1

A 34-year-old housewife was admitted to hospital with a provisional diagnosis of Cushing's syndrome. As an out-patient, her serum [cortisol] had not been suppressed when an overnight dexamethasone suppression test (1 mg dexamethasone) was performed. She was obese (weight 74 kg, height 1.7 m), hypertensive (blood pressure, 165/105 mmHg) and had wasting of the proximal limb muscles. The following results were obtained for adrenal function tests:

Test	Result			Interpretation
Diurnal rhythm of serum cortisol (nmol/L)	8 a.m.: 400			Ref. range: 150–550
	10 p.m.: 380			Ref. range: up to 200
Insulin hypoglycaemia test	Basal	Max. response		
Plasma [glucose] (mmol/L)	4.5	1.5		Should fall below 2.2
Serum [cortisol] (nmol/L)	435	480		Increment of at least 145 if response normal
Dexamethasone suppression test	Basal	After 48 h 0.5 mg q.i.d.	After 48 h 2.0 mg q.i.d.	
Serum [cortisol] (nmol/L)	420	410	500	See pages 210 and 212
Plasma [ACTH] (ng/L)	8 a.m.	<2		Ref. range: 7–51

How would you interpret these results?

Comments on Case 16.1

These results are consistent with a diagnosis of Cushing's syndrome due to an adrenal adenoma. These tumours account for 5–10 % of all cases of Cushing's syndrome.

Ultrasound examination, CT and 75Se-cholesterol scans confirmed the presence of a tumour in the right adrenal, and the patient was treated successfully by right adrenalectomy.

CHAPTER 17

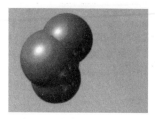

Hypothalamic and Pituitary Hormones

Hypothalamic and anterior
  pituitary hormones, 221
Thyrotrophin-releasing
  hormone and thyroid-
  stimulating hormone,
  221
Gonadotrophin-releasing

hormone (Gn-RH), FSH
  and LH, 222
Corticotrophin-releasing-
  hormone and
  adernocorticotrophic
  hormone, 222
Growth hormone, 223

Prolactin, 223
Anterior pituitary disease
  and its investigation, 225
Posterior pituitary
  hormones, 226
Vasopressin, 226

This chapter briefly describes the hypothalamic and pituitary hormones. Investigation of the function of these hormones is often intimately concerned with the investigation of the hormonal axes they control. Further information can be found in the chapters on thyroid hormones, the adrenal, and reproductive endocrinology.

Hypothalamic and anterior pituitary hormones

The hypothalamus secretes a number of hormones or factors that pass down the hypothalamo–hypophyseal portal blood vessels to the pituitary. They control the release of hormones from the anterior pituitary, in some cases by stimulating hormonal release and in others by inhibiting it (Table 17.1). The hormones produced by the target glands controlled by the anterior pituitary may exert negative feedback effects on the secretion of the corresponding hypothalamic hormone (e.g. plasma [free cortisol] influences the output of corticotrophinreleasing hormone, CRH). Release of hypothalamic hormones is also influenced by stimuli from higher central nervous system centres.

Thyrotrophin-releasing hormone and thyroid-stimulating hormone

Thyrotrophin-releasing hormone (TRH) is a tripeptide that controls the secretion of thyrotrophin or thyroid-stimulating hormone (TSH) by the anterior pituitary. Release of TRH is influenced by plasma free thyroid hormones, but thyroid hormones exert their main feedback effects directly on TSH secretion (Fig. 15.3).

TSH is a glycoprotein composed of an α-subunit that is common to luteinizing hormone (LH), follicle-stimulating hormone (FSH) and human chorionic gonadotrophin (hCG), and a β-subunit specific to TSH. The place of TSH measurements in the investigation of thyroid function is discussed in Chapter 15.

TRH test

The only indication for the TRH test is in distinguishing secondary hyperthyroidism (due to TSH-secreting tumour) from end-organ resistance to the action of thyroid hormones (due to a nuclear T3 receptor defect). Both of these conditions cause increased thyroid hormones with a slightly raised (or inappropriately normal) plasma [TSH], and the patients may appear clinically hyperthyroid.

In normal subjects, after intravenous TRH, serum [TSH] increases by more than 2 mU/L

HYPOTHALAMIC AND ANTERIOR PITUITARY HORMONES

Hypothalamic stimulating hormone or factor	Anterior pituitary hormone(s) released	Feedback control hormone or compound
Corticotrophin-releasing hormone (CRH)	ACTH, β-lipotrophin (LPH)	Cortisol
Growth hormone-releasing factor (GH-RF)	Growth hormone (GH)	GH release-inhibiting hormone
Gonadotrophin-releasing hormone (Gn-RH)	Follicle-stimulating hormone (FSH)	Gonadal steroids and inhibin
	Luteinizing hormone (LH)	Gonadal steroids
No stimulating factor identified	Prolactin	Dopamine
Thyrotrophin-releasing hormone (TRH)	TSH (and prolactin)	Free T4, free T3

Table 17.1 Hypothalamic and anterior pituitary hormones and factors.

above the basal level at 20 min and returns towards the basal value at 60 min. Patients with T3-receptor defects show a TSH response in a TRH test, and partial suppression of T4 and TSH after T3 administration. These responses are not seen in TSH-secreting tumours. Also, serum [α-subunits] of TSH are increased, often markedly, in patients with thyrotroph adenomas, whereas normal concentrations are present in patients with abnormal receptors. (See also Chapter 15.)

There is no increase in the [TSH] response to TRH in patients with primary hyperthyroidism, and an absent response may also occur in hypopituitarism. In hypothyroidism, the response is exaggerated, whilst a normal response is found in about 50% of patients with pituitary disease.

Gonadotrophin-releasing hormone (Gn-RH), FSH and LH

Gn-RH is a decapeptide released from the hypothalamus in pulses into the hypothalamic–hypophyseal portal circulation. The release of Gn-RH is modified by oestrogens, progesterone and androgens. A Gn-RH test similar to the TRH test has been used to investigate gonadotrophin reserve.

Gn-RH test

In the Gn-RH test, blood samples are obtained before, and 20 and 60 min after, giving the patient an intravenous injection of Gn-RH. This test is often normal even in the presence of clinical hypogonadism. There is no point in performing the test when there are raised basal gonadotrophin levels, indicating primary gonadal failure. Subnormal responses may be seen in Cushing's syndrome as well as in hypopituitarism. (See also Chapter 18.)

Corticotrophin-releasing-hormone and adrenocorticotrophic hormone

Corticotrophin-releasing hormone (CRH) is composed of 41 amino acids, and is the main factor involved in the control of the pituitary–adrenal axis. Its release is subject to negative feedback control by plasma [free cortisol] (Fig. 16.2).

Adrenocorticotrophic hormone (ACTH) is a polypeptide of 39 amino acids. Its biological activity is contained in the 24 amino acids at the N-terminal end. The major activity of ACTH is the stimulation of adrenal steroid synthesis, especially that of the glucocorticoid, cortisol, but it also plays a permissive role in the synthesis of aldosterone. ACTH also stimulates melanocytes to produce melanin. This is the cause of the increased pigmentation seen in patients with ACTH-driven causes of Cushing's syndrome, in adrenocortical hypofunction, and in Nelson's syndrome.

ACTH and β-lipotrophin (β-LPH) exist next to each other at the C-terminal end of a much larger precursor molecule, pro-opiomelanocortin. In ectopic ACTH production, it seems that there is abnormal processing of pro-opiomelanocortin resulting in the release of 'big ACTH'.

Growth hormone

Growth hormone (GH) is a polypeptide, structurally similar to prolactin and human placental lactogen. It stimulates protein synthesis and growth, and also has metabolic effects that oppose the action of insulin.

Release of GH is stimulated by GH-releasing hormone (GH-RH, a 44 amino acid peptide) and inhibited by somatostatin (a 14 amino acid peptide). Somatostatin inhibits the release of several pituitary hormones, including GH and TSH. GH secretion occurs in pulses, mainly at night. Only infrequent small pulses occur during the day. Measurement of basal plasma [GH] is of little value, since during much of the day levels are undetectable.

GH release is suppressed by high doses of glucose, and this response is used in the investigation of suspected acromegaly and gigantism. Conversely, increases in plasma [GH] can be caused by stress, exercise, a fall in blood [glucose], fasting and certain amino acids. This forms the basis of investigations for inadequate GH secretion.

Tests of growth hormone reserve

The insulin stress test is the traditional test for the assessment of GH reserve, as well as for the hypothalamic–pituitary–adrenal axis. It is used for the investigation of suspected hypopituitarism in adults and of short stature in children. The test is performed as described on p. 211, but the initial dose of insulin is reduced to 0.10 U/kg. Normally, hypoglycaemia causes a marked increase in plasma [GH] to more than 20 mU/L, but this increase is not observed in severe pituitary dysfunction. A limited response, with plasma [GH] rising to less than

20 mU/L, may be observed in patients with partial pituitary failure.

In an attempt to avoid insulin stress tests, a number of other physiological and pharmacological tests of GH secretion are used, especially in children. These include measurements during the hours of sleep, the response to standardized exercise, or to administration of glucagon, clonidine or arginine. All these tests are associated with rather variable responses, and their choice depends on local preferences.

Children of both sexes show subnormal responses to hypoglycaemia and other dynamic tests in the years just before puberty. The response should be restored by priming with gonadal steroids before performing the test.

Acromegaly and gigantism

These disorders are caused by adenomas of the anterior pituitary. Gigantism results if the disorder occurs before closure of the epiphyses of the long bones, acromegaly if it occurs after their closure.

Basal plasma [GH] is often very high in these patients, but the concentrations are too variable for accurate diagnosis, which should be made by measuring the response of plasma [GH] to an oral glucose tolerance test (p. 152). Normally, plasma [GH] falls to less than 2 mU/L at some time during this test. However, in patients with acromegaly or gigantism, plasma [GH] does not fall in response to the stimulus of hyperglycaemia, and may even increase.

Prolactin

This hormone is distinct from growth hormone, but the two have some common structural features. Prolactin is a single polypeptide, secreted by the lactotrophs. It is responsible for lactation, and has a role in the complex processes controlling gonadal function.

Prolactin secretion is unusual in being under inhibitory control by dopamine. There is a diurnal rhythm of prolactin secretion, with the highest levels occurring during sleep and the lowest between 9 a.m. and noon. Superimposed on these gradual changes, there are occasional sharp (pulsatile) increases in plasma [prolactin]. Prolactin secretion increases in response to oestrogens, suckling and stress. It can therefore be difficult to interpret the results of single measurements. Plasma [prolactin] is higher in women of child-bearing age, especially during pregnancy, than it is in girls before puberty, in postmenopausal women, or in males.

Stimulation or suppression tests are not required. Basal [prolactin] gives full information, but, since levels vary from day to day, two or three samples should be obtained before making a firm diagnosis or instituting treatment.

There are many causes of hyperprolactinaemia other than pituitary disease (Table 17.2). Before collecting blood for measuring plasma [prolactin], it is particularly important to enquire about the intake of drugs.

Prolactin measurements should be performed in the investigation of amenorrhoea, oligomenorrhoea and subfertility, whether or not there is galactorrhoea (pp. 233, 236). It should also be measured in any patient with spontaneous inappropriate lactation. A significant proportion of subfertile female patients have hyperprolactinaemia, and may respond to treatment with bromocriptine, a dopamine agonist.

Hyperprolactinaemia and pituitary tumours

Plasma [prolactin] greater than 700 mU/L (reference range 60–390 mU/L) may indicate the presence of a pituitary tumour. However, before this interpretation is made, the possibility of other nonpathological causes of a raised level should be considered (Table 17.2), and the measurement should be repeated, since a high result may represent a response to stress.

Pituitary tumours may secrete prolactin directly (prolactinoma) or, alternatively, a non-prolactin-secreting tumour may give rise to hyperprolactinaemia because the tumour exerts pressure on the pituitary stalk and prevents dopamine from reaching the pituitary from the hypothalamus.

Prolactin is the only hormone secreted by prolactinomas, although increased plasma

HYPERPROLACTINAEMIA

Category of cause	Examples
Physiological	Pregnancy
	Suckling
	Stress
Drugs	
(a) Dopamine receptor–blocking agents	Phenothiazines
	Butyrophenones
	Tricyclic antidepressants
	Metoclopramide
(b) Dopamine-depleting drugs	Methyldopa
	Reserpine
(c) Histamine-receptor agonists	Cimetidine
(d) Monoamine oxidase inhibitors	Phenelzine
Pathological	Prolactinoma
	Other pituitary tumours
	Idiopathic
	Chronic renal failure
	Primary hypothyroidism

Table 17.2 Causes of hyperprolactinaemia.

[prolactin] also occurs in some patients with acromegaly, when there is a tumour that secretes both GH and prolactin. Approximately one-third of prolactinomas are associated with only moderate increases in plasma [prolactin], in the range 700–1000 mU/L, but basal levels of plasma [prolactin] greater than 1000 mU/L strongly suggest that a tumour is present. If, in addition, radiological abnormalities are visible in the pituitary fossa, this supports the diagnosis of prolactinoma rather than functional hyperprolactinaemia in these patients. Also, some ectopic hormone-secreting tumours produce prolactin.

Anterior pituitary disease and its investigation

A wide range of conditions can affect the anterior pituitary and result in hypopituitarism either directly or through an effect on the hypothalamus (Table 17.3). The most common causes of hypopituitarism are pituitary tumour, particularly prolactin-secreting tumours, and therapeutic action such as the removal of a pituitary tumour or irradiation. Failure may be total (panhypopituitarism) or partial, in which case secretion of one or more pituitary hormones is retained.

Most pituitary adenomas produce a single hormone in excess. Pressure effects may decrease secretion of other pituitary hormones so in all patients where the presence of an adenoma has been established, overall pituitary function should be assessed.

Initially, impairment of function may only be revealed by the use of stimulation tests. Later, basal concentrations of the pituitary hormones in blood will be affected. In general, the secretion of GH, LH and FSH are affected relatively early in disease involving the anterior pituitary, whereas ACTH, TSH and prolactin are not affected until much later.

The wide variety of tests available, and controversy regarding the use and interpretation of some of them, mean that the way in which pituitary function is assessed is often a matter for clinical and personal judgement. The following is a suggestion for the initial investigation of a patient with suspected pituitary disease. Further tests may be required, depending on the results and the clinical circumstances.

1 Basal measurements provide useful diagnostic information, and should be performed first. A basal 9 a.m. blood sample should be obtained for measurement of cortisol, T4 (free or total), TSH, testosterone or oestradiol depending on sex, LH and FSH, and prolactin. Serum and urine osmolalities should also be measured if there is clinical suspicion of posterior pituitary dysfunction.

2 If plasma [cortisol] is less than 100 nmol/L,

Table 17.3 Causes of hypopituitarism.

HYPOPITUITARISM	
Category of cause	Examples
Tumours	Pituitary adenoma, craniopharyngioma primary or secondary cerebral tumours
Granulomatous disease	Sarcoidosis
Vascular disease	Severe hypotension, cranial arteritis, infarction, especially of pre-existing tumour, postpartum necrosis (Sheehan's syndrome)
Trauma	
Infection	Meningitis, especially tuberculous
Iatrogenic	Surgery, radiotherapy, prolonged steroid treatment causing ACTH deficiency
Hypothalamic disorders	Tumours, impaired secretion of hypothalamic releasing hormones, functional disturbances as in starvation and anorexia nervosa

as long as the patient is not on steroids, and Addison's disease is not a possibility, ACTH deficiency can be assumed, and an insulin stress test is contra-indicated.

3 Thyroid and ACTH deficiencies identified on the basal sample should be treated before any further investigation. Hypothyroidism reduces the ACTH and GH responses to an insulin stress test.

4 If the patient is of normal stature, there is no other clinical evidence of pituitary disease, the thyroid and gonadal axes and osmolalities are normal, and plasma [cortisol] is greater than 400 nmol/L, pituitary function can be assumed to be normal. If plasma [cortisol] is 100–400 nmol/L, proceed to a Synacthen test, and then to an insulin stress test if the result is equivocal.

5 If there is strong clinical evidence for pituitary disease likely to cause hypopituitarism, or there are basal deficiencies, perform an insulin stress test to assess ACTH and GH reserve, unless there is a contraindication. If there is a contraindication, or in patients with acromegaly (where GH deficiency is not a consideration), perform a Synacthen test.

6 If symptoms or basal osmolalities suggest it is needed, perform a water deprivation test. Any identified ACTH deficiency should first have been corrected by administration of cortisol.

Combined pituitary function test

When hypopituitarism is thought to be very likely, a combined test of pituitary function can be performed to assess the anterior pituitary reserve for ACTH, GH, FSH and LH production. In this test, blood is collected for measurement of glucose (to assess hypoglycaemic response in the test) and basal serum FSH, LH, oestradiol or testosterone, cortisol, TSH, T4, GH and prolactin concentrations. Insulin (0.10 U/kg), TRH (200 μg) and GnRH (50 μg) are injected, and further blood specimens are collected at 20, 30, 60, 90 and 120 minutes. Responses in this combined function test are interpreted in the same way as when the tests are performed separately. This test is now infrequently performed, with investigation being more tailored to the individual clinical circumstances and the results of basal measurements.

Posterior pituitary hormones

The posterior pituitary is an integral part of the neurohypophysis. Its secretion is directly subject to nervous control. It produces at least two hormones, vasopressin (antidiuretic hormone, ADH), and oxytocin. Oxytocin is involved in control of uterine contraction and milk release from the lactating breast. Disorders of oxytocin secretion are uncommon and not clinically important.

Vasopressin

Vasopressin has an important role in the control of the tonicity of extracellular fluid and hence of water balance. It is a nonapeptide synthesized in the hypothalamus. Neurosecretory granules containing vasopressin combined with neurophysin II migrate to the posterior pituitary. Vasopressin is released in response either to a rise in plasma osmolality or to a fall in extracellular fluid volume. It increases the permeability of the distal tubules and collecting ducts of the kidney to water.

The syndrome of inappropriate secretion of ADH (SIADH) is defined as the excessive secretion of vasopressin (or ADH) in the absence of the normal major stimuli for vasopressin secretion. SIADH is considered in more detail on p. 22.

Deficiency of vasopressin gives rise to cranial diabetes insipidus. It is either primary (idiopathic, familial) or secondary to disease or injury in or close to the pituitary. Deficiency of vasopressin may be the sole hormonal abnormality, or there may also be disturbances of anterior pituitary hormone production in patients with secondary vasopressin deficiency. Recognition of hyposecretion of vasopressin depends on urine concentration tests, i.e. the fluid deprivation test and the DDAVP test (pp. 56, 57). Measurements of plasma [vasopressin] are not usually required.

KEY POINTS

1 Pituitary function may initially be assessed by measuring basal plasma cortisol, T4, TSH, testosterone, oestradiol, LH, FSH, prolactin. If these are all normal, no further tests are usually needed, but if clinical suspicion is high or one or more abnormal results are found, stimulation tests may be necessary, e.g. Synachthen test or insulin stress test.

2 Posterior pituitary dysfunction should be investigated initially by measuring basal serum and urine osmolalities. A water deprivation test may be needed subsequently.

3 In children with short stature, the insulin stress test is usually avoided. A number of other tests of GH secretion are used instead including measurements of GH during sleep or in response to exercise, or to administration of glucagon, clonidine or arginine.

4 In acromegaly, basal plasma [GH] is often very high but the concentrations are too variable for accurate diagnosis. The failure of plasma [GH] to fall to less than 2 mU/L in an oral glucose tolerance test is a more reliable test.

5 Prolactin measurements help in the diagnosis of amenorrhoea, oligomenorrhoea and subfertility, and in spontaneous inappropriate lactation.

6 Plasma [prolactin] greater than 700 mU/L may indicate the presence of a pituitary tumour, but also may be due to stress, drugs or other causes.

Case 17.1

A 56-year-old bank manager complained to his general practitioner of excessive sweating which was embarrassing him during meetings with clients. His general practitioner had known him over many years, although had not seen him recently, and thought that his facial features had become coarser over this period. Closer questioning revealed that he had recently had to buy new shoes since his old ones were becoming tight, and that he had experienced problems with impotence over the past few months. Examination revealed hypertension and glucosuria.

He was referred to an endocrine clinic with a presumptive diagnosis of acromegaly. Basal investigations on a sample taken at 9 a.m. were as follows:

Analyte	Result	Reference range
Cortisol (nmol/L)	625	160–565
Free T4 (pmol/L)	18	9–23
TSH (mU/L)	1.3	0.15–3.5
Testosterone (nmol/L)	7	10–30
LH (U/L)	1.1	1.5–9.0
FSH (U/L)	1.4	1.5–9.0
Prolactin (mU/L)	960	60–390

A glucose tolerance test was performed:

Time (minutes)	Glucose (mmol/L)	GH (mU/L)
0	9.2	25
30	15.8	22
60	14.1	20
90	13.6	22
120	13.5	21

Continued on p. 228

Case 17.1 *continued*

Visual fields were normal, and a magnetic resonance imaging (MRI) scan revealed the appearance of a small adenoma, confined within the pituitary gland.

Comments on Case 17.1

The strong clinical suspicion of acromegaly is confirmed by the lack of suppression of GH during the glucose tolerance test. The glucose tolerance test also confirms the patient to have diabetes, due to the diabetogenic actions of GH. Abnormal glucose tolerance is seen in about a quarter of patients with acromegaly, impaired glucose tolerance being slightly commoner among these than frank diabetes.

Gonadotrophins and testosterone are low, confirming gonadal failure secondary to the pituitary lesion, rather than primary testicular failure.

The prolactin is elevated. Some GH-secreting adenomas also secrete prolactin. Alternatively, the adenoma may be interfering with the inhibitory control of prolactin secretion by dopamine.

The basal results suggest that the function of the adrenal and thyroid axes is normal.

Case 17.2

A 26-year-old woman attended an out-patient clinic with a complaint of galactorrhoea for several months. Her only other medical history was of troublesome migraines since childhood, for which she had taken a variety of medications whose names she could not remember. On examination, it was possible to express milk from her breasts.

Investigations were unremarkable apart from: prolactin 1127 mU/L (reference range 60–390 mU/L).

Comments on Case 17.2

Closer questioning revealed that her migraine treatment had been changed some months previously to a preparation that combined an analgesic (paracetamol) and anti-emetic (metoclopramide). Metoclopramide can cause hyperprolactinaemia through its antidopaminergic activity.

The patient stopped this preparation, and took paracetamol alone. The galactorrhoea and hyperprolactinaemia resolved.

Case 17.3

A 58-year-old man saw his general practitioner for review of his hypertension. He mentioned problems with impotence and decreased libido, which he ascribed to his antihypertensive medication (a β-blocker), having read the package insert containing information for patients. However, further questioning revealed that the patient was now shaving only once a week. Examination revealed pallor and loss of axillary and pubic hair.

The results of baseline blood tests were as follows:

Test	Result	Reference range
Cortisol (nmol/L)	90	160–565
TSH (mU/L)	0.3	0.3–5.0
Free T4 (pmol/L)	8	10–27
Testosterone (nmol/L)	4	10–30
LH (U/L)	1.0	1.5–9.0
FSH (U/L)	0.9	1.5–9.0
Prolactin (mU/L)	40	60–390

Continued on p. 229

Case 17.3 *continued*

What do these results show? What further investigations are required?

Comments on Case 17.3

The history, physical signs and hypofunction of multiple endocrine glands suggest hypopituitarism. In the presence of the other biochemical findings and the pallor, primary adrenal failure is unlikely to be the cause of the low plasma [cortisol]. This is due to ACTH deficiency. The thyroid function tests show insufficiency secondary to pituitary insufficiency, and the low gonadotrophins and testosterone confirm secondary gonadal failure.

The biochemical results are sufficiently informative for there to be no need for further biochemical investigation, although plasma [ACTH] or a Synacthen test could be used to confirm ACTH deficiency. Radiological investigation of the pituitary using computed tomography (CT) or MRI scanning is indicated.

The patient can be treated with cortisol, and, in due course, thyroxine and testosterone. Although there is nothing in the history to suggest posterior pituitary insufficiency (diabetes insipidus), this may be unmasked by cortisol treatment. The patient may need investigation using a water deprivation test.

CHAPTER 18

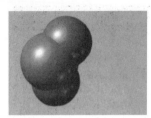

Gonadal Function, Steroid Contraceptives and Pregnancy

Male gonadal function, 230
Investigation of infertility and
   male hypogonadism, 231

Female gonadal function, 233
Pregnancy and the
   fetoplacental unit, 239

Infertility in women and menstrual irregularities are relatively common clinical problems. They often have an endocrine cause and result from abnormal ovarian, thyroid, pituitary or adrenal function. The laboratory can help with the diagnosis of these endocrine abnormalities. Biochemical tests are also useful in screening hirsute women for the presence of occult ovarian or adrenal tumours. Endocrine causes of male infertility are rare, but biochemical tests do play an important role in assessing such patients.

Biochemical tests are also used for screening for neural tube defects and Down's syndrome in pregnant women at 16–18 weeks' gestation.

This chapter outlines the function of the hypothalamic pituitary gonadal axis, and describes the biochemical tests that are required for the investigation of infertility, menstrual disorders and hirsutism. Guidance on the correct interpretation of the test employed is also provided. The role of biochemical tests in pregnancy is also discussed.

Male gonadal function

Spermatogenesis and its control

Spermatogenesis takes place in the seminiferous tubules, and requires normal functioning of both the Leydig and the Sertoli cells. Leydig cells produce testosterone, the principal androgen under the control of luteinizing hormone (LH). Sertoli cells provide other testicular cells with nutrients, and also produce several regulatory proteins, of which inhibin and androgen-binding protein (ABP) are the best characterized. Sertoli cell function is regulated by follicle-stimulating hormone (FSH).

The entire hypothalamic–pituitary–testicular axis (Fig. 18.1) must be functioning normally for spermatogenesis. Gonadotrophin-releasing hormone (Gn-RH) from the hypothalamus stimulates release of LH and FSH; its effects on LH release are more marked than on FSH release. The secretion of Gn-RH, and thus of LH, occurs in pulses; the secretion of FSH is less markedly pulsatile. The amplitude and frequency of the pulses of LH release appear to be important in exerting effects on testosterone production.

The secretion of LH is under negative feedback control from plasma [free testosterone], and the release of FSH is inhibited by inhibin. High testicular [testosterone] is ensured by the anatomical proximity of Leydig, Sertoli and spermatogenic cells, and by the local release of ABP.

Transport and metabolism of testosterone

In the circulation, about 65% of testosterone is bound to sex hormone–binding globulin (SHBG) and 30% to albumin. It is the free (unbound) fraction that gains access to tissues and exerts its biological activity. Target tissues for androgens have high-affinity cytosolic receptors that transport androgens into the

HYPOTHALMIC-PITUITARY-TESTICULAR AXIS

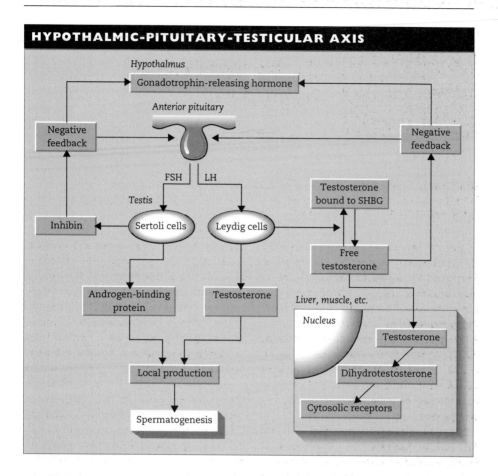

Fig. 18.1 The hypothalmic–pituitary–testicular axis. SHBG, sex hormone–binding globulin.

cell nucleus; these receptors can bind other androgens besides testosterone.

In many tissues, testosterone is converted to the more biologically active compound 5α-dihydrotestosterone (5α-DHT) by 5α-reductase.

Investigation of infertility and male hypogonadism

Endocrine causes of subfertility are rare in men. Most infertile males are eugonadal, with oligospermia due to failure of the seminiferous tubules. In the eugonadal male with a normal sperm count, no endocrine investigations are required. Causes of male hypogonadism are given in Table 18.1.

If the sperm count is low, on two occasions, measurements of plasma LH, FSH, and testosterone concentrations should be made to determine whether hypogonadism is caused by a primary defect in the testes or in the hypothalamic–pituitary region. Both forms lead to infertility (Fig. 18.2). Plasma [prolactin] should be determined (p. 223), as hyperprolactinaemia can lead to hypogonadism and impotence.

Misleadingly high values for LH and FSH might be observed because of pulsatile release. Plasma [total testosterone] results are affected by changes in plasma [SHBG], but plasma [free testosterone] or the free androgen index can

CAUSES OF MALE HYPOGONADISM

Primary hypogonadism

Congenital
Klinefelter's syndrome
Androgen resistance
Androgen synthesis defects
Anorchia

Acquired lesion
Epididimo-orchitis (e.g. mumps)
Testicular torsion
Trauma

Systemic disease
Liver disease
Renal disease
Dystrophia myotonica

Secondary hypogonadism
Hypothalamic–pituitary disease
Isolated GnRH deficiency
Panhypopituitarism
Destructive pituitary tumour
Cushing's syndrome
Hyperprolactinaemia

Table 18.1 Causes of hypogonadism in the male.

be estimated by determining both plasma [total testosterone] and [SHBG] and calculating plasma [free testosterone] from these.

Hypergonadotrophic and hypogonadotrophic hypogonadism

Primary gonadal failure: hypergonadotrophic hypogonadism

The primary abnormality is in the testes, and plasma [testosterone] is reduced whilst gonadotrophins are increased. This group of conditions includes congenital defects such as Klinefelter's syndrome (usually 47XXY) and acquired lesions due to drugs, viruses, or systemic diseases that affect testicular function.

Hypothalamic–pituitary disease: hypogonadotrophic hypogonadism

The primary abnormality is in the hypothalamus or the pituitary; the deficiency may be part of a generalized failure of pituitary hormone production. Cushing's syndrome may also be the cause. Plasma gonadotrophins and [testosterone] are both reduced.

Human chorionic gonadotrophin (hCG), injected daily for several days, can be used to help differentiate between hypergonadotrophic (primary) and hypogonadotrophic

(secondary) hypogonadism. A failure to show a rise in plasma [testosterone] suggests an absence of functioning testicular tissue.

Disorders of male sex differentiation

Many conditions have been described, all rare. In some, the gonads degenerate; in others, there is an enzyme defect affecting steroid synthesis. In a third group, there is androgen resistance at the end organ, and a fourth group consists of the true hermaphrodites.

The testicular feminization syndrome is probably due to a receptor defect or end-organ resistance to androgens; plasma [testosterone] is abnormally high. In many of the other conditions, plasma [testosterone] is low, both in childhood and in adult life.

Gynaecomastia in males

Breast development occurring in males other than during puberty usually has a pathological cause. The principal causes are conditions that lead to an imbalance of oestrogen and androgens. These include decreased androgen activity in hypogonadism, and increased oestrogen production resulting from a variety of endocrine tumours; these tumours may synthesize oestrogens or secrete hCG, which then acts as a stimulus of oestrogen production. Various drugs with anti-androgen activity or oestrogenic activity may also cause gynaecomastia.

INVESTIGATION OF MALE INFERTILITY

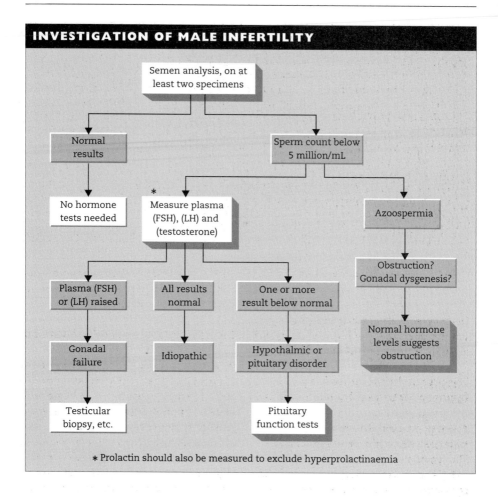

Fig. 18.2 The investigation of male infertility.
* Prolactin should also be measured to exclude hyperprolactinaemia.

These patients require full endocrine investigation, including measurement of plasma oestrogens, androgens, gonadotrophins and prolactin.

Female gonadal function

Menstrual disorders and infertility

The changes that occur in normal menstrual cycles depend on cyclical variations in the output of FSH and LH, influenced by the output of Gn-RH. The effects of Gn-RH on LH and FSH release, in terms of the amounts secreted at different stages of the menstrual cycle, are strongly influenced by negative feedback control effects exerted by oestradiol-17β and progesterone.

The developing Graafian follicles in the ovaries respond to the cyclical stimulus of gonadotrophins by secreting two oestrogens, oestradiol-17β and oestrone; these are metabolized to a third oestrogen, oestriol. After ovulation, the corpus luteum secretes progesterone as well as oestrogens. The changes in the uterus are determined by the ovarian steroid output at each stage. These changes are modified if pregnancy occurs.

Changes in plasma concentrations of FSH, LH and the principal gonadal steroids in the

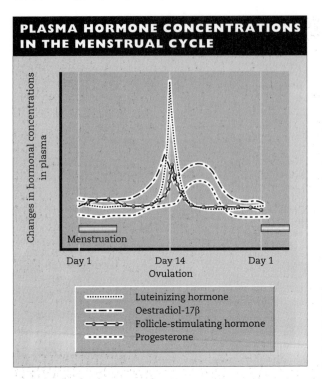

PLASMA HORMONE CONCENTRATIONS IN THE MENSTRUAL CYCLE

Menstruation

Day 1   Day 14   Day 1
                 Ovulation

.... Luteinizing hormone
— · — · —   Oestradiol-17β
—○—○—○—   Follicle-stimulating hormone
— — — — —   Progesterone

Fig. 18.3 Cyclical changes in the plasma concentrations of the pituitary gonadotrophins and the principal ovarian steroid sex hormones in a normal 28-day menstrual cycle.

normal menstrual cycle (i.e. a cycle unmodified by oral contraceptives) are shown diagrammatically in Figure 18.3. Reference ranges for these hormones are given in Table 18.2.

Oestrogens act on several target tissues, including the uterus, vagina and breast; progesterone mainly acts on the uterus, and is essential for the maintenance of early pregnancy. Both oestrogens and progesterone are important in the control of the hypothalamic–pituitary–ovarian axis. Oestradiol-17β may stimulate or inhibit the secretion of gonadotrophins, depending on its concentration in plasma; the stimulating effect of oestradiol-17β can be prevented by high plasma [progesterone].

Ovarian dysfunction and its investigation

The relationships between the hypothalamus, pituitary and ovary in the control of gonadal function mean that abnormality in any of these organs may cause abnormal menstruation and infertility. Other endocrine diseases (e.g. Cushing's syndrome, thyroid disease) can also have these effects.

Oligomenorrhoea and amenorrhoea

Women with oligomenorrhoea or amenorrhoea may present because of concerns they have regarding their bleeding pattern, infertility, hirsutism, virilism, or a combination of these.

Physiological causes of amenorrhoea (pregnancy, lactation) and anatomical abnormalities should first be excluded as the possible cause. Amenorrhoea may be primary, i.e. the patient has never menstruated, in which case abnormal development is a likely cause, or secondary to various causes (Table 18.3).

Measurements of plasma concentrations of prolactin, FSH, LH, oestradiol-17β, thyroid-stimulating hormone (TSH) and free T4 are required. In addition, plasma testosterone, androstenedione and dehydroepiandrosterone sulphate (DHAS) concentrations may need to

GONADOTROPHINS AND SEX HORMONES IN PLASMA

Hormone	Males	Menstruating female			Postmenopausal
		Early follicular	Mid-cycle	Luteal	
Follicle-stimulating hormone (IU/L)	1.5–9.0	3.0–15.0	<20	3.0–15.0	30–115
Luteinizing hormone (IU/L)	1.5–9.0	2.5–9.0	<90	2.5–9.0	30–115
Oestradiol-17β (pmol/L)	<200	110–180	550–1650	370–700	<100
Progesterone (nmol/L)		In peak luteal phase (days 18–24), a progesterone greater than 30 nmol/L indicates normal cycle; levels less than 10 nmol/L indicate anovulatory cycle			
Testosterone (nmol/L)	10–30	0.4–2.8			

Table 18.2 Reference ranges in men and women for the plasma concentrations of the pituitary gonadotrophins and of the principal sex hormones (data kindly provided by Dr J. Seth and Dr S. Gow).

AMENORRHOEA AND INFERTILITY: ENDOCRINE CAUSES

Site of lesion	Examples
Hypothalamus	Anorexia nervosa Severe weight loss Stress (psychological and/or physical) Gn-RH deficiency (Kallmann's syndrome) Tumours (e.g. craniopharyngioma, acromegaly)
Anterior pituitary	Hyperprolactinaemia Hypopituitarism Functional tumours (e.g. Cushing's disease) Isolated deficiency of FSH or of LH
Ovaries	Polycystic ovary syndrome Ovarian failure* Ovarian tumours
Receptor defect	Testicular feminization syndrome
Other endocrine diseases	Diabetes mellitus Thyrotoxicosis Adrenal dysfunction (e.g. late-onset CAH)

*Ovarian failure may be auto-immune, chromosomal, iatrogenic (e.g. after cancer therapy), or idiopathic.

Table 18.3 Endocrine causes of amenorrhoea and infertility.

be measured if there is hirsutism or virilization. Figure 18.4 summarizes the interpretation of investigations commonly performed in patients with menstrual abnormalities.

Plasma [prolactin] high. This finding needs to be confirmed by repeating the investigation. Even then, it must be interpreted with caution, since stress, certain drugs, hypothyroidism and

Fig. 18.4 The investigation of oligomenorrhoea and amenorrhoea. It is assumed that other endocrine causes of these conditions (e.g. thyroid disease) have been excluded.

chronic renal failure can all lead to marked elevations in plasma [prolactin] (p. 223). About 20% of women with secondary amenorrhoea and ovulatory failure have *hyperprolactinaemia*; some of these patients have galactorrhoea. These patients may respond to dopamine agonists.

Plasma [prolactin] normal. As indicated in Figure 18.4, the results from the measurement of plasma concentrations of FSH, LH and oestradiol-17β should then be interpreted.

1 *Plasma [FSH] and [LH] high, [oestradiol-17β] low.* There is primary ovarian failure, due to a

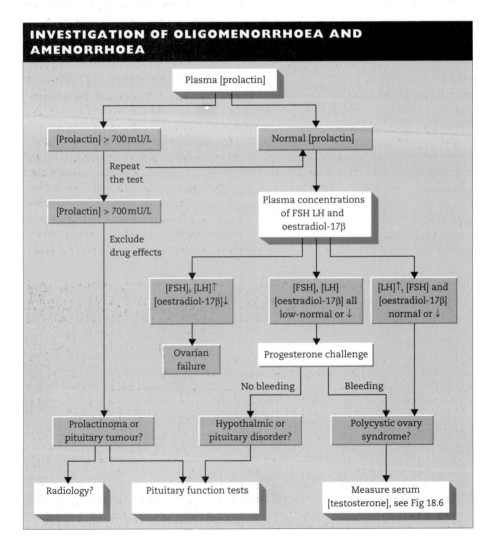

INVESTIGATION OF OLIGOMENORRHOEA AND AMENORRHOEA

Plasma [prolactin]

[Prolactin] > 700 mU/L   Normal [prolactin]

Repeat the test

[Prolactin] > 700 mU/L   Plasma concentrations of FSH LH and oestradiol-17β

Exclude drug effects

[FSH], [LH]↑ [oestradiol-17β]↓   [FSH], [LH] [oestradiol-17β] all low-normal or ↓   [LH]↑, [FSH] and [oestradiol-17β] normal or ↓

Ovarian failure   Progesterone challenge

No bleeding   Bleeding

Prolactinoma or pituitary tumour?   Hypothalmic or pituitary disorder?   Polycystic ovary syndrome?

Radiology?   Pituitary function tests   Measure serum [testosterone], see Fig 18.6

chromosomal abnormality, chemotherapy or auto-immune disease, or it may be idiopathic due to a premature menopause.

2 *Plasma [LH] high, [FSH] and [oestradiol-17β] low* or at the lower limit of their reference ranges. The patient may have the polycystic ovary syndrome (p. 239).

3 *Plasma [FSH], [LH] and [oestradiol-17β] all low*, or at the lower limits of their reference ranges. The patient may have hypothalamic, pituitary or other endocrine disease but, before this possibility is investigated, a progesterone challenge test should be performed. In this test, the patient takes 5 mg medroxyprogesterone daily for five days. Menstrual bleeding in the week following progesterone withdrawal indicates that there has been adequate priming of the endometrium by oestrogens; in these patients, polycystic ovary syndrome may be the diagnosis.

Infertility

Table 18.3 summarizes the endocrine causes of infertility that may have to be considered, especially if there are menstrual abnormalities also.

Fig. 18.5 The investigation of female infertility in patients with normal menstrual cycles. In the luteal phase of the menstrual cycle, serum [progesterone] is normally >15 nmol/L.

Once it has been established that the patient is not taking oral contraceptives, and that other endocrine diseases (e.g. diabetes mellitus, hypothyroidism) are not the cause of the infertility, investigation should proceed according to the schemes outlined in Figures 18.4 and 18.5, depending on whether or not the patient has normal menstruation.

In patients who menstruate normally (Fig. 18.5), it is important to establish whether the cycles are ovulatory or anovulatory. Serum [progesterone] should be measured on one occasion between days 19 and 23 of the cycle, and the response in three separate cycles should be monitored. If the serum [progesterone] is greater than 30 nmol/L, this indicates an ovulatory cycle, whereas levels less than 10 nmol/L strongly suggest anovulatory cycles. In patients who have a serum [progesterone] between 10 and 30 nmol/L, it is thought that the cycles are ovulatory, but that there may be a defect in the luteal phase leading to decreased fertility.

In patients who have a low luteal-phase serum [progesterone] or anovulatory cycles, clomiphene may be used for treatment. It acts by blocking oestrogen receptor sites in the hypothalamus and pituitary, thereby inhibiting the normal negative feedback control by plasma oestrogens. Normally, therefore, clomiphene stimulates release of gonadotrophins,

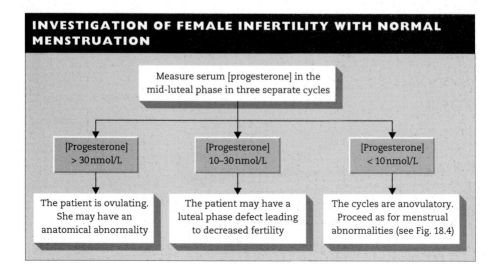

INVESTIGATION OF FEMALE INFERTILITY WITH NORMAL MENSTRUATION

Measure serum [progesterone] in the mid-luteal phase in three separate cycles

[Progesterone] > 30 nmol/L	[Progesterone] 10–30 nmol/L	[Progesterone] < 10 nmol/L
The patient is ovulating. She may have an anatomical abnormality	The patient may have a luteal phase defect leading to decreased fertility	The cycles are anovulatory. Proceed as for menstrual abnormalities (see Fig. 18.4)

and these stimulate steroid output from the ovaries.

Hirsutism and virilism

Hirsutism is a fairly common complaint among women. Most hirsute women have normal menstruation and no evidence of virilism. By itself, hirsutism rarely signifies an important disease, but it still requires investigation, because patients with ovarian or adrenal tumours have been described with normal menstrual cycles. Patients who have menstrual

Fig. 18.6 The investigation of hirsutism in females. Continus from Fig. 18.4 if the results there indicate the need to measure serum [testosterone]. Reference ranges for testosterone and for dehydroepiandrosterone sulphate (DHEAS) in females are, respectively, 0.8–2.8 nmol/L and 1.5–11.5 μmol/L.

disorders in addition to hirsutism are more likely to have endocrine dysfunction.

Figure 18.6 outlines a scheme for the investigation of female hirsutism. Serum [testosterone] and [DHAS] should be measured; in females, DHAS is a specific adrenal product. Most hirsute women have *idiopathic hirsutism* with normal levels of these steroids. Detailed investigation, however, may reveal evidence of androgen excess due, for instance, to low plasma [SHBG] accompanied by increased serum [free androgens], or to increased conversion of testosterone to 5α-DHT in the skin.

A second group of hirsute women (Fig. 18.6) have moderately increased serum [testosterone], 2.8–7.0 nmol/L, secondary to increased production by the ovaries or the adrenals, and often associated with menstrual irregularity. If the underlying cause is *late-onset congenital adrenal hyperplasia* (CAH), due to partial deficiency of 21-hydroxylase (p. 217),

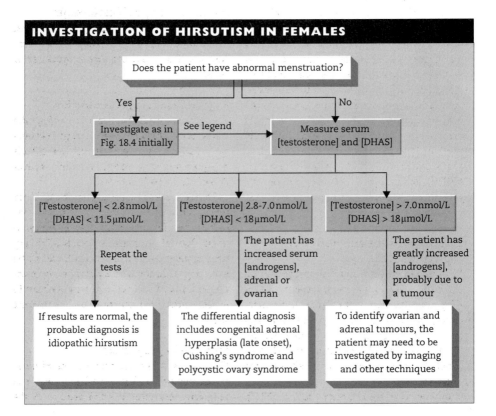

INVESTIGATION OF HIRSUTISM IN FEMALES

Does the patient have abnormal menstruation?

Yes — Investigate as in Fig. 18.4 initially | See legend → No — Measure serum [testosterone] and [DHAS]

| [Testosterone] < 2.8 nmol/L [DHAS] < 11.5 μmol/L | [Testosterone] 2.8-7.0 nmol/L [DHAS] < 18 μmol/L | [Testosterone] > 7.0 nmol/L [DHAS] > 18 μmol/L |

Repeat the tests | The patient has increased serum [androgens], adrenal or ovarian | The patient has greatly increased [androgens], probably due to a tumour

If results are normal, the probable diagnosis is idiopathic hirsutism | The differential diagnosis includes congenital adrenal hyperplasia (late onset), Cushing's syndrome and polycystic ovary syndrome | To identify ovarian and adrenal tumours, the patient may need to be investigated by imaging and other techniques this can be confirmed by injecting tetracosac-trin (Synacthen, 250 mg intramuscularly) and measuring serum [17α-hydroxyprogesterone] one hour later. In a patient with CAH, there will be an increase in serum [17α-hydrox-yprogesterone] to more than twice the upper reference value. About 5% of hirsute women have late-onset CAH. *Polycystic ovary syndrome* (Stein–Leventhal syndrome) is a more com-mon cause of hirsutism, with patients often having irregular menses, moderately increased serum [testosterone] and serum [DHAS] with increased plasma [LH].

A third group of hirsute women (Fig. 18.6) have considerably increased serum [testo-sterone] and [DHAS], and may show signs of virilism. Late-onset CAH should be excluded as should rarer causes of these abnormalities, e.g. ovarian or adrenal tumours.

Steroid contraceptives

Steroid contraceptives, principally those con-taining synthetic oestrogens, may cause diverse metabolic effects. For example, increases in plasma hormone-binding proteins and lipids may occur, and release of gonadotrophin and endogenous oestrogen will be inhibited. Contraceptives that only contain progesto-gens are largely free from these effects. Progestogens largely oppose the effects of oestrogens. Thus, in preparations containing combinations of oestrogen and progestogens, the net effect on the lipid profile and hormone-binding proteins, etc., will depend on the balance of these hormones in the individual preparations.

The menopause and hormone replacement therapy

In most women, the perimenopause can be diagnosed clinically. In women over the age of 45 years with oligomenorrhoea or amenor-rhoea, biochemical investigations will add little to the diagnosis of the perimenopause. Younger women with menstrual disturbances should be investigated as described earlier in this chapter.

In hormone replacement therapy (HRT),

natural oestrogens are often used in combina-tion with a progestogen. The effect on plasma lipids and other biochemistry will depend on the particular preparation used and also on whether the hormones are given orally or as a dermal patch.

There is little place for the measurement of reproductive hormones in patients taking HRT, except perhaps to check whether an implant containing oestradiol needs replacing.

Pregnancy and the fetoplacental unit

The placenta produces several proteins, includ-ing (human) chorionic gonadotrophin (hCG) and (human) placental lactogen (hPL). It also produces large amounts of steroid hormones, and is the main source of progesterone during pregnancy.

Proteins of trophoblastic origin

There are several pregnancy-specific proteins, all of which normally originate in the tro-phoblast. The most commonly measured is hCG.

Human chorionic gonadotrophin

Following synthesis, hCG is secreted into the maternal circulation. There is a surge in mater-nal [hCG] in early pregnancy, peak blood levels being reached at 12 weeks; thereafter, produc-tion of hCG rapidly declines.

Trophoblastic tumours secrete hCG. These tumours can occur in males and females; they include hydatidiform mole and choriocarci-noma, both of which may secrete hCG in very large amounts. A female who is found to be excreting hCG, and who is not pregnant, most frequently has a tumour of the trophoblast; in males, testicular teratoma is the commonest source.

Steroids in pregnancy

Oestrogens and progesterone are secreted by the corpus luteum during the first six weeks of pregnancy, but after this the placenta is the most important source of these steroids. Oestriol is the oestrogen produced in the greatest amounts, but oestradiol-17β and oestrone are also produced in large amounts. The placenta cannot synthesize oestriol *de novo*, but it can produce oestriol from C-19 adrenal steroids that are supplied by the fetal adrenal in the form of DHAS. The oestriol produced in this way is secreted into the maternal and fetal circulation. Oestriol production thus requires the involvement of both the placenta and the fetus, and recognition of this interdependence led to the concept of the fetoplacental unit.

Chemical tests in pregnancy

Diagnosis of pregnancy and ectopic pregnancy

In pregnancy, hCG becomes detectable in urine about 10 days after conception. This forms the basis of readily available pregnancy tests.

In ectopic pregnancy, plasma [hCG] fails to rise at the normal rate (approximately doubling every two days). In practice, the diagnosis is made on a high clinical suspicion, qualitative pregnancy tests, ultrasound and, if indicated, laparoscopy.

Assessment of fetoplacental function

Measurements of plasma [oestriol] and plasma [hPL] have been used in the past to monitor fetoplacental function. Low levels give an indication of a failing fetoplacental unit. These tests have now largely been replaced by ultrasound.

Other chemical changes in pregnancy

Hormones and binding proteins. Plasma prolactin, [oestrogens] and [testosterone] show a steady increase in pregnancy, as does the concentration of SHBG. The concentrations of growth hormone and the pituitary gonadotrophins are decreased. However, some less specific methods for the measurement of LH may show cross-reaction with hCG, leading to apparent high LH levels.

There are large increases in serum [cortisol]

due to increased plasma [cortisol-binding globulin (CBG)], but the diurnal rhythm is retained. There is also an increase in serum [free cortisol] and in the 24-hour urinary excretion of cortisol, probably due to the production of an adrenocorticotrophic hormone (ACTH)-like substance by the placenta. This may help to explain why pregnant women often show intolerance of glucose, and occasionally develop Cushingoid features.

The effects of pregnancy on *thyroid function* tests are described in Chapter 15.

Plasma [1:25-dihydrocholecalciferol] is increased, and there is enhanced absorption of calcium.

Plasma volume and renal function. During pregnancy, the plasma volume and glomerular filtration rate (GFR) increases, sometimes by as much as 50%. This is accompanied by decreases in, for example, plasma [Na$^+$], [urea], [creatinine] and [albumin].

Plasma lipids and proteins. Plasma [triglyceride] may increase as much as three-fold in pregnancy; plasma [cholesterol], low-density lipoprotein (LDL) and high-density lipoprotein (HDL) increase to a lesser extent. Plasma [albumin] and [prealbumin] fall because of the increase in plasma volume. Plasma [fibrinogen] and [ceruloplasmin] increase.

Alkaline phosphatase (ALP). In pregnancy, a placental isoenzyme is released, and total ALP activity may rise to as much as three times nonpregnant levels.

Iron and ferritin. During pregnancy, increased maternal red cell synthesis and transfer of iron to the developing fetus causes a greater demand for iron. Unless iron supplements are given, iron stores generally fall, with accompanying falls in plasma [ferritin], plasma [iron] and rises in plasma [transferrin] and total iron-binding capacity (TIBC).

Maternal complications in pregnancy

Diabetes mellitus

At the antenatal clinic, urine specimens should be routinely tested for glucose. Plasma [glucose] is usually measured at the first clinic attendance. Detection of glucosuria does not necessarily indicate the presence of diabetes mellitus, as the renal threshold for glucose is often lowered in pregnancy, and the glucosuria usually disappears after delivery. A glucose tolerance test may be needed if gestational diabetes mellitus is suspected (p. 152). Some pregnant women with impaired glucose tolerance will revert to normal after the baby is born, whilst others may remain frankly diabetic.

Pre-eclampsia

At the antenatal clinic, urine specimens should also be routinely tested for protein (p. 298). Proteinuria, if detected, may be the first evidence of pre-eclampsia and, as the condition worsens, proteinuria in excess of 1 g/24h may occur. Patients with pre-eclampsia may develop impaired renal function with increasing plasma [creatinine] and [urea] as the renal impairment worsens, or as a result of vomiting and dehydration. A plasma [urea] of 7.0 mmol/L should be regarded as definitely abnormal, since plasma [urea] is normally reduced in pregnancy due to the increase in plasma volume.

Impaired renal function causes reduced tubular clearance of urate. Plasma [urate] may be measured to assess the severity of pre-eclampsia, and to provide an index of prognosis. A plasma [urate] greater than 0.35 mmol/L before 32 weeks' gestation, or greater than 0.40 mmol/L after 32 weeks, is significantly raised.

Prenatal diagnosis of fetal abnormalities

Neural tube defects

The fetal liver begins to produce α_1-fetoprotein (AFP) from the sixth week of gestation and the highest concentration of AFP in fetal serum occurs at about 18 weeks, after which it falls progressively until term. If the fetus has an open neural tube defect, abnormal amounts of AFP are present in amniotic fluid in about 95% of cases at 16 weeks' gestation, and in maternal serum in about 80% of cases at that time.

In many countries, maternal serum [AFP] (MSAFP) is measured as a screening test for neural tube defects, carried out with a view to identifying those women who should be further investigated by ultrasound and then, in appropriate cases, by amniocentesis. If the diagnosis of open neural tube defect is confirmed before the twentieth week, termination of pregnancy can be offered.

It is essential to know the gestational date for the interpretation of results, since MSAFP concentrations vary considerably with the length of gestation. The best discrimination between normality and abnormality is obtained at 16–18 weeks' gestation, but even then, considerable overlap between [MSAFP] in normal pregnancies and in women carrying affected fetuses occurs.

Other causes of high [MSAFP] include multiple pregnancy and some rare, non-neurological fetal abnormalities (e.g. oesophageal or duodenal atresia, exomphalos).

Amniocentesis before 20 weeks' gestation. If an abnormal result for [MSAFP] is reported, it is usual to repeat the serum measurement and, if the result is again abnormal, to proceed to ultrasound examination. This detects multiple pregnancy, and will also often detect neural tube defects. Ultrasound examination helps with placental localization for subsequent amniocentesis, if this is to be performed.

Amniocentesis carries a risk to the fetus estimated to be between 0.5% and 2% loss. To justify its performance, there must be a high index of suspicion that a fetal abnormality is present. An appropriate course of action must be available in the event that an abnormality is diagnosed as a result of amniocentesis. The risks of chorionic villus sampling, important in the prenatal diagnosis of inherited metabolic disease (p. 249), are correspondingly low, but are likewise not negligible.

Amniotic fluid [AFP] is abnormal in over 95% of cases where there is a neural tube defect. However, false-positive results may be obtained when the fluid is blood-stained, or when certain other defects (e.g. exomphalos) are present. In some centres, amniotic fluid acetylcholinesterase activity may also be measured, and this is increased when the fetus has a neural tube defect.

Screening for Down's syndrome

Down's syndrome (trisomy of chromosome 21) is the commonest congenital cause of mental retardation. The overall prevalence is one in 1000 births, and affected pregnancies can be identified by chromosome analysis of cells obtained at amniocentesis in the midtrimester. The prevalence of Down's syndrome varies greatly with maternal age; women over 35 years of age have a risk of at least one in 250 of carrying an affected fetus, whereas in women aged less than 20 years, the risk is one in 2000. However, since women aged over 35 years represent only 5–7% of total pregnancies, only 30% of Down's syndrome pregnancies can be detected by performing amniocentesis in this older group.

Abnormalities in a number of maternal serum analytes are associated with Down's syndrome pregnancies. These include decreased [MSAFP] and [pregnancy-associated protein A], increased serum total [hCG], [free β subunit of hCG] and [unconjugated oestriol]. Each of these measurements shows overlap between Down's syndrome pregnancies and the normal population. However, if the distributions of the concentrations of these analytes for Down's syndrome pregnancies and normal pregnancies are known, a likelihood ratio for the risk of the fetus having Down's syndrome can be calculated for an individual woman. Patients with a high risk of carrying an affected child may then be offered amniocentesis. Individual maternity units determine what combination of analytes to measure and at what level of risk amniocentesis should be offered. Trials are underway to determine whether ultrasound may be able to replace chemical tests.

KEY POINTS

1 Endocrine causes of infertility in the male are rare.

2 Abnormal menstruation and infertility in women can arise from disease of the hypothalamus, pituitary, ovary, adrenal or thyroid.

3 Pituitary and hypothalamic causes include stress and anorexia, hyperprolactinaemia and hypopituitarism.

4 Ovarian causes include polycystic ovary disease, ovarian failure and tumours.

5 Hirsutism is common, and is usually idiopathic unless accompanied by menstrual disorder or virilism.

6 In women over 45 years, biochemical investigations will add little to the diagnosis of the perimenopause.

7 Maternal serum α-fetoprotein (AFP) is used to screen for neural tube defects at 18–20 weeks gestation. If elevated concentrations are found on two occasions, ultrasound and amniocentesis may be indicated.

8 Screening for the presence of a fetus with Down's syndrome can be performed using measurements of AFP, human chorionic gonadotrophin (hCG) and unconjugated oestriol in maternal serum.

Case 18.1

A 17-year-old boy was investigated for delayed onset of puberty. There was nothing of note in his medical history, and he had not been receiving any drugs; his 14-year-old brother was already more advanced developmentally. The patient was on the 25th centile for height, and had poorly developed secondary sexual characteristics. There were no signs of endocrine disturbances. However, it was noticed that the patient had a poor sense of smell. Hormone investigations on blood samples gave the following results:

Hormone	Result	Reference range	Units
LH	1.2	1.5–9.0	U/L
FSH	Not detected	1.5–9.0	U/L
TSH	1.3	0.3–5.0	mU/L
Free T4	21	10–27	pmol/L
Prolactin	200	60–390	mU/L
Testosterone	2	10–30	nmol/L
Cortisol (8 a.m.)	500	160–565	nmol/L

How would you interpret these results in the light of the patient's history and clinical findings?

Comments on Case 18.1

The findings suggest that the patient had hypogonadotrophic hypogonadism as the sole endocrine abnormality, but a combined test of pituitary functional reserve (p. 226) would be worth considering; it would provide information about growth hormone. The lack of a sense of smell is typical of Kallmann's syndrome, in which there is an isolated deficiency of Gn-RH. Stimulation with exogenous Gn-RH can be used both diagnostically and as treatment, but usually puberty is induced in these patients with sex steroids.

Case 18.2

A 17-year-old girl consulted her doctor because she was embarrassed about the amount of dark hair that was growing on her face. She told the doctor that her menstrual periods had never been regular (menarche age 13) and that she had not had a period for over four months. She was not pregnant.

On examination, the doctor found that the patient was slightly overweight and had an extensive growth of dark hair on her lower abdomen (an escutcheon), as well as much dark hair on her upper lip, arms and legs. The patient was referred to an endocrinologist. After it was confirmed that the patient was not pregnant, the following hormones were measured in blood (reference ranges are for the early follicular phase, where relevant):

Hormone	Result	Reference range	Units
Prolactin	450	60–390	mU/L
LH	23	2.5–9.0	U/L
FSH	2.0	3–15	U/L
Oestradiol-17β	250	110–180	pmol/L
Testosterone	3.5	0.8–2.8	nmol/L
DHAS	12	1.5–3.5	µmol/L
TSH	0.4	0.3–5.0	mU/L
Free T4	18	10–27	pmol/L

Continued on p. 244

Case 18.2 *continued*

What do you think is the most likely diagnosis? What is your differential diagnosis?

Comments on Case 18.2

This girl had the clinical and biochemical features of polycystic ovary syndrome (PCOS). The slight increase in plasma [prolactin] is not of pathological significance; it may, for instance, be due to stress. The gonadotrophin pattern excludes hypogonadotrophic

hypogonadism and ovarian failure as the cause of amenorrhoea (pregnancy had already been excluded), and the testosterone and DHAS concentrations were such as to make it most unlikely that the patient had an androgen-secreting tumour. Late-onset CAH can present with all the features of PCOS, and should be excluded by measuring the 17-hydroxyprogesterone (17-OHP) response to Synacthen stimulation (p. 239).

Case 18.3

A 24-year-old housewife was four months pregnant when she consulted her doctor because she felt extremely uncomfortable in the current warm weather. She was concerned because, 20 years before, her mother had had similar symptoms and had been found to have Graves' disease. Furthermore, she had read in a medical column in a magazine an article

concerning the potential hazards to the fetus if the mother had Graves' disease.

The patient showed no signs or symptoms of thyroid disease. However, the doctor decided to request the following thyroid function tests (reference ranges for free thyroid hormones relate to the second trimester of pregnancy):

Hormone	Result	Reference range	Units
TSH	<0.1	0.3–5.0	mU/L
Free T4	19	10–27	pmol/L
Total T4	190	70–150	nmol/L
Free T3	4.5	3.0–9.0	pmol/L
Total T3	3.0	1.2–2.8	nmol/L

How would you interpret these results? Would you request any further thyroid-related tests?

Comments on Case 18.3

Plasma [TSH] was below the limits of sensitivity of the assay. Undetectable TSH could be due to hyperthyroidism, but it could also be due to the mild thyrotrophic action of the high plasma [hCG] that is found until about the fifteenth week of pregnancy.

Plasma [TBG] increases in pregnancy. This causes increases in plasma [total T4] and [total T3], without at the same time causing raised levels of the free thyroid hormones. When interpreting results for plasma [free T4] and

[free T3] in pregnant women, it is important to use the appropriate trimester-related reference ranges. In this patient, the results for these analyses were both normal, so Graves' disease as a cause of the low plasma [TSH] is very unlikely.

As a follow-up investigation, a blood specimen was examined for TSH-receptor antibodies. As these could not be detected, this supported the conclusion that TSH was undetectable due to the effects of hCG, and did not represent evidence suggesting that the patient had Graves' disease. The patient was reassured that she was undergoing a normal pregnancy.

Case 18.4

A 22-year-old secretary presented to her doctor complaining of a white milk-like discharge from the nipple of each breast. She had had these symptoms intermittently for the previous month.

On questioning, it was found that she had also been experiencing menstrual irregularities over the previous year, and had not had a period for at least six months. She was a non-smoker, and was not taking any medication.

Plasma [prolactin] was found to be markedly elevated at 1846 mU/L (reference range 60–390), and a second sample taken two weeks later showed a similar elevation at 1240 mU/L.

She was referred to an endocrinologist. The patient was clinically euthyroid, not pigmented and had normal secondary sexual characteristics. Visual fields were normal.

The following hormones were measured in blood:

Hormone	Result	Reference range	Units
Prolactin	1400	60–390	mU/L
LH	1.6	2.5–9.0	U/L
FSH	3.5	3.0–15	U/L
TSH	2.2	0.3–5.0	mU/L
Free T4	15	10–27	pmol/L

How would you interpret these results in light of the history and clinical findings? What further investigations should be performed?

Comments on Case 18.4

The very high prolactin levels, accompanied by galactorrhoea and amenorrhoea, suggest the presence of a prolactinoma.

In patients with a prolactin level over 700 mU/L, stress, hypothyroidism and pharmacological causes of a raised prolactin level should be excluded, and the test should be repeated to confirm an elevated level. A computed tomography (CT) scan of the pituitary should be performed in patients with unexplained hyperprolactinaemia. In this patient, a CT scan showed a possible low-density lesion in the anterior pituitary, which on a magnetic resonance imaging (MRI) scan was found to be microadenoma. The patient was treated successfully with dopamine agonists.

CHAPTER 19

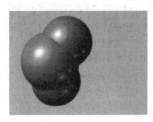

Clinical Biochemistry in Paediatrics and Geriatrics

Paediatrics, 246
  Inherited metabolic
    disorders, 247
  Some biochemical problems
    in the neonatal period and
    infancy, 252

Failure to thrive in
  childhood, 255
Miscellaneous conditions in
  paediatrics, 257
Geriatrics, 258

Reference ranges in
  geriatrics, 258
Screening for disease in
  elderly patients, 258

Disorders of *children*, particularly the neonate, are often markedly different from those in the adult. In the neonate, there are problems associated with prematurity, problems in adapting to the new external environment and problems with a variety of inherited metabolic disorders. Later in childhood, there may be disorders of growth, failure to thrive, presentation of inherited disorders, etc.

In *old age*, the differences from general adult medicine are fewer. However, multiple pathology is common, and diagnosis is often made difficult by the fact that symptoms may be minimal or atypical. For this reason, more reliance may have to be placed on laboratory tests.

Paediatrics

In this section, we discuss the following areas of diagnosis:

1 *Inherited or other congenital metabolic disorders:* diagnosing these in the neonatal period and detecting them during intrauterine life by techniques such as chorionic villus biopsy and amniotic fluid studies; the place of screening in early diagnosis.

2 *Causes and diagnosis of biochemical disturbances,* such as hypoglycaemia hyperbilirubinaemia and hypercalcaemia, which are commonly found in the *neonate* and in early childhood.

3 *Biochemical abnormalities* associated with failure to thrive, malnutrition and short stature

Specimen collection from neonates and children

This should be done expertly, and managed in such a way that only important investigations are requested and the number of collections and amount of blood taken is minimized. Capillary blood is generally preferable.

Blood specimens from babies are best obtained by heel prick, from the fleshy (lateral) parts of the heel. It is important not to use the central part of the heel, as the calcaneus is very close to the surface and injury to it by the blood-collecting lancet can cause necrotizing osteochondritis. In older children, the sides of the fingers provide the best sites, especially where repeated sample collection may be needed (e.g. in diabetics).

Reference ranges in paediatrics

Reference ranges appropriate for the age-group of the patient (Table 19.1), available from the biochemistry laboratory performing the test, should always be used.

In neonates, particularly when of low birth weight or when premature, interpretation of

AGE-DEPENDENT PLASMA REFERENCE RANGES

Constituent	Neonates	Infants	Childhood	Adults
Albumin (g/L)	30–42	34–46	36–47	36–47
Alkaline phosphatase (U/L)	70–550	70–550	125–400	40–125
Bilirubin, total (μmol/L)	<200		<26	2–17
Calcium (mmol/L)	1.60–3.00	2.10–2.80	2.12–2.62	2.12–2.62
Creatinine (μmol/L)	40–80	30–60	30–80	55–120
γ-Glutamyl transferase (U/L)	<200	<120	<35	10–55 (M)
Phosphate, fasting (mmol/L)	1.3–3.0	1.0–2.1	1.0–1.9	0.8–1.4
Potassium (mmol/L)	4.0–6.6	4.1–5.6	3.3–4.7	3.3–4.7
Protein, total (g/L)	51–68	55–78	60–80	60–80
Thyroid-stimulating hormone (mU/L)	<25		0.15–3.5	0.15–3.5
Thyroxine, free (pmol/L)	10–50		9–23	9–23
Thyroxine, total (nmol/L)	140–440	90–195	70–180	70–150

Table 19.1 Examples of plasma reference ranges that are age-dependent (data for children kindly provided by Dr A. Westwood).

results is especially difficult and requires considerable experience.

Inherited metabolic disorders

Many inherited metabolic diseases are due to an inborn error. These subdivide into two main groups:

1 *Addition or deletion of chromosomes or parts of chromosomes.* This group has an incidence of about six per 1000 live births, and the disorders lead to clinically significant abnormalities (e.g. Down's syndrome, Turner's syndrome) in about three per 1000 live births. These disorders will not be considered here.

2 *The Mendelian disorders*, in which the primary defect is probably in the structure of the gene. This group includes a wide variety of conditions, mostly very uncommon. Chemical investigations (often very specialized) are usually needed for their proper characterization.

The primary defect in each of the Mendelian disorders is probably a change in the base sequence of a gene. This change affects the synthesis of a structural or transport protein, an enzyme, etc. The consequences depend on the functions of the protein affected by the

primary alteration in the gene, and can be illustrated by discussing a defect that gives rise to a marked reduction of activity of an enzyme (E) involved in the metabolism of a compound, A, at one stage in the following reaction sequence:

$$\begin{array}{cccc} E_1 & E_2 & E_3 & E_n \\ A \rightarrow B \rightarrow C \rightarrow D \rightarrow R \end{array}$$

We shall later on make the important assumption that the defect resulting from the Mendelian disorder makes the reaction catalysed by the affected enzyme into the rate-limiting step in the pathway.

Diagnosis

An increasing number of metabolic disorders can be detected biochemically in the neonatal period. The individual disorders are rare (Table 19.2), but *collectively* they are not at all uncommon. Some are detected by screening programmes (see below). Others present acutely (Table 19.3). In one group of these, an infant assessed as normal at birth typically develops reluctance to feed, vomiting, abnormal breathing, and without treatment rapidly progresses to multiple organ failure, coma and death. A second group may have a more chronic and progressive course, with symptoms such as failure to thrive, progressive hepatomegaly or neurological deterioration developing over

METABOLIC DISEASES IN NEONATES

Disorder	Incidence
Cystic fibrosis	50
α_1-Protease inhibitor deficiency	50
Hypothyroidism	20–30
Duchenne's muscular dystrophy	20–30
Phenylketonuria	10–20
21-Hydroxylase deficiency	10
Cystinuria	5–10
Hartnup disease	5–10
Mucopolysaccharidoses	5–10
Urea cycle defects	2–5
Galactosaemia	1–2
Homocystinuria	1
11β-Hydroxylase deficiency	1
Maple syrup urine disease	1
Nonketotic hyperglycaemia	1

Table 19.2 Incidence in the United Kingdom of some metabolic diseases detectable in neonates (approximate frequency in terms of numbers of cases per 100 000 live births).

months or years. A diagnostically challenging group of children presents with repeated acute attacks of coma. Between attacks, they are clinically and biochemically normal. These patients may be classed under Reye's syndrome (p. 257) if appropriate investigations are not carried out at the time of the attack. The smallest group of children comprises those with clearly defined clinical syndromes that require biochemical confirmation, such as Zellweger's disease – a peroxisomal disorder affecting oxidation of very long chain fatty acids that typically presents at birth, or shortly after, with severe hypotonia and fits.

In families in which there has been no index case, the recognition that there is a metabolic disease present, and thereafter the precise identification of its nature, can present complex diagnostic problems. About 10% of deaths in infancy in Britain are due to genetic disorders.

The index case
Simple urine tests, e.g. for glucose, reducing substances, pH and ketones, may suggest additional more specific investigations, such as those for galactosaemia, hereditary fructose intolerance, or organic aciduria.

Depending on the infant's clinical condition, blood-gas studies and measurements of plasma concentrations of bilirubin, calcium, creatinine or urea, glucose, lactate, potassium and sodium may all be indicated. The following investigations may also be indicated (Table 19.3):

1 Blood [NH_3]. This is probably the best initial investigation if a urea cycle defect is suspected; the test should usually be available locally.

2 Urine and plasma amino acids.

3 Urinary organic acids.

4 Red cell galactose-1-phosphate uridylyltransferase.

It should be noted that the clinical management of a very sick infant using treatments such as dextrose-saline infusions or exchange transfusion, can interfere seriously with the investigation of suspected metabolic disorders. It is important, therefore, to collect appropriate specimens early, and to note the feeding regime and any drug therapy at the time of specimen collection.

Confirmation of the diagnosis
The specific recognition of an inherited metabolic disorder often cannot be made solely on the basis of blood and urine examinations. Tissue preparations or biopsy specimens for intracellular enzyme or other studies are often needed for precise diagnosis. This diagnosis is necessary both for the investigation of relatives who may be affected and for planning the management and investigation, and possibly prenatal diagnosis, in any subsequent pregnancy.

Genetic counselling may be required for parents who have had a child affected by one of the inherited metabolic disorders.

Several other inherited metabolic disorders may present less acutely than the conditions listed in Table 19.3, but may nevertheless carry a very poor prognosis; examples are given in Table 19.4.

INHERITED METABOLIC DISORDERS

Metabolic group and examples	Site of enzymic block
Amino acid disorders	
Tyrosinaemia type I	Fumarylacetoacetate hydrolase
Maple syrup urine disease	Branched-chain ketoacid decarboxylation
Nonketotic hyperglycinaemia	Glycine decarboxylase system
Carbohydrate disorders	
Galactosaemia (commonest form)	Galactose-1-phosphate uridylyltransferase
Glycogen storage disease type I (von Gierke's disease)	Glucose-6-phosphatase
Hereditary fructose intolerance*	Fructose-1-phosphate aldolase
Organic acid disorders	
Dicarboxylic aciduria*	Fatty acid β-oxidation
Isovaleric acidaemia	Isovaleryl-CoA dehydrogenase
Propionic acidaemia	Propionyl-CoA carboxylase
Urea cycle defects	
Argininosuccinic aciduria	Argininosuccinate lyase
Citrullinaemia	Argininosuccinate synthetase
Ornithine transcarbamylase deficiency	Ornithine carbamoyltransferase
Steroid synthesis defects	
Congenital adrenal hyperplasia	21-Hydroxylase, 11β-hydroxylase, desmolase, etc.

*Neonatal presentation unusual.

Table 19.3 Examples of inherited metabolic disorders that may produce acute illness, especially in the neonatal period (after Haan E.A. & Danks D.M. (1981) Clinical investigation of suspected metabolic disease. In: *Laboratory Investigation of Fetal Disease* (ed. A.J. Barson). pp. 410–28). John Wright, Bristol.

Screening for heterozygotes

This is at present mainly confined to screening the relatives of patients found to have an inherited metabolic disorder, and is normally restricted to the specific abnormality identified in the index case.

The effect of the metabolic defect can sometimes be assessed directly and quantitatively. Usually, however, the effect of the mutant gene can only be detected by investigating the metabolic reaction directly as an enzymatic assay, or indirectly by measuring the effects of the block or partial block when subjected to a loading test. For instance, an allopurinol loading test can be used to screen for heterozygotes for ornithine transcarbamylase deficiency. Heterozygote detection depends increasingly on DNA analysis, using the same techniques as those being developed for prenatal diagnosis.

Early diagnosis of inherited metabolic disease

The aim of identifying disorders that will prove to cause severe handicaps and will be untreatable and eventually fatal, is to be able to offer the mother the opportunity of a therapeutic abortion if the fetus is found to be affected in the same way as a previous child.

Prenatal diagnosis: chorionic villus biopsy

This technique allows prenatal diagnosis of inherited metabolic disorders to be made at a much earlier stage of pregnancy than amniocentesis, i.e. from the tenth week of pregnancy. The biopsy can be used for karyotyping and for gene probe diagnosis. The whole process of

LESS ACUTE INHERITED METABOLIC DISORDERS

Category and examples	Enzyme defect
Glycogen storage diseases	
Anderson's disease (type IV)	1,4-α-glucan branching enzyme
Lipid storage diseases	
Fabry's disease*,†	α-D-Galactosidase
Niemann–Pick disease*	Sphingomyelin phosphodiesterase
Gaucher's disease*	Glucosylceramidase
Tay–Sachs disease	β-N-acetyl-D-hexosaminidase (hexosaminidase A)
Krabbe's disease	β-galactocerebrosidase
Mucopolysaccharidoses (MPS)	
Hurler's disease (MPS 1H)	α-L-Iduronidase
Sanfilippo A disease (MPS IIIA)	Sulphoglucosamine sulphamidase (heparan-N-sulphatase)
Purine metabolism	
Lesch–Nyhan syndrome†	Hypoxanthine-guanine phosphoribosyltransferase
Perioxisomal defects	
Adrenoleucodystrophy†	CoA ester transfer across perioxisomal membrane

*Fabry's disease and Gaucher's diseaes are often not diagnosed until adult life.
† X-linked inheritance.

Table 19.4 Inherited metabolic diseases that may present less acutely than the examples listed in Table 19.3; some have a very poor prognosis in the index case, and termination of pregnancy may be considered for affected cases in later pregnancies.

gene probe analysis, using DNA from chorionic villus tissue, takes about 10 days. The technique has been applied particularly to the diagnosis of haemoglobinopathies, but also to several other conditions, including cystic fibrosis (p. 255) and Duchenne's muscular dystrophy (p. 103).

Prenatal diagnosis: amniotic fluid studies

Amniocentesis can be carried out at about the 15th week of pregnancy for cytogenetic reasons (e.g. to detect Down's syndrome), or to detect the appropriate *one* of a wide range of rare untreatable metabolic disorders in families in which there has already been an identified defect in an index case. Diagnosis is usually made on the basis of enzyme studies carried out on fibroblasts cultured from the amniotic fluid. Although culture and the subsequent specialized investigations take time, it

should be possible to complete them by 20 weeks' gestation.

If a pregnancy is terminated on the basis of information derived from prenatal diagnostic investigations, the correctness of the diagnosis should be confirmed by further biochemical studies carried out on the aborted fetus.

Screening of neonates: phenylketonuria (PKU)

This disease provides a good example of a potentially treatable condition that can be readily detected by neonatal screening programmes.

The first step in the major pathway of phenylalanine metabolism, its conversion to tyrosine, depends on hepatic phenylalanine hydroxylase (Fig. 19.1). In the classical form of PKU, phenylalanine hydroxylase activity is either undetectable or very much reduced. However, a minority (1–2%) of patients with inherited abnormalities of phenylalanine metabolism have defects associated with tetrahydrobiopterin (a cofactor for phenylalanine hydroxylase) metabolism. These rarer forms of PKU must be differentiated from

METABOLISM OF PHENYLALANINE

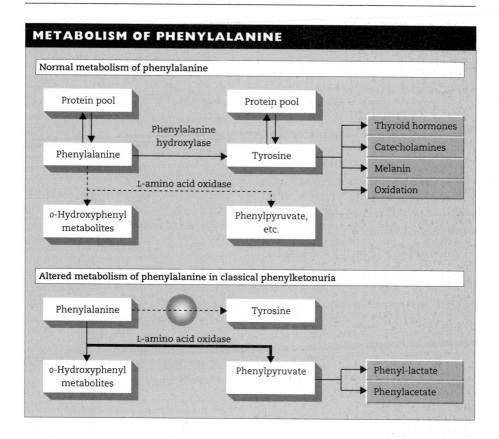

Normal metabolism of phenylalanine

Altered metabolism of phenylalanine in classical phenylketonuria

Fig. 19.1 The metabolism of phenylalanine. In the classical form of phenylketonuria (also by far the commonest form), the activity of phenylalanine hydroxylase is greatly reduced, and normally minor metabolites of phenylalanine are excreted in much increased amounts.

the classical form, as they require different treatment.

Classical PKU illustrates many of the principles that underlie the diverse effects of inherited metabolic disorders. The defect in PKU corresponds to a block at the first stage, A→B, in the general reaction sequence (A→R) shown on p. 247. The following effects may be observed:

1 *Accumulation of the substrate of the blocked reaction.* This occurs in the liver. Plasma [phenylalanine] is much increased, unless dietary phenylalanine is restricted.

2 *Reduced formation of product.* Tyrosine formation is severely affected in patients, but tyrosine deficiency can be avoided if the diet is supplemented.

3 *Alternative paths of metabolism of the precursor that accumulates.* There is increased formation and urinary excretion of phenylpyruvate, phenyllactate and phenylacetate, and of various o-hydroxyphenyl metabolites. Dietary phenylalanine restriction reduces the output of these metabolites.

4 *Effects on other reactions.* Accumulation of phenylalanine and its metabolites inhibits the transport of other amino acids into the liver and brain, and their concentrations in these tissues fall. The activity of enzymes involved in the metabolism of other amino acids (e.g. tyrosine, tryptophan) may also be inhibited.

Other inherited metabolic disorders give rise to features additional to those exemplified by PKU. Reduced formation of an important product may interfere with a negative feedback control mechanism, e.g. failure to synthesize cortisol in normal amounts in congenital adrenal hyperplasia leads to increased output of adrenocorticotrophic hormone (ACTH; p. 217).

Screening for phenylketonuria

All infants in the United Kingdom are screened for PKU (and for congenital hypothyroidism) at 6–14 days old by collection of blood samples onto filter paper that is subsequently allowed to dry and then sent to the specialist centre where the analysis is performed. The most widely employed initial screening procedure, the Guthrie test, uses a mutant strain of *Bacillus subtilis* that is incorporated into agar that includes β-thienylalanine, an analogue of phenylalanine that prevents bacterial growth unless there is excess phenylalanine available. A few laboratories use chromatographic (Scriver), enzymatic or fluorometric methods.

Threshold levels of blood [phenylalanine] in the Guthrie test need to be set sufficiently low (usually about 240 μmol/L) not to miss any cases of PKU. Because mild to moderate hyperphenylalaninaemia is more often due to other disorders than to PKU, the diagnosis needs to be confirmed by full amino acid analysis. Other appropriate tests, such as those to differentiate between classical PKU and the much rarer variants described above, are also needed. However, in the presence of high [phenylalanine] levels, a presumptive diagnosis of PKU should be made, and the child should immediately be placed on a low phenylalanine diet. Frequent monitoring of plasma [phenylalanine] is required in order to maintain the level between 120 and 360 μmol/L.

Other screening programmes in infancy

Screening programmes require considerable organization. Before embarking on them, several questions need to be considered:

1 What is the incidence of the disease?
2 Is the disease life-threatening or liable to be severe?
3 Is acceptable treatment available?
4 Is a suitable screening test available?
5 Can abnormal results be followed up?
6 Are the costs acceptable?

Screening programmes for PKU and neonatal hypothyroidism fulfil these criteria. Other conditions may be diagnosed at no great additional cost if the same sample as that obtained for PKU can be used. These include tests for maple syrup urine disease, homocystinuria, tyrosinaemia and galactosaemia. However, the screening arrangements may not be ideal for these other disorders e.g., many patients with galactosaemia will have life-threatening symptoms before the sixth day of life.

Congenital hypothyroidism

The incidence of congenital hypothyroidism is about one in 4000 live births. The condition is amenable to treatment, particularly if started early, but can be difficult to diagnose clinically. Serum [thyroid-stimulating hormone, TSH] has been found to be more reliable than serum [total T4] as a screening test.

Some biochemical problems in the neonatal period and infancy

Hypoglycaemia

Neonates

Although the neonate is at greater risk from hypoglycaemia because of its relatively large brain, the absence of neuroglycopenic symptoms led to the perception that the neonate could tolerate lower plasma glucose levels than older children. Studies have now shown that this is not so, and current recommendations are to use the same intervention limits as for older children, i.e. plasma [glucose] less than 2.0–2.5 mmol/L. Infants who are small for their dates, have a low birth weight, and those with infections are particularly at risk from the consequences of undetected hypoglycaemia.

Neonates at risk of hypoglycaemia should have their blood glucose monitored regularly on the ward. However, low ward [glucose] readings, below 2.0 mmol/L, should always be confirmed by a laboratory measurement before treatment with intravenous dextrose.

Although most common in children who are small for their gestational age, neonatal hypoglycaemia also occurs quite commonly in babies of diabetic mothers, particularly if the maternal diabetes has been poorly controlled. *Ketosis*, detectable by urine tests, is a normal accompaniment of hypoglycaemia, but is not present when there is hyperinsulinism of infancy (*nesidioblastosis*). This condition is due to hyperplasia of pancreatic β-cells, and causes intractable hypoglycaemia. Diagnosis depends on showing a high plasma [insulin] inappropriate to the hypoglycaemia.

During childhood
Recurrent hypoglycaemia of infancy and childhood may be due to any of the causes listed in Table 11.5 (p. 158) as well as several other inherited metabolic disorders (e.g. fatty acid oxidation disorders, maple syrup urine disease, tyrosinaemia), or Reye's syndrome (p. 257). Although nesidioblastosis usually presents in the first few days of life, symptoms may be delayed for up to six months.

Calcium and magnesium
Plasma [calcium] tends to fall, in normal full-term infants, by about 10–20% in the first two to three days of life. It then returns to normal (2.2–2.6 mmol/L) over the course of the next three to four days.

Neonatal hypocalcaemia within the first 48 hours, sufficient to give rise to twitching, irritability and convulsions, occurs particularly in infants who are premature, those of diabetic mothers and those who have been asphyxiated. Maternal vitamin D status may also be a factor (e.g. in Asian women). The mechanism is complex, but the hypocalcaemic tendency usually corrects itself spontaneously, although calcium gluconate may need to be given intravenously if convulsions occur, e.g. if plasma [calcium] falls to less than 1.50 mmol/L. Rarely, hypocalcaemic convulsions in the neonate are associated with maternal hyperparathyroidism, which may produce temporary hypoparathy-

roidism in the neonate due to the fetus having been exposed to maternal hypercalcaemia.

Late neonatal hypocalcaemia, between the fourth and tenth days of life, may occur in full-term as well as in premature infants. Hyperexcitability of muscles is usually also present. This is liable to occur in infants whose mothers had a low intake of vitamin D during pregnancy; these infants may also have low plasma [magnesium]. Rarely, it may also be associated with hyperphosphataemia caused by the high phosphate content of cow's milk, or be due to renal disease presenting in the neonatal period. Treatment with intravenous calcium, and often magnesium, may be required.

Neonatal rickets. Hypocalcaemia, defective bone mineralization and a raised plasma alkaline phosphatase, sometimes giving rise to rickets, may occur, especially in premature infants, because of their increased requirements for calcium, phosphate and vitamin D. It may present at any time during the neonatal period or the next two to three months, but is itself a very rare cause of convulsions or muscular hyperexcitability.

Hypomagnesaemia is an occasional cause of neonatal convulsions; it tends to occur in association with decreased plasma [calcium]. The primary defect is probably in the intestinal absorption of magnesium. In untreated infants, plasma [magnesium] may be as low as 0.1 mmol/L (reference range 0.75–1.15 mmol/L).

Respiratory distress syndrome (RDS)
Any cause of hypoxia or marked acid–base disturbance may give rise to convulsions in the neonatal period.

Respiratory difficulty in neonates is most often due to RDS. This occurs mainly in premature infants of less than 38 weeks' gestation. There is atelectasis, probably due to deficiency of surfactant activity in the alveoli, a low arterial Po_2 and high Pco_2, and often an accompanying metabolic acidosis. Treatment should be monitored by measuring blood [H+], Pco_2 and Po_2. It is possible to predict the likelihood of

RDS developing after birth by determining amniotic fluid [lecithin] late in pregnancy, and synthetic surfactant treatment can be given to the infant if necessary.

Neonatal hyperbilirubinaemia

About half of normal babies have a 'physiological' hyperbilirubinaemia, up to 200 µmol/L, during the first week of life. However, babies with plasma [bilirubin] greater than 200 µmol/L that persists beyond 10 days of life or has a significant (over 20%) conjugated bilirubin component, must be regarded as having some additional cause for the hyperbilirubinaemia.

High concentrations of unconjugated bilirubin can cross the blood–brain barrier and cause *kernicterus*. The critical plasma [bilirubin] at which this occurs in full-term infants is about 340 µmol/L, but this depends on:

1 *Plasma [albumin]*, which binds unconjugated bilirubin.
2 *The presence of drugs* (e.g. sulphonamides) that occupy albumin binding sites.
3 *Acid–base disturbances* that may affect the equilibrium between albumin-bound and unbound bilirubin.
4 *The integrity of the blood–brain barrier.*

The critical level is much lower for severely ill infants. It is also much lower for premature infants, being approximately related to birth weight; it may, for instance, be as low as 200 µmol/L for infants with a very low birth weight.

Neonatal hyperbilirubinaemia is most often associated with increased plasma [unconjugated bilirubin]. It is useful diagnostically to distinguish infants in whom conjugated bilirubin is normal from those in whom it is raised. Urine tests or inspection of the nappy may help, since urine does not contain bilirubin when there is solely unconjugated hyperbilirubinaemia. However, laboratory measurements of direct bilirubin should be carried out in all cases of prolonged jaundice.

In the neonatal period and infancy, separate measurements of conjugated and unconjugated bilirubin in plasma, for diagnosis and to follow treatment, are of much more value than in adults.

Physiological unconjugated hyperbilirubinaemia

This occurs very frequently. Factors that contribute to its development include:

1 *Overproduction of bilirubin* from haemoglobin, due to a shortened red cell life-span and ineffective erythropoiesis.
2 *Immaturity of the hepatic processes* of bilirubin uptake from plasma and conjugation in the hepatocyte.
3 *Interference with hepatic transport functions* by compounds transferred across the placenta or present in human breast milk (e.g. progesterone and steroids with progesterone-like activity, such as $3\alpha,20\beta$-pregnanediol) or by drugs.
4 *Reabsorption of unconjugated bilirubin* from the intestine. In the neonate, β glucuronidase in the small intestine releases bilirubin from its conjugates. Since the intestinal bacteria that normally then convert bilirubin to urobilinogen are not fully developed at this age, some unconjugated bilirubin can be reabsorbed and thus add to the load that the liver has to take up, conjugate and excrete.

Pathological causes of unconjugated hyperbilirubinaemia

In the neonate, these exacerbate the tendency for physiological hyperbilirubinaemia, especially in premature infants. The groupings of pathological causes are:

1 *Increased haemolysis*, due to rhesus or ABO incompatibility, or to abnormalities within the red cell (e.g. glucose-6-phosphate dehydrogenase deficiency).
2 *Defective hepatic uptake or conjugation.* This may occur in prematurity, or because of hypoglycaemia or hypothyroidism, or inherited disorders of bilirubin metabolism (Gilbert's syndrome, Crigler–Najjar syndrome, p. 116).
3 *Dehydration, intercurrent infection, bruising, polycythaemia,* other coincident disorders.

Severe unconjugated hyperbilirubinaemia carries a high risk of *kernicterus* (see above).

Rehydration, phototherapy and even exchange transfusion may be required, and plasma [bilirubin] may need to be measured every four to six hours.

Conjugated hyperbilirubinaemia

Patients in this group have increased plasma [conjugated bilirubin], but this may nevertheless constitute only 20–30% of the total bilirubin in their plasma. Normally, most of the bilirubin in plasma is unconjugated. There are several causes of conjugated hyperbilirubinaemia in infancy. These may be grouped as follows:

1 *Developmental abnormalities of the biliary tree.* The most important of these is extrahepatic biliary atresia. Intrahepatic biliary atresia also occurs.

2 *Neonatal hepatitis.* The hepatitis is caused by an ill-defined group of disorders – infective (e.g. cytomegalovirus), metabolic (e.g. α_1-protease inhibitor deficiency, p. 90, and galactosaemia, p. 159) and endocrine (e.g. congenital hypopituitarism).

Chemical tests are of little help in distinguishing infants with jaundice due to extrahepatic biliary atresia (in whom surgery is indicated) from infants with intrahepatic lesions (in whom surgery is not indicated). The commonly performed liver function tests usually show a predominantly cholestatic pattern, with large rises in plasma alkaline phosphatase activity, but plasma aminotransferase activities – alanine aminotransferase (ALT) and aspartate aminotransferase (AST) – are also increased.

Failure to thrive in childhood

Malnutrition is by far the commonest cause. Of the many inherited metabolic diseases that can cause failure to thrive, only cystic fibrosis will be discussed here.

Malnutrition in children

Protein-energy malnutrition (PEM), in its severest forms, includes kwashiorkor and marasmus; there is a range of less severe clinical presentations. There may be other impor-

tant factors, e.g. deficiency of essential fatty acids, or the consequences of immune defence mechanisms being impaired by malnutrition.

Plasma [albumin] is probably the most valuable, though insensitive, test for malnutrition. Plasma [albumin] below 30 g/L should be regarded as abnormally low; values below 25 g/L are associated with increasing degrees of oedema. Parallel changes in plasma [prealbumin] and [transferrin] also occur.

Malnutrition severe enough to cause hypoglycaemia is encountered in children with kwashiorkor and in starvation (e.g. due to gross parental neglect). If malnutrition is severe enough to cause liver failure to develop, many other chemical tests become abnormal.

Vitamin deficiency diseases make up a potentially important group of nutritional causes of failure to thrive, since the growing child has relatively greater requirements for vitamins than the mature adult. Rickets (p. 80) due to inadequate nutrition continues to occur, even in developed countries.

Cystic fibrosis (CF)

This autosomal recessive disorder is the commonest inherited metabolic disease in Caucasians; occurring in about one in 2000 live births. Abnormalities of the cystic fibrosis transmembrane conductance protein, expressed in all epithelial cells, result in failure of cyclic adenosine monophosphate (cAMP)-regulated Cl^- transport across the cell membranes. Alterations in the ion concentrations in the secreted fluid lead to abnormally thick mucus in the lung, which predisposes to chronic infection and the development of obstructive airways disease. It also produces exocrine pancreatic insufficiency and high concentrations of chloride and sodium in secreted sweat. Chemical investigations used for diagnostic purposes mostly depend on tests relating to sweat production or to pancreatic function.

Tests on sweat. The reference biochemical method for the diagnosis of CF is measurement of $[Na^+]$ and $[Cl^-]$ in sweat obtained by iontophoresis from a small area of skin under standardized conditions; sweating is induced by applying pilocarpine to the skin under a low electric current. The test demands close attention to detail if reliable results are to be obtained, and should only be carried out by staff who are experienced in performing it. It should not be performed before three weeks of age, in full-term infants, as many very young infants fail to produce sweat fast enough, even in response to pilocarpine stimulation.

In healthy children and adults, in pilocarpine-stimulated sweat, $[Cl^-]$ and $[Na^+]$ are normally below 50 mmol/L. In patients with CF, the concentrations are nearly always above 70 mmol/L.

Screening tests for cystic fibrosis

Sweat tests are too time-consuming and require too much attention to detail to be used for this purpose.

Immunoreactive trypsin (IRT) concentration, measured in dried blood spots similar to those collected when screening for PKU, is greatly increased in specimens collected from CF infants in the first month of life. It is the best CF-screening method among the tests so far evaluated, but it cannot be used after the first few weeks of life, since IRT falls as pancreatic insufficiency develops.

DNA analysis

A single mutation, ΔF_{508}, is found in about 70% of cystic fibrosis chromosomes in Northern Europe. Additional analysis for common mutations allows identification of the genotype in up to 90% of cases. In families in which an index case has been diagnosed, pre-natal diagnosis, using chorionic villus sampling at 10 weeks' gestation, is possible in most cases by direct mutation analysis, and in the remainder by linked DNA probes. Several centres carry out extended family DNA studies to determine carrier status in relatives of affected patients. Screening in the community is capable of identifying 90% of cystic fibrosis carriers, but it remains controversial whether such programmes should be set up.

Short stature

Table 19.5 lists the principal categories of disordered growth, with examples. In this section, we shall only consider the investigation of children for possible growth hormone deficiency and for coeliac disease.

Table 19.5 Disorders of growth.

GROWTH DISORDERS

Growth abnormality and category	Examples
Short stature	
Genetic	Familial short stature, delayed development
Intra-uterine	Low birth weight dwarfism
Nutritional	Inadequate food supply, malabsorption (p. 131), coeliac disease,* infections
Systemic disease	Chronic renal disease, congenital heart disease
Endocrine disease	Growth hormone deficiency,* hypothyroidism, corticosteroid excess, precocious puberty
Miscellaneous	Emotional disturbance (battered children), Turner's syndrome
Tall stature	
Genetic	Familial tall stature, advanced development
Endocrine disease	Growth hormone excess, hyperthyroidism, precocious puberty
Miscellaneous	Klinefelter's (XXY) syndrome, XYY anomaly

* Growth hormone deficiency and coeliac disease are considered here.

Growth hormone deficiency

This may be an isolated defect, partial or complete, or it may be a component of panhypopituitarism. Growth hormone (GH) is released into the circulation in pulses, mainly at night. Measurements of basal plasma [GH] in daytime specimens from normal children will often therefore be undetectable. Consequently, GH provocation tests must be used.

The *insulin hypoglycaemia test* is only safe in children if its performance can be properly supervised by staff who perform it on children regularly. It is usually preceded by other GH provocation tests such as collecting blood specimens for analysis after physical exercise, or after a meal, or soon after waking from a night's sleep. However, these tests are difficult to standardize, and the GH response to them is variable. The clonidine test is more reliable.

In the *clonidine test*, clonidine is given orally to stimulate GH release; blood specimens are collected before giving clonidine (0.15 mg/m^2 body surface area) and at 30-minute intervals for 2.5 hours afterwards. It may be considered advisable to 'prime' peripubertal children with the appropriate sex steroid, and the clonidine test can be combined with a thyrotrophin-releasing hormone (TRH) test and a gonadotrophin releasing hormone (Gn-RH) test if a combined pituitary function test (p. 226) is to be performed.

Glucagon may also be used instead of insulin to provoke GH release. As glucagon normally stimulates the release of both GH and ACTH from the pituitary, this test can be used to assess both the GH and cortisol responses to glucagon. However, whether the clonidine test or the glucagon test is used, in some children it may still be necessary to perform an *insulin hypoglycaemia test*, but modified slightly from the test as used in adults (p. 211). Specimens are taken before an intravenous injection of soluble insulin (0.15 U/kg, or 0.075–0.10 U/kg if panhypopituitarism is suspected), and at 20, 30, 45, 60 and 90 minutes after the injection. Plasma [GH] and [glucose] are measured in all the specimens, and serum [cortisol] in the 20-minute and 45-minute specimens. The test may

be combined with a TRH test and a Gn-RH test if a combined pituitary function test is to be performed. The insulin hypoglycaemia test should only be undertaken in a specialized unit with much experience of the test.

Coeliac disease

This is a common cause of growth retardation. The definitive method of diagnosis is small intestinal biopsy examination. Other diagnostic features include the improvement that is brought about by a gluten-free diet, both physically and in the severity of steatorrhoea, and the relapse that follows dietary relaxation.

Chemical tests can be valuable as preliminary investigations, jejunal biopsy being reserved for patients with abnormal results in preliminary tests such as antigliadin and anti-endomysial antibodies.

Miscellaneous conditions in paediatrics

Abnormal calcium metabolism

Hypercalciuria in childhood may be due to increased intestinal absorption of calcium (e.g. due to excessive intake of vitamin D), renal tubular disorders and, rarely, primary hyperparathyroidism (alone or part of one of the multiple endocrine neoplasia syndromes, p. 201). Children with hypercalciuria due to renal disease are best detected by measuring the urinary calcium : creatinine ratio (normally below 0.8); they have normal plasma [parathyroid hormone]. *Pseudohypoparathyroidism* (PHP) has been discussed elsewhere (p. 80). For those children with suspected (i.e. not florid) PHP, a parathyroid hormone (PTH) stimulation test can be performed. Normally, in response to the injection of PTH, plasma [cAMP] rises, but in patients with PHP there is little or no response.

Hypercalcaemia in childhood. In the neonatal period, phosphate depletion may lead to hypercalcaemia in premature neonates.

Reye's syndrome

This is a rare, acute illness with symptoms of

severe vomiting, drowsiness and behavioural changes; its onset is usually preceded by a viral illness (e.g. influenza, chickenpox). In the United Kingdom, most patients are under six, and few are over 12 years old. The encephalopathy is often fatal, and liver function tests reflect the severity of the general disturbance of mitochondrial functions.

Abnormal results of chemical investigations include increased plasma ALT and AST activities and blood [ammonia], hypoglycaemia and prolonged prothrombin time.

The cause of Reye's syndrome is unknown, but aspirin appears to have been a contributory factor in some cases. The differential diagnosis is wide, and includes several inherited metabolic disorders (e.g. urea cycle defects, hereditary fructose intolerance and fatty acid oxidation defects).

Neuroblastoma and ganglioneuroma

Neuroblastoma and related tumours, although rare, account for approximately one-third of childhood deaths from malignant disease. They are catecholamine-producing tumours, and excessive formation of dopamine is a practically constant feature. Marked pharmacological effects are uncommon, because dopamine and the catecholamines derived from it (noradrenaline, adrenaline) are largely metabolized by the tumour tissue to form inactive metabolites. Only occasionally is there hypertension.

The following tests may be performed, the measurements usually being related to urinary [creatinine] because it is difficult to obtain complete 24-hour urine collections in children:

1 *Total metadrenalines* or other index of the output of noradrenaline and adrenaline (e.g. 4-hydroxy-3-methoxymandelic acid, HMMA) are the tests most often performed initially. In children, abnormal excretion of these catecholamine metabolites nearly always points to a diagnosis of neuroblastoma or ganglioneuroblastoma rather than of phaeochromocytoma.

2 *4-hydroxy-3-methoxyphenylacetic acid* (homovanillic acid, HVA), a dopamine metabolite, is excreted in large amounts.

Geriatrics

The additional diagnostic biochemical problems in the elderly arise mainly from the increased frequency of multiorgan disease, polypharmacy and the tendency for symptoms to be absent or atypical. There are a few aspects that merit emphasis.

Reference ranges in geriatrics

These merely represent the extension of changes that have been gradually occurring throughout adult life.

Examples of the effects of ageing

Creatinine clearance tends to fall as a consequence of the progressive loss of nephrons that starts in middle age. However, the reduction in muscle mass and the smaller dietary intake of protein that tend to occur with older people may offset the effects of the loss of nephrons on plasma [creatinine].

Plasma [cholesterol], on average, increases progressively throughout adult life. In the United Kingdom, by the age of 65, mean values are 10–30% higher than in the 20–30 age group.

Plasma [glucose] tends to increase with age due to progressive impairment of glucose tolerance. However, patients do not necessarily go on to develop overt diabetes mellitus.

Plasma alkaline phosphatase activity is probably higher in healthy people over 65 than in younger adults, but it is difficult to separate the effects of disorders such as Paget's disease, which are very common in the elderly.

Some plasma constituents tend to decrease in concentration with increasing age (e.g. total protein, albumin), but these changes are unlikely to cause difficulties in interpretation.

Screening for disease in elderly patients

Because of the masking of clinical symptoms and signs, it is common practice to perform an admission biochemical screen on patients admitted to geriatric assessment units. Table

SCREENING ELDERLY PATIENTS

Examination	Abnormalities commonly detected
Side-room tests	
Urine	Glucosuria, proteinuria
Faeces	Gastrointestinal tract blood loss (e.g. haemorrhoids, carcinoma of the colon or of the rectum
Measurements on blood specimens	
Albumin, total protein	Evidence of poor nutrition
Creatinine, urea	Renal disease, postrenal uraemia
Glucose	Diabetes mellitus
Calcium (phosphate and alkaline phosphatase)	Hypocalcaemia (often due to osteomalacia)
Potassium	Hypokalaemia (often due to diuretic therapy)
Thyroid function tests	Hypothyroidism or hyperthyroidism (but see Tables 15.1 and 15.2, p. 195)
C-reactive protein (or erythrocyte sedimentation rate)	Nonspecific indicator of the presence of organic disease

Table 19.6 Admission screening of elderly patients by means of chemical tests.

19.6 lists some of the tests that are commonly used. In addition to the laboratory measurements listed in the table, side-room testing of urine specimens for glucose and protein, and faeces for occult blood (p. 299), should also form part of the initial investigation of these patients.

Inadequate nutrition
Old people living alone are particularly at risk of having an inadequate diet, especially if they are poor, or are unable or unwilling to feed themselves properly. Although plasma [albumin] may be low, its diagnostic value is limited.

Diabetes mellitus
The presence of diabetes mellitus may not be detected by side-room testing of urine for glucose, as the renal threshold for glucose tends to rise with age. Plasma glucose measurements may be needed (p. 152).

Management of elderly diabetic patients may need to depend on the help of relatives. Because of the higher renal threshold for glucose, home monitoring of blood [glucose]

will probably be needed. In these patients, examination of records of home monitoring measurements of blood [glucose] at the time of clinic attendances are usually adequate to assess treatment; there is little need for haemoglobin A_{1c} to be measured.

Bone disease
The incidence of bone disease rises markedly in old age. *Osteoporosis* is the commonest cause, especially in women, but routinely available chemical investigations are not of value in detecting it.

Paget's disease is very common. It is one of the first diagnoses to be considered when increased plasma alkaline phosphatase activity is found as an isolated abnormality in an elderly patient. It is occasionally necessary to determine whether the increased total enzymatic activity is due to the bone isoenzyme, as would be the case in Paget's disease, or to the liver isoenzyme (e.g. due to secondary deposits of carcinoma in the liver).

Osteomalacia in the elderly is usually due to lack of exposure to sunlight, combined with nutritional deficiency. Plasma [calcium] and [phosphate] may both be reduced and alkaline phosphatase activity increased in many cases. Plasma [25-hydroxycholecalciferol, HCC] is often normal, but it may be reduced due to inadequate intake of vitamin D or lack of endogenous synthesis, or both (p. 79).

Thyroid disease

Many geriatric assessment units have reported that screening for thyroid dysfunction is worthwhile, and hitherto unsuspected hypothyroidism is said to have been detected in 2–6% of patients. About 3% of patients admitted to these units may have an undetectable plasma [TSH] without there necessarily being clinical or other biochemical evidence of thyroid disease.

Many elderly patients are suffering either from nonthyroidal illnesses (Table 17.3) or are being treated with drugs that interfere with thyroid hormone tests (Table 17.4) at the time of their admission to geriatric assessment units. Abnormal results must be viewed with caution (see Chapter 15), and the following guidelines should be followed:

1 Thyroid function tests should *not* be used indiscriminately as screening investigations in otherwise fit individuals.

2 They should not be requested for patients who are severely ill (e.g. myocardial infarction), unless there are clinical indications that thyroid disease, particularly hypothyroidism, which is more common in the elderly, might be present.

3 Because hypothyroidism is relatively common and often insidious in onset, it is reasonable to request thyroid function tests in patients with nonspecific or vague symptoms, or who are for some other reason undergoing assessment in the absence of acute illness.

Measurements of plasma [TSH] provide the best screening test. The following conclusions can be drawn from its results:

1 A normal result excludes primary thyroid disease.

2 If, at the time the test is performed, the patient is not recovering from a recent nonthyroidal illness, a plasma [TSH] greater than 10 mU/L indicates that the patient has hypothyroidism and may require treatment with thyroxine, or repetition of the test after a few weeks before deciding about the need for treatment.

3 If the plasma [TSH] is less than 0.1 mU/L, plasma [free T4] or [total T4] and plasma [total T3] should be measured. If the results for either the T4 or T3 measurements are raised, the patient should be referred for specialist advice, as treatment for hyperthyroidism may be required. If, however, the results for the T4 and T3 measurements are normal or low, this suggests that the cause of the low plasma [TSH] is nonthyroidal illness or, rarely, secondary hypothyroidism.

KEY POINTS

Paediatrics

1 Prenatal diagnosis of some inherited metabolic diseases by chorionic villus sampling or by studies on amniotic fluid is possible. Other disorders, notably phenylketonuria and congenital hypothyroidism, are usually detected by neonatal screening programmes.

2 When an inherited abnormality is found, the whole family may need to be investigated to determine the likelihood of additional affected children.

3 In the neonatal period, particularly in premature babies, jaundice, hypoglycaemia and hypocalcaemia are common. These often differ in origin and treatment from the corresponding adult conditions.

4 During early childhood, failure to thrive and short stature may be due to biochemical abnormalities.

Geriatrics

1 In old age, multiple pathology in one individual is common. Furthermore, some disorders tend to present in an atypical fashion or to be asymptomatic.

2 There may be a case for more widespread use of screening programmes to detect inadequate nutrition, diabetes mellitus, and bone and thyroid disease.

Case 19.1

A 73-year-old retired schoolteacher had been admitted to hospital one month previously for an upper gastrointestinal endoscopy. She gave a history of having moderately severe hypertension, which her general practitioner had been treating with a combined preparation of atenolol and chlorthalidone for the previous two years. Endoscopy confirmed that she had a benign gastric ulcer, and she was discharged home on treatment with carbenoxolone and ranitidine. Two weeks later, she was seen by her general practitioner because her ankles had begun to swell, for which he prescribed frusemide. However, her ankle swelling persisted, and she began to complain of feeling very weak. She was readmitted to hospital, where examination of a blood specimen gave the following results:

	Plasma analyses (mmol/L)	Reference range (mmol/L)
[Urea]	5.0	2.5–6.6
[Na+]	148	132–144
[K+]	1.9	3.3–4.7
[Total CO$_2$]	30	24–30

Comment on the likely causes of this patient's hypokalaemia.

Comments on Case 19.1

There are several drug-related reasons why this patient had developed marked hypokalaemia:
1 Chlorthalidone is a thiazide diuretic. It can cause modest K+ depletion, although this is not usually sufficient by itself to require potassium supplements.
2 Carbenoxolone has marked mineralocorticoid effects, causing retention of water and Na+, and K+ loss. Its use is contraindicated in the elderly or in hypertensive patients.
3 Frusemide causes K+ loss. When using it for the treatment of oedema, it would be normal practice to use it in combination with a K+-sparing diuretic. However, it is worth noting that amiloride and spironolactone (both K+-sparing diuretics) antagonize the effects of carbenoxolone both on the kidney and on its ulcer-healing properties.

The drug treatment of this patient was changed in the light of these analytical results.

Case 19.2

A 78-year-old retired civil servant was admitted to a geriatric assessment unit with a recent history of rapidly progressing dementia. Side-room tests and the results of admission screening investigations were all normal, apart from the results of thyroid function tests, which were as follows:

Analysis	Result	Reference range
TSH (mU/L)	<0.1	0.15–3.5
Free T4 (pmol/L)	19	9–23
Free T3 (pmol/L)	3.0	3.0–9.0

Continued on p. 262

Case 19.2 *continued*

How would you interpret these results?

Comments on Case 19.2

Undetectable plasma [TSH] is reported in 1–3 % of patients admitted to geriatric assessment units if thyroid function tests are performed as part of a routine admission screening of all patients. Although undetectable plasma [TSH] is found in hyperthyroidism and in secondary hypothyroidism, in these elderly patients nonthyroidal illness and the effects of drug therapy (p. 198) are much more frequent reasons for this finding.

In this patient, the normal plasma [free T4] and the low-normal plasma [free T3] excluded hyperthyroidism and secondary hypothyroidism. The final diagnosis was multiple cerebral infarctions caused by extensive atheromatous disease of the cerebral vessels, detected by computed tomography (CT) scanning.

CHAPTER 20

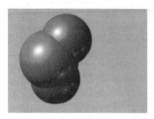

Molecular Biology in Clinical Biochemistry

Principles and applications, 263
  Complementarity, 263
  Restriction endonucleases
    and other enzymes, 264
  Gene cloning, 265
  How are genes cloned?, 266

DNA sequencing, 270
Southern blotting, 270
Restriction fragment length
  polymorphisms, 273
Polymerase chain
  reaction, 277

Molecular genetics of single-
  gene and polygenic
  disorders, 279
Single-gene disorders, 279
Polygenic disorders, 280

This chapter reviews some of the principles behind molecular biology, the methods that concern themselves with the analysis of the structure and function of deoxyribonucleic acid (DNA) and ribonucleic acid (RNA) at the molecular level. These techniques are important in the diagnosis of genetic disorders (e.g. cystic fibrosis), and are also used to diagnose certain infective disorders, such as human immunodeficiency virus (HIV) and hepatitis B and C infections. The impact on therapy is already evident in the range of genetically engineered therapeutic products (e.g. insulin, growth hormone) and viral proteins for immunization (e.g. hepatitis B). The potential for 'gene therapy' is under active investigation. The same techniques are used to investigate the molecular basis of cancer (with a view to developing cancer vaccines or cancer gene therapy, for example) and to study common polygenic disorders such as essential hypertension and diabetes mellitus.

Principles and applications

Several new techniques and discoveries have contributed to the developments in molecular biology. The details are beyond the scope of this chapter, but the principles of some of these techniques will be described.

Complementarity

One of the properties of nucleic acids that contributes to the analytical potential of molecular biology resides in the ability of complementary nucleotide sequences to hybridize with one another. In the DNA double helix, the purine base guanine always pairs with the pyrimidine base cytidine, and the purine base adenine always pairs with the pyrimidine base thymidine. Short pieces of DNA can thus act as specific probes to identify unique sequences in the genome. The genomic DNA is first dissociated by temperature or chemical means. The probe DNA sequence can subsequently be annealed to the target DNA by lowering the temperature. Careful attention to the temperature, ionic strength and other variables allows this process to be highly specific. Under stringent conditions, a suitable oligonucleotide probe of 20 base pairs can bind to its complementary DNA sequence with complete fidelity. However, a change in a single base pair in the genomic DNA in the complementary sequence will prevent hybridization. In other words, a mutation involving a single base change in the genomic DNA can be detected with suitable oligonucleotide probes.

Restriction endonucleases and other enzymes

Restriction endonucleases

A major discovery, deriving from bacterial genetics, was the isolation of enzymes that cut DNA at specific sequences. Bacteria use these enzymes to degrade the DNA of invading viruses, preventing their replication in the host. By methylating bases in the host bacterial DNA, the same enzymes can be prevented from degrading host DNA. A battery of such enzymes is now available to cut human (or other) DNA at precisely defined sites. A useful feature of some of these endonucleases is their ability to recognize palindromic sequences in DNA and generate single-strand overhangs or 'sticky ends' that are complementary to other fragments generated by the same enzyme. This allows DNA from two different sources, yet cut with the same enzyme, to hybridize together and to be covalently linked by a DNA ligase (Fig. 20.1). Other important enzymes are:

1 *DNA ligases.* These allow pieces of DNA to be covalently inserted at specific locations. For example, circular DNA from a plasmid may be opened at a discrete location using a restriction endonuclease, and then closed with a ligase enzyme. If the closure is carried out in the presence of linear pieces of foreign DNA that can hybridize with the open ends of the plasmid DNA, some recombinant plasmids will be produced containing the inserted DNA. The hybridization is made possible if the same restriction endonuclease is used to open the plasmid and to cleave the foreign DNA, provided the endonuclease also produces 'sticky ends'.

2 *Reverse transcriptase.* This allows single-stranded DNA to be synthesized from an RNA template. If the source of RNA is messenger RNA (mRNA) from a particular cell type, then it is possible to generate copy DNA (cDNA) from all the representative mRNA species that are being expressed in that cell type.

3 *DNA polymerase I.* The large fragment,

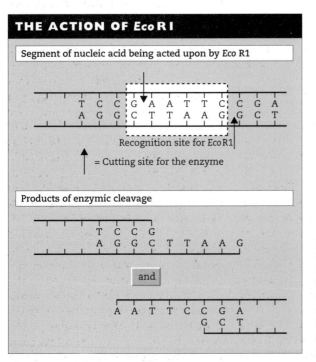

Fig. 20.1 The action of the restriction endonuclease *Eco* R1. Note how *Eco* R1 recognizes a palindromic nucleotide sequence, producing daughter molecules with 'sticky ends'. In this and later figures: A, adenine; C, cytosine; G, guanine; and T, thymidine.

lacking exonuclease activity, can be used to label a DNA probe by synthesizing a complementary labelled strand from ^{32}P-labelled nucleotides, provided short oligonucleotides are provided as primers.

4 *Taq polymerase.* This DNA polymerase, isolated from a bacterial species thriving at high temperature, *Thermus aquaticus*, is the basis of a method that *repeatedly* replicates defined segments of DNA by using oligonucleotide primers to each complementary strand of DNA. This is the polymerase chain reaction (PCR).

Gene cloning

This is a method for isolating and replicating the DNA sequence corresponding to a particular gene. The two basic types of clone are the so-called genomic clone and the copy DNA (cDNA) clone.

A *genomic clone* is generated by directly cloning the DNA from the organism of interest, and thus consists of the true sequence of nucleotides corresponding to the cloned gene. It therefore includes noncoding regions of the gene (introns) as well as the coding regions (exons), which are ultimately transcribed into mRNA and encode the amino acid sequence of the gene product. The precise functions of the introns, a feature of most eukaryotic genes, are unknown. Both the introns and exons are transcribed as RNA during gene expression, but the intron sequences are cleaved from the resultant product, and the exon sequences are spliced together to form the mRNA product. Further modification to the mRNA occurs before translation; it is 'capped', and a series of adenine (A) residues added to its tail. A genomic clone may also contain important 'upstream' sequences (before the 5′ and of the gene) and 'downstream' sequences (beyond the 3′ end of the gene), which may be important in regulating gene expression.

cDNA is generated by the action of reverse transcriptase on the mRNA coding for the protein of interest, and can also be cloned. In this regard, cDNA clones contain only the corresponding coding regions of the gene, and lack sequences that regulate gene expression.

Cloned genes are powerful analytical tools. The genomic clone provides detailed sequence information about the gene itself, and allows characterization of a mutant gene, from simple point mutations to deletions and mutations in regulatory elements. Used as a probe, or as specific oligonucleotide sequences directed at the mutation site, it can be used to identify the mutant gene by specific DNA–DNA hybridization using a method called Southern blotting (see below). Although cDNA clones may be less informative, they permit deduction of the parent protein amino acid sequence, and can be used as probes to isolate the genomic clone. The cDNA clone will also specifically hybridize to cytoplasmic mRNA, and can be used to quantify gene transcription in another technique, known as 'Northern' blotting.

When incorporated into a suitable 'expression vector', the cloned gene can be expressed from within the genomic DNA of foreign hosts, whether bacteria, yeasts, or higher animals. The gene product can be made available in large quantities (e.g. for therapeutic purposes) if a rapidly growing bacterial culture, for example, is used to express it. A cloned gene can be injected into a single fertilized egg or the early embryo stage of a foreign species, and may become incorporated into the host chromosome. A suitable promoter may be included that enables the gene to be expressed in specific cell types in the developing embryo or mature adult. When at least some of the germ cells of the developing embryo contain the foreign gene, it can be transferred to the next generation, thereby producing an established transgenic line. Such animals can serve as models of human disease and for gene therapy.

Sequence information about mRNA also allows the construction of 'anti-sense' oligonucleotides. These are single-stranded lengths of DNA (15–30 nucleotides in length) complementary to part of the specific mRNA under study. If these oligonucleotides can be made to enter cells, they hybridize there with the specific mRNA. The double-stranded regions formed by this process cannot be translated and, furthermore, they initiate degradation of the mRNA. By this means, it is possible to suppress the synthesis of a particular protein uniquely, and to examine the consequences.

How are genes cloned?

The DNA sequence of interest, whether genomic DNA or cDNA, must be part of a conveniently-sized recombinant DNA that has the ability to replicate. Several suitable vectors have been extensively characterized and widely used for this purpose. Plasmids are simple, self-replicating DNA sequences that infect bacteria. In clinical practice, they are important in carrying genes for antibiotic resistance in the host bacterium. One of the best characterized plasmid-cloning vehicles is pUC19 and its derivatives, a circular double-stranded DNA carrying antibiotic-resistance sites and known

STRUCTURE OF THE PLASMID, pUC19

Polylinker
Also called the multiple cloning site (MCS), it contains many useful restriction enzyme sites (see below) for inserting exactly that piece of DNA that you want in this plasmid

Amp
Gene that confers resistance to the antibiotic ampicillin, permitting selection for bacteria that contain the plasmid (see selection)

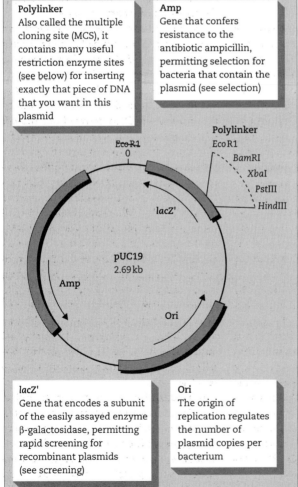

lacZ'
Gene that encodes a subunit of the easily assayed enzyme β-galactosidase, permitting rapid screening for recombinant plasmids (see screening)

Ori
The origin of replication regulates the number of plasmid copies per bacterium

Fig. 20.2 Map of the important parts of a plasmid, the workhorse of molecular biology. Shown is the plasmid pUC19, a late-generation cloning vector of 2686 bp (2.69 kb) that was constructed from parts of previous plasmids using recombinant DNA technology. The '0' point at the top is where the numbering of the base pairs starts, proceeding clockwise. An Eco R1 restriction enzyme site that was originally at this position was deleted during construction, as indicated by the line through the name, to maintain the uniqueness of the Eco R1 site in the polylinker.

endonuclease restriction enzyme sites (Fig. 20.2). One of the limitations of these plasmids is that the size of the foreign DNA insert cannot be much more than 10–20 kb (1 kb = 1000 nucleotide bases). Bacteriophage vectors (e.g. lambda) have also been widely used in cloning, and artificially engineered cosmids (consisting of plasmid DNA packaged into a phage) allow cloning of fragments of DNA up to 50 kb. More recently, bacterial artificial chromosomes (BACs) and yeast artificial chromosomes (YACs) have permitted cloning and characterization of DNA fragments of 100 000–1 million bases. The ultimate prospect is to construct artificial chromosomes that will allow many megabases of DNA to be introduced and propagated in the cell.

Many ingenious strategies for cloning have been used, and it is beyond the scope of this chapter to consider these in detail. Inevitably, there is a hit-and-miss component to cloning. In general, the more abundant the protein and the more that is known about it, the more straightforward the procedure for cloning its corresponding gene. On the other hand, many years of patient endeavour may be required to clone the gene of a low-abundance protein. It is often possible to clone the gene using a functional or complementation assay, before anything is known about the protein. This has been the case in cystic fibrosis (CF), for example, where the structure and properties of the mutant protein have been inferred from the cloned gene for CF.

A technique for cloning a cDNA copy of the coding region of a gene using a plasmid is illustrated in Figure 20.3. A cell type is first chosen on the basis that the gene is expressed in that particular cell; for instance, to clone the cDNA coding for an enzyme of the urea cycle, liver cells would be chosen. The mRNA is extracted from liver cells, and cDNA is synthesized using reverse transcriptase; included amongst the cDNA formed will be one that codes for the protein of interest. Reverse transcriptase creates a double-stranded cDNA–RNA hybrid, from which double-stranded cDNA can be generated (Fig. 20.3). In this process,

RNAase H degrades the mRNA strand to give short complementary RNA primers that are used by DNA Pol I for second strand synthesis. Synthetic oligonucleotide adaptors, each with one Eco RI compatible overhanging end, can then be added. The 'sticky ends' created in this way are able to hybridize with the corresponding 'sticky ends' created when the plasmid vector is opened using the same Eco RI restriction enzyme. The cut plasmid and cDNA are then mixed together and ligated. This procedure results in the re-formation of the original plasmid, and also in the formation of recombinant plasmids containing inserts of cDNA. Included among the recombinant plasmids should be some that contain cDNA synthesized from the desired message.

The recombinant plasmids that result can be replicated by transformation into a suitable bacterial host, and the transformed bacteria can then be specifically isolated by their antibiotic resistance, conferred by the plasmid. The collection of recombinant plasmids, containing portions of cDNA derived from liver cell mRNA, is known as a 'liver cell cDNA library'. This is the starting point for screening for the particular cDNA; in practice, it is often possible to obtain such a cDNA library commercially. It is also possible to construct genomic libraries in which the recombinant clones are constructed not with cDNA, but with suitably sized fragments of genomic DNA. Fragments of about 20 kb can be generated with an appropriate endonuclease, isolated, and inserted into a cosmid or lambda phage that can then be replicated following infection of a suitable host. By producing a large number of recombinants, the statistical probability that the library will contain almost the whole of the genome, distributed among the recombinants, can be made very high.

A method has to be devised to isolate plasmid or phage recombinants that contain the relevant cDNA of interest. One possible strategy depends on having some information about the primary amino acid sequence of the corresponding protein. If a sequence of six amino acids (or more) is known, it is possible

PREPARING CLONED cDNA

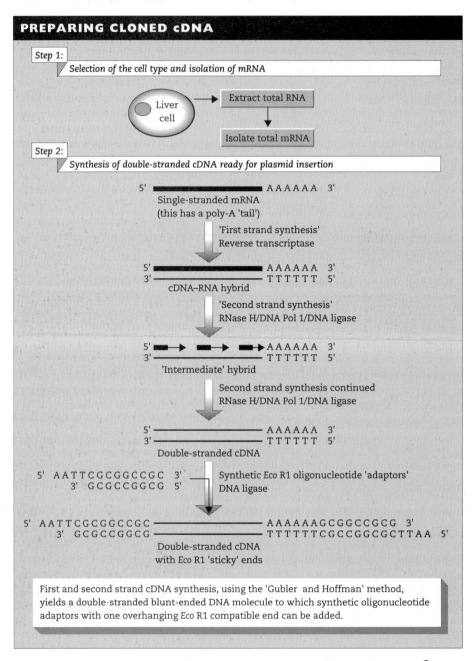

Step 1:

Selection of the cell type and isolation of mRNA

Liver cell → Extract total RNA

↓

Isolate total mRNA

Step 2:

Synthesis of double-stranded cDNA ready for plasmid insertion

5' ▬▬▬▬▬ A A A A A A 3'
Single-stranded mRNA
(this has a poly-A 'tail')

'First strand synthesis'
Reverse transcriptase

5' ▬▬▬▬▬ A A A A A A 3'
3' ─────── T T T T T 5'
cDNA–RNA hybrid

'Second strand synthesis'
RNase H/DNA Pol 1/DNA ligase

5' ▬▶ ▬▶ ▬▶A A A A A A 3'
3' ─────── T T T T T 5'
'Intermediate' hybrid

Second strand synthesis continued
RNase H/DNA Pol 1/DNA ligase

5' ─────── A A A A A A 3'
3' ─────── T T T T T 5'
Double-stranded cDNA

5' A A T T C G C G G C C G C 3' ┐   Synthetic Eco R1 oligonucleotide 'adaptors'
   3' G C G C C G G C G 5' ┘   DNA ligase

5' A A T T C G C G G C C G C ─────── A A A A A A G C G G C C G C G 3'
   3' G C G C C G G C G ─────── T T T T T C G C C G G C G C T T A A 5'
Double-stranded cDNA
with Eco R1 'sticky' ends

First and second strand cDNA synthesis, using the 'Gubler and Hoffman' method, yields a double-stranded blunt-ended DNA molecule to which synthetic oligonucleotide adaptors with one overhanging Eco R1 compatible end can be added.

Fig. 20.3 Example of a cloning strategy for preparing cloned cDNA for a liver-specific protein. ●, clones with required cDNA insert; ○, other clones.

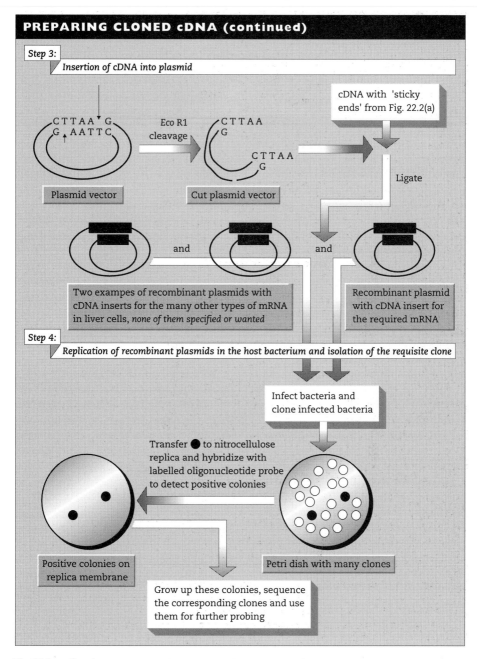

PREPARING CLONED cDNA (continued)

Step 3:

Insertion of cDNA into plasmid

cDNA with 'sticky ends' from Fig. 22.2(a)

CTTAA G
G AATTC

Eco R1 cleavage

CTTAA
G

CTTAA
G

Plasmid vector

Cut plasmid vector

Ligate

and

and

Two examples of recombinant plasmids with cDNA inserts for the many other types of mRNA in liver cells, *none of them specified or wanted*

Recombinant plasmid with cDNA insert for the required mRNA

Step 4:

Replication of recombinant plasmids in the host bacterium and isolation of the requisite clone

Infect bacteria and clone infected bacteria

Transfer ● to nitrocellulose replica and hybridize with labelled oligonucleotide probe to detect positive colonies

Positive colonies on replica membrane

Petri dish with many clones

Grow up these colonies, sequence the corresponding clones and use them for further probing

Fig. 20.3 *continued.*

to predict (from the genetic code) the corresponding sequence of bases in DNA that would code for this amino acid sequence. The precise oligonucleotide sequence (18 bases in length) cannot be known because of redundancy in the genetic code (e.g. the triplets -CCC-, -CCA-, and -CCG- all code for proline in mRNA), so it is necessary to synthesize a mixture of oligonucleotide probes to cover these various permutations. The number in the mixture can be reduced by choosing residues such as phenylalanine or tyrosine, which use only two different triplet codons.

By plating out bacteria infected with an antibiotic-resistant plasmid cDNA library at an appropriate dilution onto antibiotic-containing plates, individual bacterial colonies develop. These colonies will be 'clonal' as a result of being derived from a single bacterial ancestor, therefore containing only one unique antibiotic-resistant plasmid. After replica transfer to a nitrocellulose membrane and DNA denaturation, radiolabelled oligonucleotide or DNA probes can be incubated under appropriately stringent conditions to label colonies that contain the complementary DNA sequence. These clones are subsequently detected by autoradiography. At least some of these clones should contain recombinant plasmids containing the cDNA sequence corresponding to the protein studied. The chosen clones can be isolated and grown, and the DNA sequence of the recombinant phage can be determined. It is possible to use the DNA from these plasmids to screen the library further to obtain a clone (or clones) covering the full length of the appropriate gene. Knowing the primary amino acid sequence is also a great help in identifying the correct cDNA clones.

It must be emphasized that a variety of other strategies exist for cloning new genes, taking advantage, for example, of a functional property of the encoded protein when no protein sequence information is available.

DNA sequencing (Fig. 20.4)
The ability to sequence DNA is fundamental to the success of much of molecular biology. Two methods are used, the Maxam–Gilbert method and the Sanger method; both depend on an initial fractionation of the DNA into manageable pieces. In the Sanger method, DNA synthesis occurs from the cloned DNA template and is carried out in the presence of chemically modified and radiolabelled nucleotides, the incorporation of which leads to chain termination. Four incubations are set up; each contains tracer amounts of only one of the four possible nucleotide analogues (the other three nucleotides are present, but unmodified). If the analogue is incorporated, then the newly synthesized strand fails to elongate further. Since the unmodified counterpart of the analogue is also present, all possible lengths of newly synthesized strand, terminating at the selected base, occur. All four incubations are then subjected to electrophoresis using a polyacrylamide gel system that separates the fragments on the basis of molecular mass (and therefore length). The sequence of nucleotides can then be read directly from the gel.

The Sanger method, which is the principal sequencing technique used, has now been automated so that thousands of bases per day can be sequenced. This development has made feasible the possibility of sequencing the whole of the human genome (the 'human genome project').

Southern blotting (Fig. 20.5)
The Southern blot allows detection of DNA fragments by hybridization to a suitable probe. If genomic DNA is cut using a restriction enzyme, a series of fragments is produced; the number depends on the frequency with which the particular restriction endonuclease recognition site occurs throughout the DNA. A cDNA probe or a genomic DNA probe may therefore hybridize with a number of fragments if, for example, the complementary stretch of DNA has been internally cut by the restriction enzyme. In this technique, the cleaved DNA fragments are first separated on the basis of size using agarose gel electrophoresis. After alkaline denaturation, the DNA fragments are replica-transferred to a

SANGER METHOD OF DNA SEQUENCING

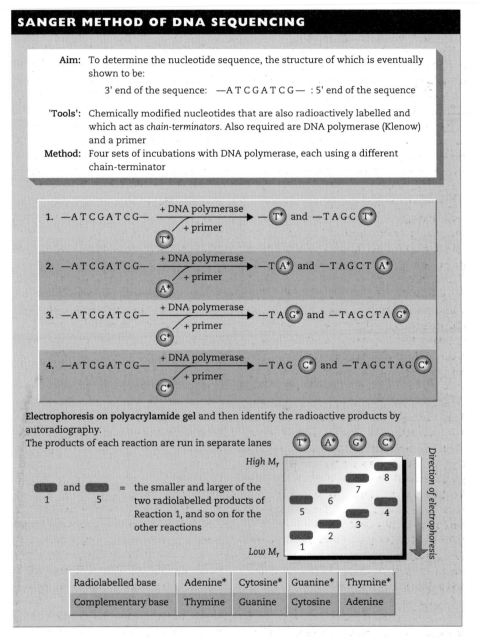

Aim: To determine the nucleotide sequence, the structure of which is eventually shown to be:

3' end of the sequence: —A T C G A T C G— : 5' end of the sequence

'Tools': Chemically modified nucleotides that are also radioactively labelled and which act as *chain-terminators*. Also required are DNA polymerase (Klenow) and a primer

Method: Four sets of incubations with DNA polymerase, each using a different chain-terminator

1. —A T C G A T C G— + DNA polymerase / + primer T* → —T* and —T A G C T*

2. —A T C G A T C G— + DNA polymerase / + primer A* → —T A* and —T A G C T A*

3. —A T C G A T C G— + DNA polymerase / + primer G* → —T A G* and —T A G C T A G*

4. —A T C G A T C G— + DNA polymerase / + primer C* → —T A G C* and —T A G C T A G C*

Electrophoresis on polyacrylamide gel and then identify the radioactive products by autoradiography.

The products of each reaction are run in separate lanes   T*   A*   G*   C*

High M_r

■■ and ■■ = the smaller and larger of the
1   5   two radiolabelled products of
                  Reaction 1, and so on for the
                  other reactions

Low M_r

Direction of electrophoresis

Radiolabelled base	Adenine*	Cytosine*	Guanine*	Thymine*
Complementary base	Thymine	Guanine	Cytosine	Adenine

Fig. 20.4 The Sanger method of DNA sequencing. Read the *complementary* nucleotide sequence 5'-TAGCTAGC-3' from the gel, in ascending numerical order of the radiolabelled products.

SOUTHERN BLOTTING

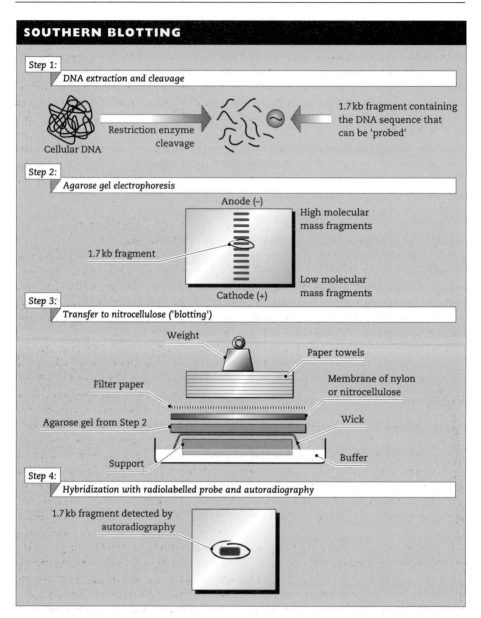

Step 1: DNA extraction and cleavage

Cellular DNA → Restriction enzyme cleavage → 1.7 kb fragment containing the DNA sequence that can be 'probed'

Step 2: Agarose gel electrophoresis

Anode (−)

High molecular mass fragments

1.7 kb fragment

Cathode (+)

Low molecular mass fragments

Step 3: Transfer to nitrocellulose ('blotting')

Weight

Filter paper

Paper towels

Membrane of nylon or nitrocellulose

Agarose gel from Step 2

Wick

Support

Buffer

Step 4: Hybridization with radiolabelled probe and autoradiography

1.7 kb fragment detected by autoradiography

Fig. 20.5 Steps in the technique of Southern blotting. The 'blot' is a replica on nitrocellulose or nylon of the DNA fragments that have been separated by electrophoresis on an agarose gel. Specific DNA sequences of interest are identified by hybridization to a specific radiolabelled probe. Fragment(s) containing the particular sequence are identified by autoradiography.

nitrocellulose membrane (the blot). This is achieved by layering the nitrocellulose membrane over the gel (which rests in buffer) and overlaying the membrane with absorbent paper that acts as a wick to draw buffer through the gel and encourage DNA transfer to the membrane. The membrane is much easier to handle than the fragile agarose, and allows the hybridization to be carried out in a stringent fashion. The labelled probe identifies those fragments of DNA that contain sufficient complementary sequence; the labelled fragments are detected by autoradiography.

In the clinical laboratory, this method is very important in the diagnosis of single-gene defects. The precise way in which it can be applied depends on how much detailed knowledge is available about the mutation event. Where this is known in detail, the technique can be made highly specific. In sickle-cell anaemia, for example, the single amino acid substitution of valine for glutamic acid is the result of a single-base change in which thymine (T) replaces adenine. This single base change leads to the loss of the recognition sequence for a restriction endonuclease termed MstIII in the mutant gene. When the genomic DNA is cut with this enzyme and subjected to Southern blotting using a probe specific for the β-globin gene, the length of DNA containing the appropriate complementary sequence differs between the sickle cell and normal specimens; this is readily detected on the Southern blot.

An alternative method uses labelled oligonucleotide probes to detect normal and mutated sequences. Labelled oligomers of about 19 nucleotides in length are constructed, one complementary to the normal sequence and the other to the mutated sequence. Under strict hybridization conditions, the 'normal' oligomer will hybridize only with the normal gene, and vice versa. The technique has been applied to the detection of α_1-antiprotease (α_1-antitrypsin) variants. In the example shown (Fig. 20.6), α_1-antiprotease deficiency results from homozygosity of the Pi^Z allele.

A further possibility is to use the technique of single-strand chain polymorphism. Single-stranded DNA folds into a complex structure that is dictated by the nucleotide sequence of the strand. In turn, the complex secondary structure influences the mobility of the single-stranded DNA on a gel. Two DNA fragments differing by a single base change are amplified (by the PCR technique; see p. 277) and run on a gel. The single base change is sufficient to lead to a difference in the complex secondary structure and a different mobility on the gel (Fig. 20.7).

Restriction fragment length polymorphisms (Fig. 20.8)

Even if the particular gene responsible for a single-gene defect is unknown, the Southern blot technique can still be used to follow the segregation of the mutated gene by detection of a DNA polymorphism that segregates with the defective trait.

At the molecular level, inherited differences in the structure of DNA will be reflected in changes in the nucleotide sequence. Where these changes involve a coding region of DNA or a region that regulates gene expression, the consequences may be serious. Nevertheless, about 50% of the human genome consists of repetitive sequences of uncertain function. If the introns and noncoding flanking sequences are included, there is clearly the possibility of inherited differences in DNA structure that have no known serious clinical consequences. These individual differences lead to altered patterns of DNA fragments when the genome is subjected to digestion by specific restriction endonucleases, and they are known as restriction fragment length polymorphisms (RFLPs).

If a particular RFLP is closely linked to a mutant gene of interest, it can be used to follow the segregation of that gene across different generations. As with all linkage analysis, the method is not foolproof, since crossing-over between the mutant gene and the RFLP site will destroy the linkage and potentially lead to misdiagnosis. By choosing RFLP sites that are very close to the mutant gene, this probability can be kept as low as possible. Moreover,

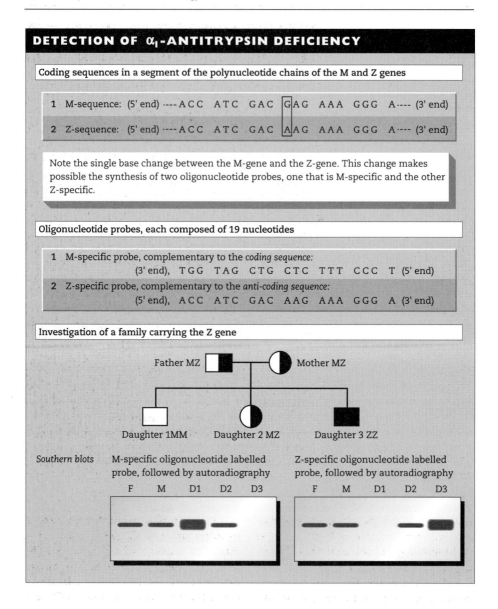

DETECTION OF α_1-ANTITRYPSIN DEFICIENCY

Coding sequences in a segment of the polynucleotide chains of the M and Z genes

1 M-sequence: (5' end) ----A C C   A T C   G A C |G|A G   A A A   G G G   A ---- (3' end)

2 Z-sequence: (5' end) ----A C C   A T C   G A C |A|A G   A A A   G G G   A ---- (3' end)

Note the single base change between the M-gene and the Z-gene. This change makes possible the synthesis of two oligonucleotide probes, one that is M-specific and the other Z-specific.

Oligonucleotide probes, each composed of 19 nucleotides

1 M-specific probe, complementary to the *coding sequence*:
                    (3' end),   T G G   T A G   C T G   C T C   T T T   C C C   T (5' end)
2 Z-specific probe, complementary to the *anti-coding sequence*:
                    (5' end),   A C C   A T C   G A C   A A G   A A A   G G G   A (3' end)

Investigation of a family carrying the Z gene

Father MZ   Mother MZ

Daughter 1MM   Daughter 2 MZ   Daughter 3 ZZ

Southern blots   M-specific oligonucleotide labelled   Z-specific oligonucleotide labelled
                    probe, followed by autoradiography   probe, followed by autoradiography

        F   M   D1   D2   D3   F   M   D1   D2   D3

Fig. 20.6 Detection of homozygous ZZ α_1-protease inhibitor (α_1-antitrypsin) deficiency by means of Southern blots, using specific oligonucleotide probes and autoradiography.

several linked RFLPs, generated using different restriction endonucleases, can be used to follow the segregation of the gene (Fig. 20.8).

If the mutant gene is unknown, 'random' genomic DNA probes must be used initially to search for any RFLP. The method can be made less hit-and-miss by using genomic probes that do not contain repetitive sequences and presumably detect structural loci. If the chromosomal location of the mutant gene is known, then probes derived from libraries made exclusively from the DNA of this chromosome can be used. In this way, it is possible to refine the analysis progressively to obtain probes closer and closer to the mutant gene. The technique is

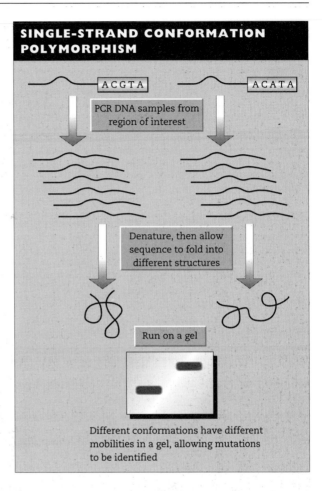

SINGLE-STRAND CONFORMATION POLYMORPHISM

ACGTA   ACATA

PCR DNA samples from region of interest

Denature, then allow sequence to fold into different structures

Run on a gel

Different conformations have different mobilities in a gel, allowing mutations to be identified

Fig. 20.7 Single-strand conformation polymorphism.

such that it is possible eventually to obtain genomic probes that contain the coding region of the mutant gene itself, even before knowledge of the gene-derived polypeptide product is available. In this way, it has been possible to clone the gene responsible for cystic fibrosis (CF).

In studies of CF, random screening techniques located the gene to chromosome 7. Once the general location of the gene was known, further refinements with different batteries of probes produced polymorphic markers with progressively closer linkage, based on family studies, to the putative gene. Eventually, it was possible to obtain sequence information on the gene itself. As a result of

this work, it is now known that a number of mutations within the CF gene occur, although about 70% of cases of CF are accounted for by deletion of a single base in codon 507 and two bases in codon 508. This results in a deletion of phenylalanine at position 508 of the CF gene product, a membrane protein that is involved in cellular chloride transport.

Hypervariable regions and RFLP

Another application of RFLP is in connection with the so-called hypervariable regions of DNA present in the genome of mammals, other animals and plants. These regions are made up of short DNA sequences, perhaps 6–8 base pairs in length and often rich in

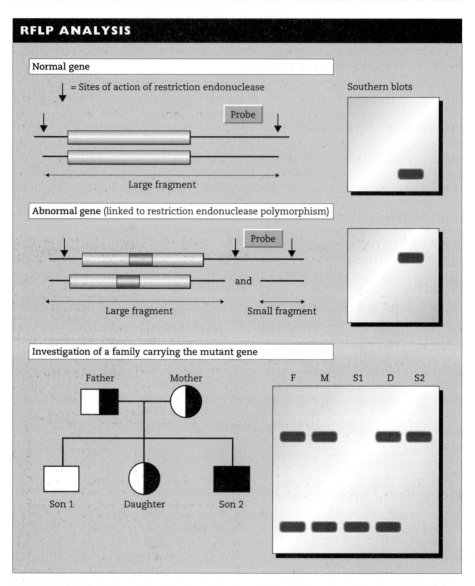

Fig. 20.8 Restriction fragment length polymorphism (RFLP) analysis. An additional restriction endonuclease site linked to the mutant gene is present in affected individuals. When the DNA is cut using the appropriate restriction endonuclease, fragments of different size are produced from normal and affected individuals. Although the probe is not directed at the gene itself, it is able to detect the different fragments thereby produced.

guanine (G) and cytosine (C), which are repeated in tandem. Polymorphism arises because the number of tandem repeats of the core DNA sequence varies between individuals. Moreover, the same tandem repeat can be found scattered throughout the genome in hypervariable regions of different lengths. The repeat structure of these regions has led to their being described as 'mini-satellite' DNA. If a restriction enzyme digest is used to cut on each side of the hypervariable region, a Southern blot analysis can be carried out to identify the different lengths of hypervariable region using the appropriate mini-satellite probe. The 'DNA fingerprint' obtained in this way is unique to a particular individual. Although there is considerable variability in the lengths of these segments of DNA, it is not so great as to prevent the pattern being used in segregation studies. A band that appears to segregate with a disease in a large pedigree study, for example, can be isolated and cloned to search for a locus-specific probe. One application of this technique has been in paternity disputes and in other forensic work.

Polymerase chain reaction (Fig. 20.9)

This reaction is a means of greatly amplifying selected portions of DNA. Its specificity for the particular length of DNA (usually from 100 to several thousand nucleotides in length) depends on the use of two oligonucleotide probes (each typically 20 nucleotides in length) that are complementary to the two ends of the

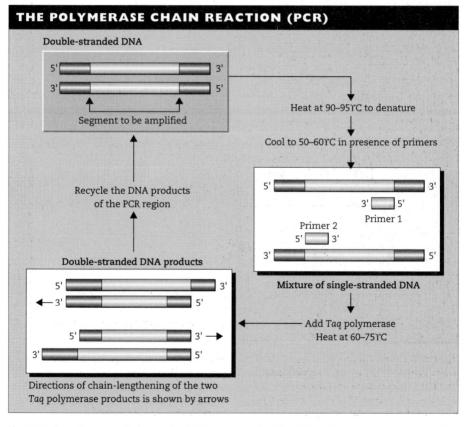

THE POLYMERASE CHAIN REACTION (PCR)

Double-stranded DNA

Segment to be amplified

Heat at 90–95˚C to denature

Cool to 50–60˚C in presence of primers

Recycle the DNA products of the PCR region

Primer 1

Primer 2

Double-stranded DNA products

Mixture of single-stranded DNA

Add Taq polymerase
Heat at 60–75˚C

Directions of chain-lengthening of the two Taq polymerase products is shown by arrows

Fig. 20.9 The polymerase chain reaction (PCR). The two double-stranded products of the first PCR cycle are subjected to a repeat cycle of denaturation, primer annealing and primer-directed extension and these processes are then repeated again and again. After three of these cycles, one-quarter of the DNA is present as short products and thereafter these products begin to accumulate exponentially. After 30 or more cycles, the vast majority of the DNA is present as short products. Amplification is sufficient to allow direct visualization of the product on a gel after staining with ethidium bromide.

sequence to be amplified; the probes are also made to hybridize to opposite strands. In PCR, the template DNA to be amplified is first heated to 90–95 °C, to cause strand separation, and then cooled to 50–65 °C in the presence of the two primers to allow annealing of the primers to their respective DNA sequences. The reaction temperature is then adjusted to 60–75 °C in the presence of heat-stable *Taq* polymerase. The *Taq* polymerase leads to a primer-mediated extension of both strands of the template DNA, in the region between the two primers. The three reactions of denaturation, primer-annealing and primer-directed extension are then repeated, leading to a *geometric* increase in the DNA between the two primers, whereas the single-stranded long products accumulate arithmetically (Fig. 20.9). The theoretical amplification achieved is 2^n, where n is the number of cycles of denaturation–annealing–extension, though the amplification is usually somewhat less, as the reaction is less then 100% efficient. Using this reaction, specific lengths of DNA can be amplified a million-fold, to an extent that the amplified product can be directly visualized on an agarose gel without the need for a Southern blot to be carried out using a labelled probe. The amplified DNA band is visualized on the gel by staining with ethidium bromide, a compound that binds avidly to DNA and fluoresces.

The PCR is a very powerful diagnostic and research tool. In microbiology, for example, it can be used to pick out and amplify DNA sequences that are unique to invading organisms, and enable their identification. It can also be used to amplify DNA for the purposes of DNA fingerprinting in the forensic laboratory. In clinical biochemistry and molecular biology, it is used, like Southern blotting, in the antenatal diagnosis of single-gene mutations and in studying structural gene polymorphisms. Thus, an amplified DNA sequence can be subject to digestion by a restriction enzyme that recognizes an allele which is linked to, or causes, an inherited disorder. Its use in the detection of the commonest mutation responsible for CF

is illustrated in Fig. 20.10, in which a modification of the PCR is used – the so-called amplification refractory mutation system (ARMS).

Oligonucleotides with single 3′-mismatched residue fail to act as primers, and so fail to amplify a particular segment of DNA by PCR, and the ARMS is based on this fact. For example, in screening for the ΔF_{508} mutation in CF, one primer is constructed that matches the normal nucleotide sequence at this site, and a second primer is constructed that matches the mutated sequence at this site. Amplification by PCR is then tested, in turn, with each primer (the primer on the other strand remains the same in both incubations). Provided this mutation alone is responsible for the CF gene defect, it can be used successfully in antenatal diagnosis (Fig. 20.10).

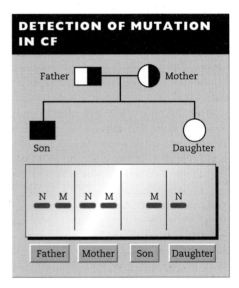

Fig. 20.10 Detection of the mutation in cystic fibrosis by an amplification-refractory mutation system. Each individual is tested in a PCR with 'normal' (N) and with a 'mutant' (M) primer; these symbols denote the PCR products in the members of the family. They are visualized on the gel with ethidium bromide. Mismatches prevent PCR amplification, and are shown by the absence of a band from the gel. The designation of the mutation in cystic fibrosis is ΔF_{508}.

Molecular genetics of single-gene and polygenic disorders

The diagnostic aspects of single-gene defects are mostly carried out in molecular genetics units. Clinical biochemistry departments in the United Kingdom as yet undertake only a limited amount of diagnostic work on single-gene defects (e.g. α_1-antiprotease deficiency, monogenetic apolipoprotein abnormalities). It is likely that, as these newer techniques are applied to diseases such as diabetes mellitus and cardiovascular disease, there will be an increasing use of DNA-based tests in the routine diagnostic laboratory. The application of these methods to research and development in clinical biochemistry will also increase.

Single-gene disorders

Several examples of the way in which molecular biology has been used in the diagnosis of single-gene defects have already been mentioned. These techniques have greatly improved our understanding of the molecular events underlying many of these single-gene defects.

Point mutations within the coding region of a protein can lead to defective protein formation. The best known example of this is haemoglobin S, but the two most important allelic variants for α_1-antiprotease deficiency, Pi^Z and Pi^S, are also point mutations. These mutations probably interfere with the tertiary folding of the newly synthesized protein, and this, in turn, prevents the processing of the enzyme that is needed for secretion to occur. As a consequence, the protein accumulates in the liver cell.

Several point mutations associated with defective receptor function have been described. In the case of the low-density lipoprotein (LDL) receptor, these mutations can lead to reduced transport from the endoplasmic reticulum to the Golgi apparatus, to reduced LDL binding, and to a failure of the receptor–LDL ligand complex to cluster in coated pits. Some point mutations lead to defective enzymes, with the accumulation of toxic precursors or metabolic by-products (e.g. phenylketonuria, Tay–Sachs disease) and others to defective membrane proteins (e.g. hereditary spherocytosis).

Molecular biology techniques have characterized the basis of other types of mutation. Genes or portions of genes may be deleted or fused with other genes. Regions of DNA can become inverted, or additional DNA can become inserted into coding regions. These types of mutation may be associated with a failure of transcription, or can lead to defective products. More unusual mutations may involve the promoter site, or recognition sites for splicing, or the initiation or termination codons of the gene.

At the time of writing, over 2000 single-gene defects with an established mode of inheri-

GENETIC DISORDERS
Single-gene defects
Acute intermittent porphyria
α_1-Protease inhibitor deficiency
Congenital adrenal hyperplasia
Cystic fibrosis
Galactosaemia
Gaucher's disease
Growth hormone deficiency
Homocystinuria
Hurler's disease
Hyperlipidaemias
Multiple endocrine neoplasia
Phenylketonuria
Tay–Sachs disease
Wilson's disease
Polygenic disorders
Cancer susceptibility
Coronary heart disease
Diabetes mellitus
Epilepsy
Manic depressive psychosis
Schizophrenia

Table 20.1 Examples of single-gene and polygenic disorders that impinge on the practice of clinical biochemistry.

tance have been described. Table 20.1 lists some of the single-gene defects associated with biochemical abnormalities that have been discussed elsewhere in this book. In all cases, these defects have been mapped to particular chromosomal locations and, in most of the examples, carrier detection and antenatal screening is feasible.

Polygenic disorders

The analytical and diagnostic power of molecular biology has been maximally exploited in single-gene defects. Some of these defects are relatively common, notably the haemoglobinopathies and cystic fibrosis; many are rare. However, most common diseases – those with the greatest impact on morbidity and mortality – are not the result of single-gene defects. Nevertheless, serious public health problems such as ischaemic cardiovascular disease, hypertension, diabetes mellitus and cancer do run in families. Environmental factors undoubtedly exert an important effect in the development of these diseases (e.g. smoking and cancer, diet and cardiovascular disease) but, at the same time, inherited factors also contribute significantly.

The genetic study of disorders in which multiple-gene (polygenic) inheritance contributes is complex. One approach is to make a calculated guess that particular genes might influence susceptibility to a disease. For example, in the study of cardiovascular disease due to atheroma, where epidemiological studies indicate a clear association between plasma [cholesterol] and ischaemic heart disease (Fig. 12.2), and where cholesterol is known to be a major component of the atheromatous plaque, a study of polymorphism among the apolipoproteins would be a rational approach. Remnant hyperlipidaemia (p. 172) is an example of an association of an apolipoprotein polymorphism with environmental factors in the genesis of atheroma. These studies may also reveal monogenetic contributions to the susceptibility to atheroma, as in familial defective apolipoprotein B (apoB) in which an abnormal apoB100 is produced that reduces the binding of LDL to its receptor, leading to elevated plasma [LDL cholesterol].

If probes exist to putative candidate genes, they can be used in RFLP analysis either to investigate large families over several generations, or to compare affected with unaffected siblings; alternatively, a range of probes can be used to look for RFLP in these groups. Whichever method is chosen, the aim is to discover RFLPs that segregate with the disease, as any such RFLP linkage would indicate a potentially important gene, or gene cluster, that influences the development of the disease under investigation.

Inheritance is known to be important in the development of diabetes mellitus, contributing more in type II than type I (p. 152). RFLP polymorphism in a hypervariable region upstream of the insulin gene has been described for both types of diabetes mellitus, but it is not yet known whether there is a gene close to the insulin gene that influences susceptibility to diabetes mellitus. In the case of type I diabetes mellitus, where auto-immune factors are important, RFLP analysis has shown linkage of polymorphisms within the class II (or DR) major histocompatibility complex, which is involved in cell-surface antigen recognition by helper T cells, with both susceptibility and resistance to type I diabetes mellitus.

Table 20.1 lists some of the more common polygenic diseases that are amenable to study using the techniques described in this chapter. For most of the polygenic diseases listed, the risk for a first-degree relative of contracting the disorder is broadly in the region 5–15%.

KEY POINTS

1 The new techniques of molecular biology have had a major impact upon clinical medicine. On the diagnostic side, accurate detection of single-gene defects for a wide range of inherited single-gene disorders is now possible (e.g. for cystic fibrosis). Molecular techniques can also be used to identify certain infectious agents, especially viruses (e.g. human immunodeficiency virus, HIV). On the therapeutic side, gene cloning and expression has allowed the synthesis of human proteins in bacteria (e.g. insulin) and the development of vaccines (e.g. hepatitis B).

2 Future developments are likely to be equally significant. Gene therapy for single-gene defects and the identification of candidate genes contributing to polygenic disorders are active areas of study. Molecular techniques are also contributing to our understanding of cancer genetics.

3 Many of these advances have depended on some very powerful analytical techniques. Deoxyribonucleic acid (DNA) can be precisely cut (using restriction endonucleases), specifically ligated to other pieces of DNA (e.g. to plasmid DNA) and cloned (e.g. by growing the plasmid in its bacterial host). Specific (including mutant) sequences of DNA can be identified by hybridization techniques on Southern blotting. DNA can be amplified (by polymerase chain reaction, PCR) and its nucleotide sequence can be determined (DNA sequencing).

CHAPTER 21

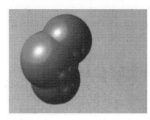

Central Nervous System and Cerebrospinal Fluid

Cerebrospinal fluid, 282
  Examination of CSF, 282

Many neurological disorders have a biochemical basis, or are associated with disturbances of metabolism. However, neurochemistry is a specialized subject that is beyond the scope of this book. Many generalized disorders of metabolism affect the central nervous system (CNS), e.g. Hartnup disease, Wilson's disease, phenylketonuria (PKU) and these are considered elsewhere. In this chapter, we discuss the information to be gained from examining the cerebrospinal fluid (CSF).

Cerebrospinal fluid

The CSF approximates to an ultrafiltrate of plasma. There are, however, differences between the relative concentrations in plasma and CSF of both low molecular mass and high molecular mass substances. For example:

1 Low molecular mass substances.

    (a) *Differential rates of diffusion.* Dissolved CO_2 diffuses into CSF more rapidly than HCO_3^-, so CSF [H^+] (which depends on the HCO_3^- : H_2CO_3 ratio) may be significantly different from plasma [H^+].

    (b) *Effects of ultrafiltration.* Bilirubin is nearly all protein-bound in plasma, and normally very little crosses the blood–brain barrier. Calcium is only partly protein-bound, and Ca^{2+} readily cross into the CSF.

2 High molecular mass substances

    (a) *Differential rates of diffusion.* Albumin is present in CSF in relatively higher concentration than larger proteins. However,

because of the blood–brain barrier, plasma [total protein] is about 200 times greater than CSF [total protein].

    (b) *Secretion of proteins.* Some proteins, e.g. immunoglobulins, are secreted into the CSF.

Examination of CSF

CSF is normally clear and colourless. Turbidity is usually due to leucocytes, but it may be due to micro-organisms. Blood-stained CSF may indicate recent haemorrhage, or damage to a blood vessel during specimen collection. Xanthochromia (yellow colour) is most often due to previous haemorrhage into the CSF, but it may indicate that CSF [protein] is very high. The CSF may be yellow in jaundiced patients.

Xanthochromia

As indicated above, this was originally a test performed by inspecting CSF for a yellow colour, particularly useful for detecting subarachnoid haemorrhage. However, the test can be made much more sensitive, and more useful clinically, by performing a spectrophotometric scan of CSF that has been obtained more than 12 hours after the clinical episode and centrifuged in the laboratory as soon as possible after the specimen has been taken. The presence of a characteristic spectral band, due to haemoglobin or its breakdown products, indicates that there has been a recent haemorrhage into the CSF.

CSF glucose

Lumbar CSF [glucose] is normally 0.5–1.0

mmol/L lower than plasma [glucose], whereas CSF [glucose] in specimens obtained from the cerebral ventricles and from the cisterna magna normally differs little from plasma [glucose]. In hypoglycaemia, CSF [glucose] may be very low; it is raised when there is hyperglycaemia.

CSF [glucose] may be low or undetectable in patients with acute bacterial, cryptococcal, tubercular or carcinomatous meningitis, or in cerebral abscess, probably due to consumption of glucose by leucocytes or other rapidly metabolizing cells. In meningitis or encephalitis due to viral infections, it is usually normal.

CSF total protein

Lumbar CSF protein (reference range 100–400 mg/L) is normally almost all albumin. Ventricular and cisternal CSF [protein] is lower than lumbar CSF [protein]. Much higher CSF [protein] may have no pathological significance in the neonatal period – for example, lumbar CSF [protein] may then be as much as 900 mg/L.

CSF [protein] is increased in a large number of pathological conditions. Whenever it is increased, organic disease of the CNS is probably present. In acute inflammatory conditions of the CNS, the increase may be very marked due to increased capillary permeability.

In the *demyelinating disorders*, there is often a moderate increase in CSF [protein], usually in the range 500–1000 mg/L.

Primary and secondary neoplasms involving the brain or the meninges can cause very large increases in lumbar CSF [protein] if spinal block occurs. Values over 5000 mg/L may be observed. These specimens may be xanthochromic, and a protein clot may form on storage after a few hours.

CSF immunoglobulin (Ig)

CSF normally contains small amounts of IgG (reference range 8–64 mg/L), a trace of IgA and minute amounts of IgM. Increases in CSF [Ig], particularly CSF [IgG], may be due to increased ultrafiltration of plasma immunoglobulins into the CSF, or to increased local synthesis of immunoglobulins.

Whenever there is increased local synthesis of IgG, the ratios CSF [IgG] : CSF [albumin] and CSF [IgG] : CSF [total protein] are higher than normal. This occurs in multiple sclerosis, neurosyphilis, subacute sclerosing panencephalitis, and some other conditions. In all these conditions, limited numbers of clones of B-cells produce immunoglobulins, and discrete oligoclonal bands are demonstrable by isoelectric focusing of CSF.

Multiple sclerosis. It can be difficult to confirm a diagnosis of multiple sclerosis in its early stages. The following tests may help:

1 *CSF [IgG]*. This lacks specificity, since any cause of increased CSF [total protein] will also tend to cause an increase in CSF [IgG].

2 *CSF [IgG] : CSF [albumin]*. This ratio renders the CSF [IgG] measurement more specific for CNS immunoglobulin synthesis, but is only abnormal in about 60–70 % of clinically definite cases of multiple sclerosis.

3 *Isoelectric focusing* for the presence in CSF of oligoclonal bands that are not present in serum. This test is abnormal in over 90 % of cases of clinically definite multiple sclerosis.

CHAPTER 22

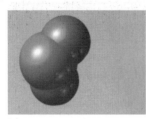

Therapeutic Drug Monitoring and Chemical Toxicology

Therapeutic drug
monitoring, 284
Chemical toxicology, 288

Industrial and occupational
hazards, 291

Poisoning is one of the commonest causes of emergency admission to hospital. Of the numerous potentially fatal chemicals and drugs, only a limited number are encountered in practice. It may be important to know the nature and blood levels of the poison, as this may help management and determine prognosis.

Drug therapy should usually be monitored on clinical grounds rather than on blood levels. However, for a few drugs, measurement of drug levels in blood is essential to ensure a therapeutic effect without toxicity.

Drug abuse is an increasing social and medical problem. Urinary drug measurements have an important part to play in the management of a number of these individuals.

This chapter outlines the important role that clinical biochemistry departments play in monitoring the therapeutic use of certain drugs, investigating patients when drugs and poisons may have been taken in overdose, and in screening for drugs of abuse.

Therapeutic drug monitoring

When is therapeutic drug monitoring required?

For many drugs, the dose given correlates well with a pharmacological effect, and the correct dosage can be satisfactorily determined by clinical assessment or the measurement of a biochemical response. For example, the pharmacological actions of anticoagulants and of antihypertensive drugs can be assessed, and dosage adjusted, on the basis of prothrombin time and blood pressure measurements, respectively.

Measurement of plasma or blood drug levels is required:
• For drugs that have a narrow therapeutic range, e.g. lithium.
• For drugs which in overdose may produce symptoms that are similar to those of the disease being treated, e.g. phenytoin, cyclosporin.
• Where the drug may produce abnormalities in hepatic or renal clearance.
• Where drug absorption may vary with dose or other circumstances.

Table 22.1 lists the drugs for which the case for therapeutic drug monitoring (TDM) has been clearly established. Regular monitoring of patients taking these drugs is not usually required once the patient has been stabilized on a dose of drug that has produced the desired clinical effect.

TDM is important if there is a particular clinical problem to be addressed, such as:
• Establishing a dose regimen when therapy has just begun, or when it needs to be changed.
• Failure to achieve therapeutic control, although dosage is apparently adequate.
• Loss of control in a patient previously stabilized on treatment. This may, for example, be due to partial compliance or altered metabolism.

THERAPEUTIC DRUG MONITORING

Drug	Therapeutic range in plasma*		Time to collect blood	Half-life (hours)	Reason †
	Level	Units			
Aminoglycoside antibiotics	Peak 5–10	mg/L	30 min to 1 h after last dose		2, 3, 4, 5
Gentamycin/ tobramycin	Trough <2	mg/L	Just before next dose	2–3	2, 3, 4, 5
Carbamazepine	4–10 17–42	mg/L μmol/L	Just before next dose	8–24	3
Cyclosporin	120–300	nmol/L	Just before next dose	6–24	3
Digoxin	0.8–2.0 1.0–2.6	ng/mL nmol/L	6–18 h after last dose	36–48	1, 2, 3, 4
Lithium	416–694 0.6–1.0	mg/100 mL mmol/L	12–18 h after last dose	10–35	1, 2, 5
Phenytoin	10–20 40–80	mg/L μmol/L	Long half-life –not critical	20–40	1, 3
Theophylline	10–20 55–110	mg/L μmol/L	Not critical‡	3–13	1, 2, 3, 4

*For conversion factors for numerical values from mass units into molar units, see p. 304.
† Key to the reasons for performing therapeutic drug monitoring:
1. Wide inter-individual variation.
2. Low therapeutic index.
3. Therapeutic effect or signs of toxicity difficult to recognize.
4. Administration of a potentially toxic drug to a seriously ill patient.
5. Very toxic in overdose.
‡ Timing of peak levels will depend on formulation, e.g. slow-acting preparations.

Table 22.1 Therapeutic drug monitoring: the principal drugs for which it is indicated.

• To check for toxicity, especially if several drugs are being given.

When should the blood sample be taken?

When a single dose of drug is taken for the first time, plasma levels will initially rise rapidly and then decline in a curvilinear manner similar to that shown in Figure 22.1. The characteristics of this curve provide essential details about the kinetics of the drug and the information needed to calculate the approximate dose and frequency of the drug for the desired therapeutic concentration in plasma. For any drug given at regular intervals, a steady-state relatively constant concentration in plasma is reached after about five half-lives (Fig. 22.1). However, peak levels (achieved just after administration) and trough levels (achieved immediately prior to the next dose) may still be recognized. For most drugs, it is important that trough levels are adequate to achieve the desired therapeutic effect. Thus, blood samples are often withdrawn just before a dose of the drug is taken, but at any rate samples should be taken after the initial peak has subsided, unless toxicity is suspected.

In all cases, the time of blood sampling and of the last dose of the drug must be given.

Interpretation of drug levels

Therapeutic ranges. If the blood has been taken at the appropriate time, the plasma level can be

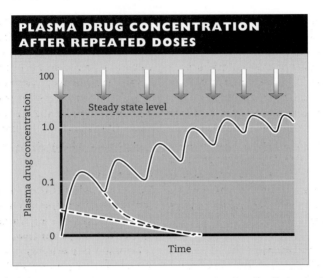

PLASMA DRUG CONCENTRATION AFTER REPEATED DOSES

Fig. 22.1 The effect on plasma drug concentration of giving repeated regular doses of a drug. As can be seen, after approximately five doses of the drug, a steady state level is reached, with peak and trough values being found.

– – –: Line showing the elimination half-life.
- —-—: Line showing the plasma drug concentration profile if a single dose of the drug had been given. Arrows show the time of each dose of the drug.

compared with published therapeutic ranges (Table 22.1). These published ranges indicate the range of plasma drug levels which in the majority of the population have been shown to provide the desired therapeutic effect without a high risk of toxicity. Published ranges offer little more than guidelines, because of inter-individual variation in the clinical response to drugs.

Interpretation of a result requires:
• *Correct timing of blood sampling in relation to the dose.* If specimens are collected too soon after the start of treatment, or after dosage has been changed (i.e. before a steady-state concentration of drug has been achieved), TDM results will be misleading.
• *Clinical information.* Published therapeutic ranges cannot make allowance for the possible effects of hepatic or renal disease in individual patients, or for the consequences of drug interactions that might stem from particular prescribing combinations. For example, in patients with renal impairment, drugs will be eliminated from the circulation at a rate that may be much slower than normal. Alternatively,

in patients taking drugs that result in the induction of hepatic drug-metabolizing enzyme systems, the clearance of other drugs being taken simultaneously by the patient may be enhanced.

Other important issues in therapeutic drug monitoring

Free and bound drugs

Most drugs circulate partly bound to plasma proteins, the bound and unbound forms being in equilibrium. The pharmacological response is usually determined by the tissue concentration which, in turn, is related to the plasma [unbound drug]. However, plasma [free drug] is difficult to measure, and TDM depends on measurements of plasma [total drug].

The importance of drug metabolites

Most drugs are metabolized to inactive products, although some are inactive when taken, and are converted to active drug in the liver or gastrointestinal tract. For example, primidone is converted to active metabolites, principally phenobarbitone. If primidone therapy is to be monitored, plasma [phenobarbitone] is the measurement required.

A number of different analytical methods are sometimes used for measurement of a single drug (and possibly of its metabolites). This explains the differences that may be found between results from different laboratories. It also explains why some less specific methods may give rise to misleading results if there are high concentrations of *inactive metabolites* in plasma. Even specific methods may give rise to misleading results if they fail to measure *active metabolites*.

Units of measurement

Plasma drug concentrations may be expressed in mass (gravimetric) or molar units of concentration (Table 22.1) The practice of referring to numerical values of drug measurements without mentioning the units is dangerous, since it can lead to serious – and sometimes fatal – mistakes.

Specific drugs

Aminoglycoside antibiotics. These antibiotics have a very short half-life of two to three hours if renal function is normal, but in patients with renal impairment the half-life is prolonged (up to 100 hours). In addition, tissue pools of gentamycin may become saturated if treatment is for more than a week, and then plasma levels may start to rise sharply. Gentamycin is *nephrotoxic* and *ototoxic*. Therefore, TDM is particularly important in patients with impaired renal function who receive the drug for more than seven days, or those on high loading doses for serious infection. Peak and trough levels should be measured.

Anticonvulsants

Carbamazepine. Carbamazepine has fewer side-effects, mainly neurotoxic, than phenytoin. Monitoring is of value in patients with poor control, since there is a variable relationship between dose and plasma concentration. The sample should be taken just before a dose.

Phenytoin. Phenytoin has a low therapeutic ratio and is subject to variable rates of hepatic metabolism, leading to a nonlinear relationship between dose and plasma concentration. Because of its undesirable side effects, which include neurotoxicity and increased frequency of fits, TDM is required in new patients, where there is an unexpected loss in control, in pregnancy, or when other drugs that interact with phenytoin are added or withdrawn.

Cyclosporin

This drug is widely used to prevent graft rejection following transplantation. It is nephrotoxic, with signs that may mimic rejection in patients with renal transplants.

Tacrolimus is a relatively new immunosuppressive drug that has replaced cyclosporin in some transplant centres. It is less toxic than cyclosporin, but TDM is still recommended to ensure efficacy.

Digoxin

Digoxin has little clinical effect at plasma concentrations below 1 nmol/L, whereas toxicity (often manifest as cardiac arrhythmia and vomiting) is common when plasma levels rise above 3.8 nmol/L. Digoxin results should always be interpreted together with a plasma potassium concentration, since hypokalaemia potentiates the effect of digoxin. Thus, toxic effects of the drug may occur in a hypokalaemic patient who has a plasma digoxin within the therapeutic range. A similar effect may be seen in hypercalcaemia, hypomagnesaemia and hypothyroidism. Equilibration of digoxin with cardiac tissue takes some time, and thus blood should not be taken for at least six hours after the dose.

Lithium

Lithium is used for the treatment of depressive illness. It has a short half-life, and plasma levels should be determined 12 hours after the last dose. TDM is essential because the drug is toxic, producing a range of symptoms including polyuria, hypothyroidism and, in severe cases, renal failure and coma. Patients with plasma [lithium] above 1.4 mmol/L are at risk of oliguria and acute renal failure. TDM may also be necessary in order to monitor compliance.

Methotrexate

Methotrexate is a dihydrofolate reductase inhibitor, and therefore reduces intracellular folate, which in turn inhibits DNA synthesis. The drug is cytotoxic; high-dose regimens are used in the treatment of some cancers, and lower-dose regimens are used for immunosuppression. TDM is of value in patients receiving high doses of methotrexate, to identify those at risk of toxic effects and to provide a guide to the dose and timing of leucovorin (a drug that restores the pool of reduced folate) rescue.

Theophylline

This drug is a vasodilator and central nervous system stimulant used to prevent or treat bronchoconstriction in some children or elderly patients who cannot easily use an inhaler. The drug commonly produces minor side-effects such as nausea and headache, even at concentrations within the therapeutic range. Serious toxicity leading to cardiac arrhythmia can occur with plasma levels above 110 mmol/L. TDM is particularly valuable to optimize the dose, confirm toxicity, or demonstrate poor compliance.

Chemical toxicology

Poisoning is one of the commonest causes of emergency admission to hospital. Although accidental poisoning does occur, intentional drug overdose is more common. If the patient is conscious and presents with specific signs and symptoms of toxicity, then a reliable history, with the clinical examination, will usually suggest which drug or drugs have been taken. This can be confirmed by laboratory investigations. Unfortunately, few of the drugs commonly taken in overdose have specific clinical signs. It is quite common for a combination of drugs to have been taken, sometimes with large amounts of alcohol.

Problems arise when the patient is unconscious and the history is unavailable or likely to be inaccurate. In such a situation, the laboratory may be asked to perform a drug screen to identify which drugs and poisons may have been taken.

Other important tests that should be performed on the patient with suspected poisoning include:

• Urea and electrolytes.
• Liver function tests.
• Blood glucose.
• Blood gases.

Treatment

A few drugs have a specific antidote (Table 22.2), but some antidotes may themselves have unpleasant side effects. For the majority of poisons no antidote is available, and the patient is treated conservatively until the drug has been eliminated from the body. If there is poor renal or liver function, it may be necessary to use haemodialysis or charcoal haemoperfusion to eliminate the drug, and in such a case measurement of plasma levels is very important.

Online computer databases are now readily available to aid the doctor with advice regarding both the diagnosis and treatment of the poisoned patient.

Specific drugs and poisons
Paracetamol

Overdose with paracetamol is common. During the first few hours there may be few symptoms, unless these arise from another drug that has been taken simultaneously. A very large overdose may produce symptoms of depressed consciousness and metabolic acidosis. In patients presenting after 20 hours, biochemical evidence of liver dysfunction is often apparent.

Approximately 8% of ingested paracetamol is converted in the liver to a toxic metabolite, N-acetyl-p-benzoquinoneimine (NABQI), which is usually detoxified by conjugation with glutathione. If large amounts of paracetamol are taken, the hepatic stores of glutathione become depleted, and NABQI binds irre-

PRINCIPAL CAUSES OF ACUTE POISONING

Substance	Active treatment of overdose or toxin
Drugs commonly taken as overdose	
Benzodiazepines	Flumazenil
Ethanol	No specific treatment available
Paracetamol	N-acetylcysteine
Salicylates	Sodium bicarbonate, haemodialysis, repeated oral activated charcoal
Tricyclic antidepressants	No specific treatment available
Drugs less commonly taken as overdose	
Carbamazepine	Repeated oral activated charcoal
Digoxin	Antidigoxin antibody
Iron	Desferrioxamine
Lithium	Saline
Opiates	Naloxone
Phenobarbitone	Repeated oral activated charcoal
Phenytoin	Repeated oral activated charcoal
Quinine	Repeated oral activated charcoal
Toxic substances	
Carbon monoxide	Oxygen
Cyanide (nonfatal dose)	Cobalt edetate, hydroxocobalamin
Ethylene glycol	Ethanol, haemodialysis
Methanol	Ethanol, haemodialysis
Organophosphorus agents	Pralidoxime, atropine
Paraquat	No specific treatment available

Table 22.2 The principal examples of substances that cause acute poisoning in the United Kingdom.

versibly to proteins within the hepatocyte, producing centrilobular necrosis. In some cases, renal damage is also produced by a similar mechanism. Increased production of NABQI occurs in patients with a chronic alcohol problem and patients taking certain enzyme-inducing drugs such as phenytoin and phenobarbitone; these patients are at risk of hepatotoxicity at lower doses of paracetamol (Fig. 22.2).

If paracetamol overdose is diagnosed quickly, a specific treatment is available (intravenous N-acetylcysteine or oral methionine). The decision to treat is based on the plasma paracetamol concentration related to the time from overdose (Fig. 22.2), although four hours should elapse from the time of ingestion to take into account drug absorption. These treat-ments show most benefit if instituted within 12 hours of the overdose, and are unlikely to be effective if used after 24 hours.

Because effective treatment is available for paracetamol poisoning if diagnosed within 12 hours of ingestion, it is necessary to measure plasma paracetamol in:

• Patients who have taken paracetamol or combined formulations containing the drug.

• Patients who have taken unidentified tablets.

• All unconscious patients.

Salicylates

Patients often present with nausea, vomiting and increased rate of respiration. Dehydration, due to vomiting, is often severe. Acid–base disturbances are common – usually a mixed respiratory alkalosis and metabolic acidosis – but if vomiting is severe, a metabolic alkalosis can develop.

The diagnosis is confirmed by measuring plasma [salicylate]. Blood gas analysis may

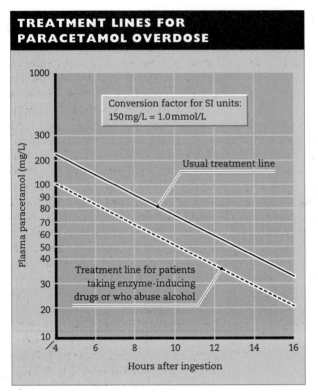

TREATMENT LINES FOR PARACETAMOL OVERDOSE

Conversion factor for SI units:
150 mg/L = 1.0 mmol/L

Usual treatment line

Treatment line for patients
taking enzyme-inducing
drugs or who abuse alcohol

Plasma paracetamol (mg/L)

Hours after ingestion

Fig. 22.2 The decision to give antidote treatment depends on the time since the overdose and on the paracetamol concentration. The timing of specimen collection is important. Specimens need to be taken 4–16 hours after suspected overdose. At less than 4 hours, the drug may not have been fully absorbed; at over 16 hours, the concentration is no longer a reliable indicator of whether to administer antidote.

also be indicated. In patients with plasma [salicylate] above 3.6 mmol/L, treatment with repeated oral administration of activated charcoal and intravenous infusion of sodium bicarbonate is often used to increase the excretion of the drug into urine. Haemodialysis may also be required in the severely poisoned patient, or if renal function is impaired.

Ethanol
The acute effects of over-indulgence in ethanol sometimes lead to admission to hospital. If the diagnosis is in doubt, plasma [ethanol] should be measured. Some patients may have drunk methylated spirits rather than ethanol, and rapid identification of both methanol and ethanol is then needed.

Methanol and ethylene glycol
Urgent measurement of plasma concentrations of these substances is required if poisoning is suspected. Methanol is metabolized to formaldehyde and formic acid, whilst ethylene

glycol is metabolized to a number of products including glycoaldehyde, glyoxylic and oxalic acids. Many of these are toxic, and also give rise to a metabolic acidosis. Severe methanol poisoning frequently leads to permanent visual impairment or complete blindness. Hypocalcaemia occurs with ethylene glycol poisoning. Treatment consists of giving ethanol, to prevent metabolism of the methanol to toxic metabolites, and haemodialysis.

Poisoning in children
Diagnosis is often more difficult than in the adult, since the range of substances that may have been taken or administered is very large, symptoms may be atypical and often more severe, and the child may not be able to give useful information. The history obtained from parents may be vague or misleading, especially if one or both parents has been responsible for unauthorized drug administration, a problem that is now recognized as being much more common than previously thought. There are a

number of urine drug-screening methods available which may, if necessary, be followed up by more accurate and specific methods such as gas chromatography–mass spectrometry (GC–MS).

Drug abuse

The marked growth in drug misuse has resulted in increasingly frequent requests for the screening of urine specimens from patients suspected of being drug abusers, for the possible presence of opiates, cocaine, lysergic acid diethylamide (LSD), benzodiazepines, methadone, buprenorphine, amphetamines and amphetamine derivatives such as ecstasy, etc.

It is important to screen for drugs of abuse:
• To corroborate claims that drugs are being misused when patients request maintenance therapy.
• To determine whether prescribed drugs (e.g. methadone) are being taken.
• To determine whether drug abuse is continuing.
• To monitor changing patterns of drug abuse.
• For medicolegal reasons.
Most drug-screening procedures are performed on urine specimens. It is essential to ensure that the sample has not been tampered with by the patient, for example with the sample being diluted or exogenous drugs added. The preliminary drug screen uses immunoassays that are sensitive, but may lack specificity due to cross-reaction with related compounds. Confirmatory tests using specific chromatographic methods with mass spectrometry are required as a follow-up to positive results because of the possibly very serious implications for patients that can stem from being identified, correctly or incorrectly, as abusers of drugs.

Industrial and occupational hazards

Metal poisons

Mercury, cadmium and lead (p. 182) are all highly toxic to humans. Their effects depend partly on the type of compound involved, whether inorganic or organometallic, and partly on the route of absorption. In all cases, the kidney is liable to be severely damaged, and often also the liver and the nervous system. Whole blood and urine measurements of the metal are important to confirm diagnosis and assess the severity of the poisoning.

Patients with chronic renal failure maintained on haemodialysis regimes are particularly at risk from poisoning by dialysis fluid constituents. Aluminium toxicity leading to *dialysis dementia* and to *metabolic bone disease* has been described. Prevention of toxicity requires periodic checks of aluminium content in the water supply and in the effluent from deionizers used with dialysers.

Organic solvents

Many organic solvents used in industry are toxic (e.g. chlorinated hydrocarbons, ethylene glycol). Toxicity may be due to accidental exposure, or sometimes to solvent abuse. The toxic agent can usually be identified specifically (e.g. by gas chromatography). Other chemical investigations may be needed, to assess hepatic and renal function.

Pesticides and herbicides

Organophosphates (e.g. parathion, malathion) may cause poisoning among farm workers by inhibiting acetylcholinesterase; plasma cholinesterase (ChE) is also inhibited. Other causes of low plasma ChE activity are summarized in Table 7.1 (p. 105). Measurements of plasma ChE activity can help in the recognition of excessive exposure to organophosphates.

Paraquat and diquat are extremely dangerous herbicides, if ingested. Paraquat has severe effects, especially on the lungs and kidneys. Clinical features usually suggest the diagnosis before the onset of complications, and the diagnosis can be confirmed by chemical examination of blood or urine for the presence of these herbicides or their metabolites. These measurements may help determine the prognosis.

KEY POINTS

1 Therapeutic drug monitoring is required for drugs with a narrow therapeutic window, such as aminoglycoside antibiotics, phenytoin, carbamazepine, digoxin, lithium and cyclosporin. The time of the last dose of the drug should always be given.

2 Paracetamol overdose is common, and may cause potentially fatal liver damage. Treatment with intravenous N-acetylcysteine is likely to be effective if started within 12 hours of the overdose. Plasma [paracetamol] should be measured in patients who have taken paracetamol, either alone or in combined formulations, or unidentified tablets and in all unconscious patients.

3 Salicylate overdose often causes nausea, vomiting and increased respiration. Dehydration and acid–base disturbances are common. If plasma [salicylate] is above 3.6 mmol/L, treatment with oral activated charcoal and intravenous sodium bicarbonate or haemodialysis may be required to increase the rate of elimination of the drug.

4 In suspected poisoning with methanol or ethylene glycol, urgent measurement of these substances is required.

5 Urinary tests for [drugs of abuse] are often required in order to monitor compliance in drug addicts on treatment and in employment screening

Case 22.1

A 19-year-old student was admitted to an accident and emergency (A&E) department after calling his doctor to state that he had taken an overdose of aspirin three hours previously. On admission, it was found that he had been vomiting and was now hyperventilating.

The following results for blood tests were found:

Analyte	Result	Reference range
[Urea] (mmol/L)	7.3	2.5–6.6
[Na+] (mmol/L)	140	132–144
[K+] (mmol/L)	3.3	3.3–4.7
[Total CO$_2$] (mmol/L)	10	24–30
[Salicylate] (mmol/L)	3.8	
[Paracetamol]	Not detected	

Comment on these results.

Comments on Case 22.1

The results and presenting features are consistent with a salicylate overdose. There is an acidosis, and salicylate is present in plasma. Paracetamol was measured, as some preparations of salicylate also contain paracetamol.

The patient was treated conservatively, and made a full recovery.

Case 22.2

A 23-year-old woman was admitted to an A&E department after being found by a flatmate lying unconscious on her bed. Next to the patient was an empty bottle of vodka, and on the bedside table there was a bottle of paracetamol tablets that appeared about half-full. The patient had appeared normal when seen by the flatmate six hours earlier. On admission, the patient's breath smelt strongly of alcohol, and the plasma paracetamol level was found to be 105 mg/L. Liver function tests were normal, as was the prothrombin time.

Comment on these results, and what treatment should be given.

Comments on Case 22.2

The patient had taken a paracetamol overdose with vodka. The time of the paracetamol overdose was not known accurately, and the patient was therefore treated with intravenous N-acetylcysteine.

No abnormalities were found in liver function tests on admission. Plasma alanine aminotransferase activity showed a transient increase over the next few days, with levels peaking at 400 U/L and then gradually falling back to reference values. These results indicate that some mild degree of liver damage had occurred.

Case 22.3

A 65-year-old woman presented to her general practitioner complaining of nausea. She had been treated with digoxin and diuretics for cardiac failure, and had tolerated the drugs well, with no previous evidence of poor compliance or poor therapeutic control. On examination, she was found to have bradycardia.

The following results were found (sampling at 14 h after last digoxin dose):

Analyte	Result	
Plasma [digoxin]	2.3 nmol/L	(therapeutic range 1.0–2.6 nmol/L)
Plasma [K⁺]	3.1 nmol/L	(reference range 3.3–4.7 nmol/L)

What is the most likely cause of the patients symptoms?

Comments on Case 22.3

The patient is likely to be suffering from digoxin toxicity. Although the plasma level of digoxin is within the therapeutic range, it is at the upper limit. However, more importantly, the patient has hypokalaemia, which will potentiate the pharmacological effect of digoxin. Plasma digoxin concentrations are a poor guide to toxicity if there is hypokalaemia. A common cause of digoxin toxicity is concurrent administration of diuretics, which cause potassium depletion.

The patient was treated successfully by giving potassium supplements to restore her plasma [potassium] to normal.

APPENDIX A

Collection of Specimens

Most quantitative chemical investigations are carried out on blood, less often on urine and other materials such as cerebrospinal fluid (CSF), intestinal secretions, faeces, calculi, sweat, amniotic fluid and fluids obtained by paracentesis, and occasionally saliva.

It is extremely important to collect, store and transport specimens correctly.

Identification of patients and specimens

The correct patient must be appropriately identified on the specimen and request form, as follows:

1 *Patient identification data (PID)*. This usually comprises name plus unique number.

2 *Test request information*. This includes relevant clinical details (including any 'risk of infection' hazard), the tests to be performed and where the report is to be sent.

3 *Collection of specimens*. In the correct tube and the appropriate preservative.

4 *Matching of specimens to requests*. Each specimen must be able to be easily and unequivocally matched to the corresponding request for investigations.

Collection and preservation of blood specimens

Lack of thought before collecting specimens or carelessness in collection may adversely affect the interpretation or impair the validity of the tests carried out on the specimens. Some factors to consider include:

1 *Diet*. Dietary constituents may alter the concentrations of analytes in blood significantly (e.g. plasma [glucose] and [triglyceride] are affected by carbohydrate and fat-containing meals, respectively).

2 *Drugs*. Many drugs influence the chemical composition of blood. Such effects of drug treatment, e.g. anti-epileptic drugs, have to be taken into account when interpreting test results. Details of relevant drug treatment must be given when requesting chemical analyses, especially when toxicological investigations are to be performed (p. 285).

3 *Diurnal variation*. The concentrations of many substances in blood vary considerably at different times of day (e.g. cortisol). Specimens for these analyses must be collected at the times specified by the laboratory, as there may be no reference ranges relating to their concentrations in blood at other times.

Care when collecting blood specimens

The posture of the patient, the choice of skin-cleansing agent, and the selection of a suitable vein (or other source) are the principal factors to consider before proceeding to collect each specimen:

1 *The skin must be clean* over the site for collecting the blood specimen. However, it must be remembered that alcohol and methylated spirits can cause haemolysis, and that their use is clearly to be avoided if blood [ethanol] is to be determined.

2 *Limbs into which intravenous infusions* are being given must not be selected as the site of venepuncture unless particular care is taken. The needle or cannula must first be thoroughly flushed out with blood to avoid dilution of the specimen with infusion fluid.

3 *Venepuncture technique should be standardized* as far as possible, to enable closer comparison of successive results on patients.

4 *Venous blood specimens should be obtained*

with *minimal stasis.* Prolonged stasis can markedly raise the concentrations of plasma proteins and other nondiffusible substances (e.g. protein-bound substances). It is advisable to release the tourniquet before withdrawing the sample of blood.

5 *Posture should be standardized if possible.* When a patient's posture changes from lying to standing, there may be an increase of as much as 13% in the concentration of plasma proteins or protein-bound constituents, due to redistribution of fluid in the extracellular space.

6 *Haemolysis should be avoided,* since it renders specimens unsuitable for plasma K+, magnesium and many protein and enzyme activity measurements.

7 *Infection hazard.* High-risk specimens require special care in collection, and this danger must be clearly indicated on the request form.

Care of blood specimens after collection

Blood specimens should be transported to the laboratory as soon as possible after collection. Special arrangements are needed for some specimens (e.g. for acid–base measurements, p. 38, or unstable hormones) because of their lack of stability. Most other analytes are stable for at least three hours in whole blood, or longer if plasma or serum is first separated from the cells. As a rule, *whole blood specimens for chemical analysis must not be stored in a refrigerator,* since ionic pumps that maintain electrolyte gradients across the cell membrane are inactive at low temperatures. Conversely, separated serum or plasma is best refrigerated, to minimize chemical changes or bacterial growth.

Several changes occur in whole blood specimens following collection. The commoner and more important changes that occur prior to the separation of plasma or serum from the cells are:

1 Glucose is converted to lactate; this process is inhibited by fluoride.

2 Several substances pass through the erythrocyte membrane, or may be added in significant amounts to plasma as a result of red cell destruction insufficient to cause detectable haemolysis. Examples include K+ and lactate dehydrogenase.

3 Loss of CO_2 occurs, since the P_{CO_2} of blood is much higher than in air.

4 Plasma [phosphate] increases due to hydrolysis of organic ester phosphates in the red cells.

5 Labile plasma enzymes lose their activity.

Collection and preservation of urine specimens

Depending on the test, either a *random* or a *complete timed collection* of urine is needed. The *timed collection* is obtained as follows:

1 Just before the collection period is due to start, the patient empties his/her bladder. *This urine must be discarded.*

2 Thereafter, from the start (e.g. at 8 a.m.) to the end of the collection period, *all urine passed by the patient must be added to the container.* If this contains preservative, the specimen must be mixed gently each time more urine is passed and added to the collection.

3 At the end of the period (e.g. 8 a.m. the next day, in the case of a 24-hour collection), the patient empties his/her bladder. *This urine must be included* in the collection.

4 The period over which the collection was made must be recorded and written on the specimen container and the request form.

For large volumes, an aliquot (e.g. 25 mL) may be sent to the laboratory, but the complete specimen must first be mixed and its volume recorded on the container and the request form.

Urine specimens tend to deteriorate unless the correct preservative is added from the start, or the specimen is refrigerated throughout the collection period. The changes include:

1 Destruction of glucose by bacteria.

2 Conversion of urea to ammonia, by bacteria, with fall in [H+] and precipitation of phosphates.

3 Oxidation of urobilinogen to urobilin and porphobilinogen to porphyrins.

Collection and preservation of faecal specimens

Quantitative work with faecal specimens can only be performed with patients who are fully co-operative, and who are preferably being looked after by trained staff in a metabolic unit. Even then, it can be difficult to ensure complete faecal collections. Faecal specimens should be refrigerated prior to their transport to the laboratory.

APPENDIX B

Near-Patient Testing

Simple side-room tests on urine and faeces have been performed for many years. However, an increasing number of chemical tests on blood can now be performed outside the main laboratory. Some use visual inspection of dipsticks, while others are performed on simple, small analysers. More specialized analysers, simple enough to be used by a wide range of staff, are used in the ward or outpatient clinic.

Their use eliminates the need to send the specimen to the laboratory, and will usually allow a more rapid turnaround time. Thus, they are particularly suitable for use in intensive care units, high-dependency units, and accident and emergency departments. Limited use of more specialized equipment may be of value in specialist clinics (e.g. glucose and HbA_{1c} in a diabetic clinic), but should generally be operated by trained technical staff. Simple analysers are sometimes used in general practice surgeries.

The above advantages of near-patient testing must be offset against need for training and re-training the operators of such equipment, the added risks of infection and the greater likelihood of error and damage to the instruments even when the operators have been trained.

Side-room tests on urine and faeces

The tests described below are subject to interference, and may give rise to unreliable results if the instructions associated with the test are not followed exactly.

Urine tests

Glucose and reducing substances

It is worth testing the urine of any patient who complains of weight loss, or excessive thirst or undue frequency of micturition, for the presence of glucose and protein. These tests should also be performed as part of any full clinical examination.

Tests for glucose in urine (glucosuria) all depend on the use of dipsticks impregnated with glucose oxidase, an enzyme that is specific for glucose. Tests for reducing substances are much less specific, and give positive results with a number of other sugars and other substances.

The recognition of renal glucosuria requires the testing of urine specimens passed during a glucose tolerance test (p. 152).

It is worth testing the urine of neonates routinely for reducing substances, as many inborn errors of metabolism give rise to urinary metabolites that react positively in this test.

Protein

Tests for proteinuria are best carried out on an early-morning specimen of urine, as this is normally the most concentrated specimen that can be readily obtained. The test materials do not detect all proteins with equal sensitivity; for instance, they often fail to detect Bence Jones protein, whereas they detect albumin in concentrations greater than 100 mg/L.

Special tests are required in order to detect Bence Jones protein (p. 94) and microalbuminuria, an early sign of diabetic nephropathy (p. 154).

Ketones

The tests for ketones in urine are most sensitive for acetoacetic acid, but they also detect acetone. However, they do not react with 3-hydroxybutyric acid, the ketone body that is present in urine in greatest amount in poorly controlled diabetes mellitus, starvation, hyperemesis gravidarum, etc.

Testing urine for ketones is important in the recognition of diabetic ketoacidosis (p. 155). Some inborn errors of metabolism give rise to the excretion of ketones in urine, and it is worth testing for these at the same time as testing for reducing substances in neonatal urine.

Urobilinogen and bilirubin

The presence of these in urine, when considered in relation to a patient's history and the findings on clinical examination, are potentially helpful in distinguishing pre-hepatic jaundice from hepatocellular and post-hepatic jaundice (Table 8.2, p. 115). They may also help with the recognition of acute hepatitis before the onset of jaundice, and in following the subsequent course of the disease.

It is essential to have a fresh specimen of urine when testing for urobilinogen.

Specific gravity

It is now more appropriate to measure urine osmolality than specific gravity when an indication of urine concentrating power is required.

pH

This is not usually a very useful measurement when performed as a side-room test.

Drugs of abuse

There are now dipsticks available to screen urine for the commoner drugs of abuse (Chapter 22).

Faeces

The detection of gastrointestinal blood loss may be very important for clinical diagnosis. The simple chemical tests depend on the pseudoperoxidase activity of haem. Unfortunately, interpretation of results is not simple, because:

1 Up to 2 mL blood may be lost normally in the faeces each day.
2 The various side-room tests differ widely in their sensitivity.
3 Meat and some vegetables, and certain iron preparations, may cause false-positive results, as they also have pseudoperoxidase activity.
4 Reducing agents (e.g. ascorbic acid) cause false-negative results if ingested in sufficient quantity.
5 Bleeding from tumours into the gut lumen is often intermittent.
6 Blood lost into the lumen of the gastrointestinal tract is unlikely to be evenly dispersed.
7 Unless faecal specimens are homogenized, sampling errors are likely.

All chemical tests for faecal occult blood yield some false-positive and some false-negative results.

False-positive results often occur with the more sensitive methods of blood detection and are serious, as they cause unnecessary further investigation, with all the attendant worry for the patient.

False-negative results occur with the less sensitive tests. Such results are dangerous, since they may cause a serious and potentially treatable condition to be missed.

However, these tests are cheap and easy to perform. There is now firm evidence that population screening for occult blood in the faeces allows earlier detection of colon cancer, and can reduce death rates from this disease by 15–20%.

Measurements on blood or urine specimens in ward, clinic and other areas

Examples of equipment that can be operated satisfactorily by clinical staff in intensive-care units, and by other nonlaboratory personnel, include the following:

1 *Bilirubinometers.* Their main use is in obstetric units for measuring plasma [bilirubin] in

jaundiced infants, to help with decisions about treatment.

2 *Blood gas analysers.* Particularly in obstetric and neonatal units, operating theatres, accident and emergency, intensive-care and high-dependency units.

3 *Blood glucose analysers.* Very widely used throughout hospitals, general practice surgeries, etc.

4 *Other ion-selective electrode systems.* These have been developed mainly for the measurement of plasma [Na$^+$] and [K$^+$] on whole blood specimens, i.e. there is no need to centrifuge these specimens prior to analysis. However, seriously misleading results for plasma [K$^+$] will be obtained if the specimen is even only slightly haemolysed; with these analysers, haemolysis is liable to go undetected. They are mostly used in intensive-care areas in support of major surgery (e.g. cardiac bypass, organ transplant operations).

5 *Cholesterol* (and other lipid) analysers in lipid clinics and primary care (Chapter 12).

Recent developments

It seems likely that simple analysers for an increasing number of analytes will be developed in the future. It is at present uncertain how extensively they will be used outside the above-mentioned critical-care units. The main reasons for this are:

1 Doubts about the reliability of the results if analyses are incorrectly performed.

2 Relatively high running costs of the equipment.

3 Need to involve medical, nursing or other staff in the testing—which is time-consuming.

4 Recent improvements in turnaround times achieved by most laboratories.

5 Dangers in handling and testing blood specimens in relatively uncontrolled environments (danger of infection with hepatitis virus, etc.)

Many of these potential dangers are discussed more fully in relation to blood [cholesterol] screening (Chapter 12).

Requirements for performing extra-laboratory blood tests

The requirements for the satisfactory performance of chemical analyses on blood specimens in the ward or clinic (including general practitioners' surgeries) are more demanding than for side-room tests on urine and faeces. This is particularly true if these measurements are to be performed by other than professionally trained laboratory staff. These requirements will be briefly reviewed here.

Health and safety

Working with blood specimens carries a significant risk of acquiring infection with, for instance, hepatitis B or human immunodeficiency virus.

It is essential that a *workable* code of safe practice be drawn up by professional laboratory staff, and that all clinic staff who will use the equipment be given appropriate instruction before undertaking specimen handling and analytical operations. These staff must be made to appreciate the need to conform thereafter to the code of practice *every time* they perform analyses.

Training

Nonlaboratory staff require to be properly trained in the operation of chemical analysers purchased for ward or clinic use. Such training should be undertaken, for each member of staff, by professional laboratory staff.

Only properly trained staff should be permitted to use the equipment, following their training. There must be simple sets of written instructions, which must include simple quality control procedures and what to do when the instrument seems to be performing unreliably.

Record-keeping

There must be a record book for entering results from patients and quality controls.

Involvement of laboratory staff

In general, laboratory staff should always be

consulted about the selection, purchase, installation and use of all near-patient analysers. Laboratory staff should also be responsible for the training of nonlaboratory users, for drawing up the appropriate protocols for use and for routine maintenance. They should also operate in-house quality assurance programmes (e.g. for ward glucose analysers).

APPENDIX C

SI Units and 'Conventional' Units

Système International (SI) units express concentrations for substances of known atomic or molecular mass in molar units. In 1974, SI units were adopted in the UK for reporting the results of chemical investigations, and many other countries world-wide have also made the change from 'conventional' to SI units for these analyses. Mass units continue to be used for the results of analyses of mixtures and proteins, and some clinical pharmacologists in the UK retain a preference for mass units. The litre (L) is the systematic SI unit of volume in medicine.

In the United States and in parts of Europe, SI units have not been universally adopted, and 'conventional' mass units are still used. Thus, glucose concentrations are expressed as 'mg/dl' or 'mg/100 mL'. Some direct read-out chemical equipment used in side-rooms presents results in these units.

In this book, we have used SI units for nearly all values, and have not used conventional units.

It is unsatisfactory, and potentially dangerous, to report results in two different sets of units, whether in SI units (with the corresponding result in 'conventional' units in brackets) or *vice versa*. However, in view of the continued use of both sets of units, conversion tables are presented in this Appendix.

Table C1 lists the reference ranges for most of the analytes for which data in SI units are given elsewhere in this book, together with the corresponding values for these reference ranges expressed in 'conventional' units.

Table C2 gives examples of conversion factors. The general formulae governing these numerical interconversions are as follows:

1 X (result, in mmol/L)×factor in column B = Y (result, in mg/100 mL).

2 Y (result, in mg/100 mL)×factor in column C = X (result, in mmol/L).

Relative molecular mass is given in Column A, and the factors derived from this shown in Columns B and C.

SI AND CONVENTIONAL REFERENCE RANGES

Plasma constituent	SI units	Conventional units
Albumin	36–47 g/L	3.6–4.7 g/100 mL
Bilirubin (total)	2–17 µmol/L	0.1–1.0 mg/100 mL
Blood urea nitrogen (BUN) (males below 50)	2.6–6.6 mmol/L	7.0–18.5 mg/100 mL
Calcium	2.12–2.62 mmol/L	8.5–10.5 mg/100 mL
Cholesterol (total)	3.6–6.7 mmol/L	140–260 mg/100 mL
Copper	12–26 µmol/L	76–165 µg/100 mL
Cortisol (total)	160–565 nmol/L at 8–9 a.m.	5.8–20.3 µg/100 mL at 8–9 a.m.
	<2.05 nmol/L at 10–12 p.m.	<7.4 mg/100 mL at 10–12 p.m.
Creatinine	55–120 µmol/L	0.6–1.3 mg/100 mL
Glucose (fasting)	3.6–5.8 mmol/L	65–105 mg/100 mL
Iron (males)	14–32 µmol/L	80–180 µg/100 mL
Iron (females)	10–28 µmol/L	60–170 µg/100 mL
Iron-binding capacity (total)	47–72 µmol/L	250–400 µg/100 mL
Magnesium	0.7–1.0 mmol/L	1.6–2.4 mg/100 mL
Phosphate (fasting, as P)	0.8–1.4 mmol/L	2.5–4.5 mg/100 mL
Protein (total)	63–83 g/L	6.3–8.3 g/100 mL
Tri-iodothyronine (total T3)	1.2–2.8 nmol/L	78–182 ng/100 mL
Thyroxine (total T4)	70–150 nmol/L	5.5–11.7 µg/100 mL
Urate (males)	0.12–0.42 mmol/L	2.0–7.0 mg/100 mL
Urate (females)	0.12–0.36 mmol/L	2.0–6.0 mg/100 mL
Urea (males below 50)	2.5–6.6 mmol/L	15–40 mg/100 mL
Zinc	10–20 µmol/L	650–1300 µg/100 mL
Constituent (arterial blood)	**SI units**	**Other units**
Hydrogen ion	36–44 nmol/L	7.35–7.45 pH units
P_{CO_2}	4.5–6.1 kPa	34–46 mmHg
P_{O_2}	12–15 kPa	90–112 mmHg

Table C1 Examples of reference ranges in SI and equivalent conventional units.

SI CONVERSION FACTORS

Plasma constituent	Relative mol. mass (Da) A	Factor (approx.) to convert numerical values expressed in:	
		SI units to conventional B	Conventional to SI units C
Albumin	66 000	0.1	10
Bilirubin	584.67	0.06	17
Blood urea nitrogen (BUN)	28.01	2.8	0.38
Calcium	40.08	4	0.25
Carbamazepine	236.26	0.24	4.2
Cholesterol (unesterified)	286.66	39	0.026
Copper	63.54	6.4	0.16
Cortisol	362.47	0.036	28
Creatinine	113.12	0.011	88
Digoxin	780.92	0.78	1.28
Glucose	180.16	18	0.055
Iron	55.84	5.6	0.18
Iron-binding capacity (total)		5.6	0.18
Lead	207.19	21	0.048
Lithium	6.94	694	0.0014
Magnesium	24.31	2.4	0.41
Phenytoin	252.26	0.25	4
Phosphate (as P)	30.97	3.1	0.32
Protein (total)	A mixture	0.1	10
Theophylline	180.17	0.18	5.55
Tri-iodothyronine (T3)	650.98	65	0.015
Thyroxine (T4)	776.87	0.078	12.9
Urate	168.11	17	0.06
Urea	60.06	6	0.17
Zinc	65.38	6.5	0.15
Constituent (arterial blood)		SI units to mmHg	mmHg to SI units
P_{CO_2}		7.5	0.13
P_{O_2}		7.5	0.13

Table C2 Examples of conversion factors between SI units and conventional units (as in Table C1).

Reference Books and Further Reading

General

Axford, J. (ed.) (1996) *Medicine*. Blackwell Science, Oxford.

Gosling, P., Marshall, W.J. & Clapham, M.C. (1994) *Intensive Care and Clinical Biochemistry*. ACB Venture Publications, London.

Hooper, J., McCreanor, G., Marshall, W. & Myers, P. (1996) *Primary Care and Laboratory Medicine*. ACB Venture Publications, London.

Marshall, W.J. & Bangert, S.K. (1995) *Clinical Biochemistry: Metabolic and Clinical Aspects*. Churchill Livingstone, Edinburgh.

Weatherall, D.J., Ledingham, J.G.G. & Warrell, D.A. (1996) *Oxford Textbook of Medicine*, 3rd edn. Oxford University Press, Oxford.

Requesting and Interpreting Laboratory Tests

Jones, R. & Payne, B. (1996) *Clinical Investigation and Statistics in Laboratory Medicine*. ACB Venture Publications, London.

Calcium Metabolism

Aviolini, L.V. & Crane, S.M. (1990) *Metabolic Bone Disease*, 2nd edn. Saunders, Philadelphia.

Favus, M.J. (1996) *Primer on the Metabolic Bone Diseases and Disorders of Mineral Metabolism*, 3rd edn. Lippincott–Raven, New York.

Tumour Markers

Sell, S. (1992) *Serological Cancer Markers*. Human Press, Ottawa.

Kidney, Electrolyte and Water Balance

Becker, G.J., Whitworth, J.A. & Kincaid-Smith, P. (1992) *Clinical Nephrology in Medical Practice*. Blackwell Science, Oxford.

Schrier, R.W. & Gottschalk, C.W. (1993) *Diseases of the Kidney*, 5th edn. Little, Brown, Boston.

Liver and Gastrointestinal Disease

Bouchier, I.A.D., Allan, R.N., Hodgson, H.J.F. & Keighley, M.R.B. (eds) (1993) *Digestion and Malabsorption of Nutrients: Gastroenterology, Clinical Science and Practice*. Saunders, London.

McIntyre, N., Benhamou, J.-P., Bircher, J., Rizzeto, M. & Rodes, J. (1991) *Oxford Textbook of Clinical Hepatology*. Oxford University Press, Oxford.

Sherlock, S. & Dooley, J. (eds) (1996) *Diseases of the Liver and Biliary System*, 10th edn. Blackwell Science, Oxford.

Stendal, S. (1997) *Practical Guide to Gastrointestinal Function Testing*. Blackwell Science, Oxford.

Nutrition

Morrison, G. & Hark, L. (1996) *Medical Nutrition and Disease*. Blackwell Science, Oxford.

Truswell, A.S. (1992) *ABC of Nutrition*, 2nd edn. British Medical Journal, London.

Lipids

Durrington, P.N. (1995) *Hyperlipidaemia: Diagnosis and Management*. Butterworth, London.

Endocrine Diseases

Alberti, K.G.M.M., Zimmet, P. & DeFronzo, R.A. (1997) *International Textbook of Diabetes Mellitus*, 2nd edn. Wiley, Chichester.

Braverman, L.E. & Utiger, R.D. (1997) *Werner and Ingbar's The Thyroid*, 7th edn. Lippincott-Raven, New York.

Brook, C.G.D. & Marshall, N.J. (1996) *Essential Endocrinology*, 3rd edn. Blackwell Science, Oxford.

Grossman, A. (1997) *Clinical Endocrinology*, 2nd edn. Blackwell Science, Oxford.

James, R.T. (1992) *The Adrenal Gland*, 2nd edn. Raven Press, New York.

Pickup, J.C. & Williams, G. (1996) *Textbook of Diabetes*. Blackwell Science, Oxford.

Paediatrics

Green A. & Morgan, I. (1993) *Neonatology and Clinical Biochemistry*. ACB Venture Publications, London.

Molecular Biology

Bradley, J., Johnson, D. & Rubenstein, D. (1995) *Molecular Medicine*. Blackwell Science, Oxford.

Hall, P.W. (1996) *Essential Molecular Biology Review*. Blackwell Science, Oxford.

Toxicology and Therapeutic Drug Monitoring

Hallworth, M. & Capps N. (1993) *Therapeutic Drug Monitoring and Clinical Biochemistry.* ACB Venture Publications, London.

Proudfoot, A.T. (1993) *Acute Poisoning: Prognosis and Management,* 2nd edn. Butterworth Heinemann, Oxford.

Vale, J.A. & Proudfoot, A.T. (1995) Paracetamol (acetaminophen) poisoning. *Lancet* **346**, 547–52.

Index

α_1-antitrypsin, detection 91, 274
α_1-fetoprotein 91
  and hepatocellular carcinoma 100
  neural tube defects 241
α_1-protease inhibitor (API) 90–1
α_2-macroglobulin 91
α-amylase (amylase) 104
abbreviations ix-xi
acetoacetate 155
acid–base assessment 37–9, 42–4
  indications for measurements 46
  mixed disturbances 43–4
  plasma [H+] decrease 43
  plasma [H+] normal 43
  temperature effects 38
  summary 47
acid–base disorders 39–44
  and oxygen transport, respiratory insufficiency 46
  renal failure 61
  treatment 46–7
acidosis
  [H+] vs $P\text{CO}_2$ 42
  metabolic 27–9, 40–3, 49
  respiratory 29, 39–40, 49
acrodermatitis enteropathica 140
acromegaly and gigantism 223
acute-phase plasma proteins 88–9
  response to injury 90
Addison's disease 29
  adrenocortical hypofunction 213–15
  cortisol and ACTH measurements 213–15
  depot (long) Synacthen test 215
  mineralocorticoid deficiency 29
  short tetracosactrin (Synacthen) test 213–15
adenylic acid, IMP, AMP and GMP synthesis 187
adrenal antibodies 215
adrenal cortex
  steroid hormone synthesis and secretion 205–8
  structure 206
adrenal disorders 205–20
  adenoma vs hyperplasia 216–17
  congenital hyperplasia (CAH) 217–18, 238
  Conn's syndrome 215
  enzyme defects, inherited 217–18
  hyperfunction 208–12
  hypofunction 212–15

adrenaline
  and hypokalaemia 27
  metadrenalines 258
adrenocortical hyperfunction *see* Cushing's syndrome
adrenocortical hypofunction *see* Addison's disease
adrenocorticotrophic hormone (ACTH) 205–6, 222–3
  deficiency 229
  measurements 207–8
agammaglobulinaemia 95
ageing effects *see* geriatrics
alanine aminotransferase (ALT) 103, 113
  neonates 255
albumin
  abnormal, and thyroid hormones 199
  in blood transport 87–8
  and calcium ions 74
  CSF Ig ratio 283
  impaired synthesis 113
  malnutrition 255
  measurement 25
  microalbumin 154
  oncotic pressure 15, 16, 87
  reference range 247
alcohol, intoxication 31, 290
alcoholic liver disease 119
aldosterone, secretion 206–7
alkaline phosphatase (ALP) 75, 103–4, 113
  geriatrics 258
  hypophosphatasia 81
  pregnancy 240
  reference range 247
alkalosis
  metabolic 27–8, 41, 43
  respiratory 40, 43
allopurinol 189–90
aluminium toxicity 291
amenorrhoea, and gonadal function 234–7
amino acid absorption
  gastrointestinal disease 128
  TPN 147
amino acidurias, renal disease 58
aminoglycoside antibiotics, therapeutic drug monitoring 285, 287
amniocentesis 241, 250
amniotic fluid, abnormal 241

amylase, pancreatic 127
anaemias, megaloblastic anaemia 108
angiotensin-converting enzyme (ACE) 18
angiotensin-converting enzyme inhibitors 29
anion gap 44–5
anterior pituitary
    combined function test 226
    see also adrenocorticotrophic hormone; follicle-
        stimulating hormone; growth hormone;
        luteinizing hormone; prolactin; thyroid–
        stimulating hormone
antidiuretic hormone, syndrome of inappropriate
        secretion of ADH (SIADH) 22
antimitochondrial antibodies, primary biliary
        cirrhosis 113–14, 121
API (α_1-protease inhibitor) 90–1
apolipoproteins 166–7
arterial disease, and hyperlipidaemia 173
ascites 113, 120
ascorbic acid (vitamin C) 141, 145
aspartate aminotransferase (AST) 103, 113
    neonates 255
aspirin, Reye's syndrome, paediatrics 257–8
asthma, hypoxia 48
atrial natriuretic peptide (ANP) 19
audit 12–13
audit cycle 13
autoantibodies, thyroid disease 200

Bartter's syndrome 28
basal metabolic rate (BMR) 136
Bence Jones protein 94
β_2-globulins 89–90
β_2-microglobulin 63, 91, 95
bicarbonate
    in acidosis 157
    blood 35
    buffering 37–8
    reabsorption and H+ excretion, renal
        mechanisms 36–7
    treatment of acid–base disturbances 46
biliary disease, malabsorption 131
bilirubin
    conjugation 111
    measurements 112, 115, 299–300
        reference range 247
    production 111–12
    transport 110–11
    urobilinogen measurements 115
    see also hyperbilirubinaemia
biotin 141, 144
blood tests 25
    acid–base assessment 37–9, 42–4
    acid–base and oxygen measurements 46
    myocardial infarction 105–7
    near-patient tests 299–301
    specimen collection 295–6
body mass index 136
bone disease 80, 82
    geriatrics 259–60

breath tests, gastrointestinal disease 130–1
buffy layer ascorbate 145

C-reactive protein 89
calcitonin 73–4
    and multiple endocrine neoplasia 201
calcitriol see 1:25-dihydroxycholecalciferol
calcium
    cytosolic 70
    extracellular fluid 70
    metabolism 71, 74
        paediatrics 257–8
    paediatrics 253–4
    and phosphate
        biological functions 69–71
        renal failure 61
    plasma 71, 74
        reference range 74, 247
    summary 84
calcium balance 69–72
    absorption 82
    daily homeostasis 70
capillary wall, oncotic pressure effects 15, 16
carbamazepine, therapeutic drug monitoring 285,
        287
carbohydrate absorption tests, gastrointestinal
        disease 128
carbohydrate metabolism disorders 149–61
carbohydrate-deficient transferrin (CDT) 119
carbon dioxide
    total
        investigation 44
        in K+ disorders 30
    transport 35–6
carboxyhaemoglobin (COHb) 183–4
carcinoembryonic antigen (CEA) 97
    colonic tumour 96
carcinoid syndrome 132–3
carcinoid tumours 132–3
cardiac failure, congestive 23
case-finding programmes, requesting and
        interpreting tests 2
catecholamines, metabolites 218–19
cell necrosis 29
cerebrospinal fluid (CSF) 282–3
    CSF glucose 282–3
    CSF immunoglobulin (Ig) 283
    CSF total protein 283
ceruloplasmin
    reference range 119
    Wilson's disease 91
chemical toxicology 288–90
children see paediatrics
chloride, plasma 25, 45
cholecalciferol 71–3
cholecystokinin–pancreozymin 127, 133
cholesterol 165
    geriatrics 258
    and ischaemic heart disease 170, 173
    total 169–70

treatment of hyperlipidaemia 173–4
cholinesterase (ChE) 104, 105
choriocarcinoma, hCG 97
chorionic villus biopsy 249–50
chromium 138, 140
chronic obstructive airways disease, respiratory
     insufficiency 46
chylomicrons, metabolism 165–8
cirrhosis
     liver disease 113, 118
     primary biliary, antimitochondrial antibodies
          113–14, 121
clonidine test 257
cloning of cDNA 268–9
cobalt 138
coeliac disease, paediatrics 257
colloid osmotic pressure 15, 16
colonic tumour, carcinoembryonic antigen (CEA)
     levels 96
coma, nonketotic, hyperglycaemic 157
Conn's syndrome, primary hyperaldosteronism
     215–17
conventional units 303–4
copper 138, 139
     in liver disease 119
Cori disease, types I and II 159
coronary heart disease, and cholesterol 170, 173
corticotrophin-releasing hormone (CRH) 209–12,
     222–3
cortisol
     Addison's disease 213–15
     measurements 207–8
     secretion 205–6, 207–8
          rhythm 208
cortisol-binding globulin 206
[51Cr]-EDTA test 128
creatine kinase (CK) 102–3
     CK-MB and CK-MM 106–7
     isoforms 102–3
     muscle disease 103
     tests in coronary unit 8, 11
     tests in general unit 11
creatinine 25, 51–4
     abnormal 53
     clearance 51–2
          elderly 258
     high 25, 53–4
     low 53
     reference range 53, 247
Crigler–Najjar syndrome, liver disease 116–17
crush injuries, rhabdomyolysis 33, 66
Cushing's syndrome 27, 208–12, 220
     algorithm 209
     carcinoid tumours 133
     causes 211
     CRH stimulation test 212
     dexamethasone suppression test 210, 212
     glucose tolerance test 212
     insulin hypoglycaemia test 211
     pituitary function tests 212
     plasma ACTH 211

potassium test 212
screening tests 208–11
selective venous sampling 212
urinary free cortisol 210
cyanocobalamin 141, 144
cyclosporin, therapeutic drug monitoring 285, 287
cystic fibrosis (CF)
     DNA analysis, paediatrics 255–6
     mutation detection 278
     screening tests 256
cystine, xanthine and oxalate excretion, renal
     disease 64
cystinuria 128
cytokines, acute-phase response 89

DDAVP test 57
dehydroepiandrosterone sulphate (DHEAS) 234,
     238, 239, 240
dexamethasone suppression test, Cushing's
     syndrome 210, 212
1:25-DHCC (1:25-dihydroxycholecalciferol) 71–3,
     78, 82
diabetes insipidus 57, 66, 226
diabetes mellitus 149, 151–7
     diagnostic criteria 153
     geriatrics 259
     lactic acidosis 157
     metabolic complications 154–5
     non-insulin dependent 137
     nonketotic hyperglycaemic coma 157
     pregnancy 152, 240–1
     secondary, and impaired glucose tolerance 151
     types I and II 151
     uncontrolled 29
diabetic ketoacidosis 162
     assessment and management 155, 157
     metabolic and clinical abnormalities 156
dialysis fluid 82
     and dementia 291
dietary constituents, principal 137–45
digoxin
     poisoning 29, 293
     therapeutic drug monitoring 285, 287
1:25-dihydroxycholecalciferol 71–3, 78–9, 82
     formation 73
     pregnancy 240
diquat 291
disaccharidase deficiency 128
diuresis and water retention 17–18
diuretic phase, renal failure 59–60
diuretics, K+-sparing 27, 29
DNA, see also molecular biology
DNA polymerases 264–5
DNA sequencing 270
dopamine, action 19
Down's syndrome, screening in pregnancy 242
drug abuse 291
drug intoxication, active treatments 289
drugs
     combination causing hypokalaemia 261

free and bound 286
metabolites 286–8
plasma concentration 286, 287
therapeutic drug monitoring (TDM) 284–8
therapy, plasma concentration effects 286
Dubin–Johnson syndrome, liver disease 117

ECF see extracellular fluid
ectopic pregnancy 240
electrocardiogram (ECG), enzyme tests 107
electrolyte balance, see also hypernatraemia;
    hyponatraemia
electrophoresis, serum protein separation 87, 94–5
enteroglucagon 133
enzymes
    activity, IU 102
    block sites, in metabolic disorders 249
    molecular biology 264–5
    release from cells 101
    tests, plasma 101–2
erythrocyte transketolase 143
erythropoiesis, ineffective 108, 111
erythropoietic porphyrias 180
ethanol, intoxication 31, 290
ethylene glycol, intoxication 290
extracellular fluid (ECF) 21 3
    calcium 70
    fluid gain 18
    hyponatraemia effects 21–3
    summary 31
    tonicity 16

faecal fat 129
Fanconi's syndrome 58
fat absorption 128–9
fatty acids 137–8, 165
ferritin 178, 240
fetal abnormalities, prenatal diagnosis 241–2
fluid balance disorders
    blood specimens 25
    chemical investigations 24–6
    fluid gain/loss, effects 18–19
    surgical patients 30
    urine specimens 25
fluorescein dilaurate tests 127
folic acid 141, 144
follicle-stimulating hormone (FSH) 222, 231, 233–4,
    236–7
    reference ranges 235
fructose intolerance 160
fructosuria 161

galactorrhoea, and hyperprolactinaemia 228
galactosaemia, metabolic disorders 159–60
galactose, enzymatic conversion to glucose 161
gamma-glutamyltransferase (GGT) 104, 113
    activity 7
    alcohol abuse 119

cirrhosis 118
reference range 247
ganglioneuroma 258
    paediatrics 258
gastric acid production, pentagastrin test 124–5
gastrin, peptic ulceration 125
gastrointestinal disease 124–33
    breath tests 129–30
    carbohyrate absorption tests 128
    carcinoid tumours/carcinoid syndrome 132–3
    fat absorption 128–9
    gastrinoma 125–6
    malabsorption 130–3
    tests 125
    Zollinger–Ellison syndrome 125
    summary 134
gastrointestinal fluid losses 28
gastrointestinal peptides 133
Gaussian distribution, variations in test results 4, 9
gene cloning 265–70
    plasmids 266
genetic disorders
    polygenic 280
    single gene 279–80
genomic cloning, cDNA 268–9
gentamicin, therapeutic drug monitoring 285, 287
geriatrics 250–60
    ageing effects 258
    bone disease 259–60
    diabetes mellitus 259
    inadequate nutrition 259
    thyroid disease 260
germ-cell tumours, AFP and hCG 97
gigantism 223
Gilbert's syndrome, liver disease 116, 121
glomerular filtration rate (GFR) 19, 51, 61
glomerular function tests 51–5
    plasma creatinine 53
    renal concentration 55–6
    tubular function 55–8
    urine osmolality 55–6
glucagon test 257
glucocorticoids
    deficiency 22
    secretion 205–6
glucose
    blood and plasma 152
    cerebrospinal fluid 282–3
    homeostasis 149–50
glucose tolerance test 152–3, 228
glycogen, synthesis and breakdown 160
glycogen storage diseases, metabolic disorders 159
glycosuria, causes 160–1
goitre 204
gonadal function
    female 233–9
    male 230–1
gonadotrophin-releasing hormone (Gn-RH), test
    222
gout
    primary 189–90

secondary 190
Graves' dsease 200, 202, 203
growth disorders, paediatrics 256–7
growth hormone 223
    deficiency 257
growth hormone releasing factor 222
guanylic acid, IMP, AMP and GMP synthesis 187
Guthrie test 252
gynaecomastia in males 232–3

haem formation 176, 181
haemochromatosis, genetic (primary) 180
haemodialysis, in poisoning 290
haemoglobin
    abnormal derivatives 183
    glycated 154
    oxygen dissociation curve 45
haptoglobins 89–90
Hashimoto's disese 200
heavy metal poisoning 291
heavy-chain disease 94
hepatic disorders see liver disease
hepatorenal failure (Wilson's disease) 91, 98, 119
herbicides 291
heterozygote screening, paediatrics 249
HGPRT 187
HGPRT deficiency 190
hirsutism, gonadal function, female 238–9
HLA system 91
HMG-CoA reductase 165
hormone replacement therapy (HRT) 239
human chorionic gonadotrophin (hCG)
    germ-cell tumours 97
    pregnancy and the fetoplacental unit 239
hydrogen ions
    buffering 37–8
    excretion 37
4-hydroxy-3-methoxymandelic acid (HMMA) 218,
    258
4-hydroxy-3-methoxyphenylacetic acid (HVA) 258
3-hydroxybutyrate 155
25-hydroxycholecalciferol (25-HCC, calcidiol)
    71–3, 79–80
21-hydroxylase deficiency 207, 217–18, 238
11β-hydroxysteroid dehydrogenase, deficiency
    218
5-hydroxytryptamine (5HT), carcinoid tumours
    132–3
hyperaldosteronism 27
    adenoma vs hyperplasia 216–17
    primary (Conn's syndrome) 215–17
    secondary 215–16
hyperbilirubinaemia 114
    cholestatic 115
    congenital 115–17
    conjugated 255
    hepatocellular 115
    neonatal 254–5
    paediatrics 254–5
    pathological unconjugated 254–5

physiological unconjugated 254
    prehepatic 115
hypercalcaemia 69, 75, 287
    causes 76–8
    clinical features 76
    familial hypocalciuric 78
    of malignancy 77
hypercalciuria
    childhood 257
    renal disease 64
hypercholesterolaemia
    primary 171
    screening 173
hypergammaglobulinaemia 93
    polyclonal/monoclonal 93
hyperglycaemic coma, nonketotic 157, 163
hyperglycaemic drugs, poisoning 164
hypergonadotrophic hypogonadism, male 232
hyperkalaemia 15, 28–31
    causes 28–31
        artefact 29–30, 34
        external
            decreased excretion of K+ 19, 29
            increased intake of K+ 19, 29
        internal distribution of K+ 19
        pseudohyperkalaemia 30
hyperlipidaemia
    arterial disease 173
    familial combined 171–2
    secondary 172
    treatment 173–4
hyperlipoproteinaemias
    hyper-α-lipoproteinaemia 172
    primary 171–2
    remnant 172
hypermagnesaemia 83
hypernatraemia 15, 23–4
    causes 21
    increased/decreased body sodium 23–4
hyperosmolar hyponatraemia 23
hyperoxaluria 64
    primary, renal disease 64
hyperparathyroidism 75–7
    primary, management 77, 84–5
    tertiary, management 78
hyperphosphataemia 75
hyperprolactinaemia, and pituitary tumours 224–5,
    228
hyperproteinaemia 25
hypertension, phaeochromocytoma 218–19
hyperthyroidism, management 200
hypertriglyceridaemia 25
    familial 171
hyperuricaemia 186, 188–90
    causes 188
hypervariable regions and RFLP, molecular biology
    275–7
hypoalbuminaemia 87–8
    causes 89
hypocalcaemia 69
    causes 78–81

clinical features 79
  ethylene glycol intoxication 290
  neonates 253
  vitamin D deficiency 79–80
hypogammaglobulinaemia, primary/secondary 95
hypoglycaemia 149, 158–9, 160
  childhood 253
  fasting 158, 159
  neonates 252–3
  reactive 158
hypogonadism, male 231–3
  hypogonadotrophic 232, 243
hypoinsulism of infancy 253
hypokalaemia 15, 26–8, 133
  causes 27–8
  deficient intake of K+ 27
  excessive losses of K+ 27–8
hypolipidaemia, secondary 173
hypolipoproteinaemias, primary 172–3
hypomagnesaemia 287
  and magnesium deficiency 83
  neonates 253
hyponatraemia 21–4
  artefact 23
  hyperosmolar 23
  increased ECF volume 23
  low ECF volume 21
  normal body sodium 24
  normal ECF volume 22
  pseudohyponatraemia 23
hypoparathyroidism 80
hypophosphataemia 75
hypophosphatasia 81
hypopituitarism, causes and examples 225
hypoproteinaemic states 23
hypothalamic and anterior pituitary hormones
    221–9
  combined function test 226
  Gn-RH test 222
  hypopituitarism, causes and examples 225
  prolactin 223–4
hypothalamic stimulating hormones and factors,
    list 222
hypothalamic–anterior pituitary–adrenal axis,
    adrenal disorders 207
hypothalamic–pituitary disease 232
hypothalamic–pituitary–testicular axis 231
hypothyroidism 287
  congenital 252
  management 199–200
hypoxanthine–guanine phosphoribostransferase
    (HGPRT) 187, 190
hypoxia, asthma 48

immunoglobulins 91–5
  cerebrospinal fluid 283
  classified 92
  liver disease 113
  structure 92
indican, urinary 130

infertility
  female 235–8
  male 231–3
inosinic acid, IMP, AMP and GMP synthesis 187
insulin 149–58
  antagonists 150
  dosage 157
  effects 150
  and hypokalaemia 27
insulin hypoglycaemia test 257
insulinoma 158
intestinal permeability tests 128
intracellular fluid (ECF)
  fluid gain 18
  summary 31
intravenous feeding 146
iodine 138
iron 175–9
  absorption 175–6
  deficiency and overload 179
  metabolism, disorders 175–84
  plasma 178
  poisoning 180
  pregnancy 240
  recommended amount 138
  saturation 178–9
  secretion, sources of loss 177
  status 177
  total iron-binding capacity (TIBC) 177, 178–9
  transport, storage and utilisation 177
ischaemic heart disease, and cholesterol 170, 173

jaundice 115, 121, 122–3
  investigations 114–16

Kallman's syndrome 243
Kayser–Fleischer rings 98, 119
kernicterus 254
Keshan disease 139
ketones
  synthesis 155
  tests 299
Klinefelter's syndrome 232
kwashiorkor 137, 255

laboratory data, interpretation and use 3–4
lactate dehydrogenase (LD) 102
lactic acidosis, diabetes mellitus 157
lead poisoning 182–3
lecithin cholesterol acetyltransferase (LCAT) 167
Lesch–Nyhan syndrome 190
lipid disorders 165–74
lipids 165–6
  plasma, abnormalities 169–74
  transport, enzymes 167
lipoprotein lipase 167
  deficiency 172
lipoprotein X, cholestasis 114

lipoproteins 166–7
  apolipoproteins 166, 167
  cholesterol 165, 169–70
  chylomicrons 165, 166, 167–8
  disorders 166–69
  HDL metabolism 169
  IDL and VLDL metabolism 168
  LDL metabolism 168
  metabolism 167
lithium 287
  and diabetes insipidus 57, 66
  therapeutic drug monitoring 285, 287–8
liver, ultrastructure 111
liver disease 110–23
  alcoholic 119
  API 91, 274
  ascites 113, 120
  cholestasis
    enzyme tests 109, 121, 122
    and hepatocellular damage 118
    lipoprotein X 114
  cirrhosis 113, 118–19
    primary biliary 113–14, 121
  copper in 119
  Crigler–Najjar syndrome 116
  diagnostic chemical tests 114–17
  disordered metabolism 114
  Dubin–Johnson syndrome 117
  Gilbert's syndrome 116, 121
  hepatitis 117, 122
  hepatitis A 122
  hepatitis B, and hepatocellular carcinoma 100
  hepatocellular damage 112–13, 117, 121
    and cholestasis 118, 121
  hepatolenticular degeneration see Wilson's
      disease
  infiltrations 118
  jaundice 115, 121, 122–3
  porphyrias 181
  prothrombin synthesis 113
  Rotor's syndrome 117
  summary 120
liver function tests 110–14
  prothrombin time 113
  TPN 147
liver structure 110
low-renin hyperaldosteronism see Conn's syndrome
luteinizing hormone (LH) 222, 231, 233–4, 236–7
  reference ranges 235

magnesium
  deficiency 83
  metabolism 82–3
  paediatrics 253–4
malabsorption
  causes 131
  investigations 131–3
malignant hyperpyrexia 103
malnutrition
  paediatrics 255

protein energy (PEM) 136–7
manganese 138, 140
marasmus 137, 255
medullary carcinoma of the thyroid 201
megaloblastic anaemia 108
Ménétrier's disease 124
Menkes' syndrome 139
menopause and hormone replacement therapy
      (HRT) 239
menstrual disorders 233–4
metabolic acidosis and alkalosis 27–8, 40–1, 47–8
metabolic disorders
  bone disease 80, 82
  see also acidosis; alkalosis
metabolic disorders, inherited 159–61
  congenital hypothyroidism 252
  early diagnosis 249–52
  enzyme block sites 249
  galactosaemia 159–60
  glycogen storage diseases 159
  infant screening programmes 252
  less acute 250
  metabolism of phenylalanine 251
  neonates 248
    screening for phenylketonuria (PKU) 250–2
  prenatal diagnosis
    amniotic fluid studies 250
    chorionic villus biopsy 249–50
  screening for heterozygotes 249
metadrenalines, neuroblastoma 258
metal poisons 291
metallothionein 139
methaemoglobin 183
methanol intoxication 290
methotrexate, therapeutic drug monitoring 288
β_2-microglobulin 63, 91, 95
milk–alkali syndrome 78
mineralocorticoid deficiency 29
molecular biology 263–80
  DNA sequencing 270
    Sanger method 271
  gene cloning 265–70
  genetic disorders 279
  hypervariable regions and RFLP 275–7
  plasmids 266
  polygenic disorders 280
  polymerase chain reaction (PCR) 277
  restriction endonucleases 264–5
  restriction fragment length polymorphisms
      (RFLPs) 273–6
  single gene disorders 279–80
  single-strand conformation polymorphism 275
  Southern blotting 270–3
molybdenum 138, 140
monoclonal (discrete) hypergammaglobulinaemia
      93
multiple endocrine neoplasia (MEN)
  insulinoma 158
  MEN syndrome 77
  tumours 201
multiple myeloma 93, 94, 99

muscle disease, creatine kinase (CK) 103
muscular dystrophy 103
myeloproliferative disorders 190
myocardial infarction
    biochemical tests 105–7
    enzyme activity 106
    non-enzyme tests 107
    plasma vs ECG 107
    plasma changes 106
    thrombolytic therapy 105
myoglobin 107

N-acetyl-p-benzoquinoneimine (NABQI),
        intoxication 288–9
natriuresis 25–6
near-patient tests 3, 298–301
neonates
    hyperbilirubinaemia 254–5
    hypoglycaemia 252–3
    hypoinsulinism 253
    inherited metabolic disorders 248
    rickets 253
    screening for phenylketonuria (PKU) 250–2
    screening tests 12
    specimen collection 246
    thyroid disease 197
nephrotic syndrome 62–3, 68
neural tube defects
    and folic acid 141, 144
    pregnancy 241–2
    prenatal diagnosis 241
neuroblastoma 258
neuron-specific enolase 97
niacin 141, 143
nonketotic hyperglycaemic coma 157, 163
nutrition
    biochemical assessment 145–8
    biochemical measurements 136–48
    carbohydrates 137
    fats 137–8
    proteins 138
    trace elements 138
    summary 148
nutritional support 145–8

obesity 137
oestradiol
    in pregnancy 240
    reference ranges 235
oligomenorrhoea and amenorrhoea, gonadal
        function, female 234–7
oncotic pressure 15, 16, 87
organic solvents 291
organophosphates 291
osmolality 15
    defined 16
    plasma 25, 31
    urine 25, 55
osmolarity, defined 16

osteomalacia 80–1, 82, 85, 259–60
osteoporosis 81–2, 259–60
ovarian cancer, CA-125 97
ovarian dysfunction 234
ovary, polycystic ovary syndrome 239, 244
oxalate, cystine and xanthine excretion, renal
        disease 64
oxygen, indications for measurements 46
oxygen dissociation curve 45
oxygen transport 45

paediatrics 246–58
    calcium and magnesium 253–4
    calcium metabolism 257–8
    coeliac disease 257
    cystic fibrosis (CF) 255–6
    growth disorders 256–7
    hyperbilirubinaemia 254–5
    hypoglycaemia
        childhood 253
        neonates 252–3
    inherited metabolic disorders 247–50
    malnutrition 255
    neuroblastoma and ganglioneuroma 258
        poisoning 290–1
    reference ranges 246–7
    respiratory distress syndrome (RDS) 253–4
    Reye's syndrome 257–8
    screening tests, cystic fibrosis (CF) 256
    short stature 256–7
    specimen collection, neonates and children 246
Paget's disease 80, 81, 259
pancreatic disease
    acute pancreatitis 126–7
    carcinoma 123
    chronic pancreatitis 127, 134–5
    malabsorption 131
    plasma amylase 127
para-aminobenzoic acid (PABA) 127
paracetamol overdose, treatment 288–90
paraproteinaemias 93–4
    investigations 94–5
paraquat 291
parathyroid hormone (PTH) 71
    assay 76–7
pentagastrin test, gastric acid production 124–6
pentosuria 161
peptic ulcer 124
    plasma gastrin 125
peptides, gastrointestinal 133
pesticides, poisoning 291
phaeochromocytoma 218–19
    plasma catecholamines 219
    urine tests 218–19
phenylketonuria (PKU) screening 250–2
phenytoin, therapeutic drug monitoring 285, 287
phosphate
    biological functions 69–71
    plasma 74–5
    reference range 74, 247

retention 82
phosphate binders 82
phospholids 165–6
pituitary hormones
    anterior 221–6
    function tests 222, 226
    posterior 226–7
plasma, osmolality 25
plasma changes, effects 74
plasma constituents, variation, requesting and
        interpreting tests 6
plasma enzymes
    clinically important examples 102–4
    diagnostic tests 101–7
plasmids 266–7
poisoning 253–91
    acute, treatments 289
    children 290–1
    pesticides and herbicides 291
polyclonal (diffuse) hypergammaglobulinaemia 93
polycystic ovary syndrome 239, 244
polygenic disorders, molecular biology 280
polymerase chain reaction (PCR) 277
porphyrias
    chemical investigations 181–2
    hepatic 181
porphyrin metabolism 180–4
posterior pituitary hormones 226–7
potassium balance
    concentration abnormalities 26–30
    excretion in renal disease 59
    hyperaldosteronism 216
    reference range 26, 247
    renal excretion 59
    screening studies 216
    TPN 147
    see also hyperkalaemia; hypokalaemia
potassium EDTA, artefact hyperkalaemia 29–30
pre-eclampsia, pregnancy 241
pregnancy
    abnormal TSH results 197
    alkaline phosphatase 240
    chemical tests 240
    diabetes mellitus 240–1
    ectopic 240
    fetoplacental unit 239–42
    maternal complications 240–2
    neural tube defects 241–2
    pre-eclampsia 241
    prenatal diagnosis of fetal abnormalities 241–2
    screening for Down's syndrome 242
pregnancy-specific proteins 239
progesterone, reference ranges 235
prolactin
    hyperprolactinaemia 224–5, 228, 245
    menstrual disorders 236
prolactinoma 245
prostatic cancer, PSA 97, 99
protein–energy malnutrition (PEM) 136–7
proteins, plasma 86–97
    acute phase 88–9

and disease 86–91
    glycation 154
    immunoglobulins 91–5
    investigation methods 86
    list and types 88
    metabolism 167–9
    reference range 247
    role and functions 86, 88
    transport functions 87
    trophoblastic origin, pregnancy and the
        fetoplacental unit 239
    tumour markers 95–7
proteinuria 61–3
    glomerular and tubular 62
    orthostatic 63
    overflow 62
    tests 298
    tubular 63
prothrombin synthesis, liver disease 113
pseudohyperkalaemia 30
pseudohyponatraemia 23
pseudohypoparathyroidism 80, 257
pulmonary emphysema, API 91
purine metabolism 186
    disorders 186–90
pyridoxine 141, 143

reference ranges 6–7
    age dependent, paediatrics 247
    paediatrics 246–7
    SI and conventional units 303
renal disease 51–68
    abnormal plasma urea 54
    amino acidurias 58
    cystine, xanthine and oxalate excretion 64
    glomerular function tests 55–6
    glomerulonephritis 63
    high plasma urea 54–5
    hypercalciuria 64
    hypocalcaemia 80
    nephrotic syndrome 62–3
    oxalate, cystine and xanthine excretion 64
    plasma urea 54–5
    potassium excretion 59
    primary hyperoxaluria 64
    sodium excretion 58
    xanthine, oxalate and cystine excretion 64
renal failure 23, 56, 59–61
    acid–base disturbances 61
    acute, defined 59
    calcium and phosphate 61
    chronic 22, 61, 67, 190
    diuretic phase 59, 60
    oliguric phase 59–60
renal function
    HCO$_3$ reabsorption 36
    hydrogen ion excretion 36–7
    sodium and potassium 58–9
    tests 55–8
renal osteodystrophy 81–2

renal stones 63–5
    chemical investigations 64–5
renal tubular acidosis 28, 58
renal tubule
    function tests 55–8
    hydrogen ion excretion 37
    reabsorption of bicarbonate 36
renin 206, 216
renin–angiotensin–aldosterone system 18–19
respiratory acidosis 39–40
respiratory alkalosis 40
respiratory distress syndrome (RDS), paediatrics
        253–4
respiratory insufficiency, COPD types I and II 46
restriction endonucleases, Eco R1, action 264
restriction fragment length polymorphisms
        (RFLPs) 273–5
    analysis 276
Reye's syndrome, paediatrics 257–8
rhabdomyolysis, crush injuries 33, 66
riboflavin 141, 143
rickets 80–1, 82
    neonates 253
Rotor's syndrome, liver disease 117

salicylates 189
    intoxication 289–90
sarcoidosis 78
scoline apnoea 104
screening tests
    advantages and disadvantages 2–3
    Cushing's syndrome 208–11
    cystic fibrosis (CF) 256
    diseases in elderly patients 258–9
    interpreting tests 2
    neonates 12
    rare diseases 11–12
    unexpected test results 3
    well population 2
    see also tests
secretin/CCK-PZ test 127
selenium 138, 139
serotonin, carcinoid tumours 132–3
sex differentiation, male disorders 232–3
sex hormones, gonadal function, female 235
SI conversion factors 304
SI units 302–3
'sick cell' syndrome 23, 32
sick euthyroid syndrome 197–8
single-strand conformation polymorphism,
        molecular biology 275
small intestinal disease 127–32
    bacterial colonization 132
    stasis 129–30
small-cell lung cancer, neuron-specific enolase 97
sodium balance 15–19
    depletion and excess 20
    disorders 19–24
    regulation 18–19
    renal excretion 58–9

TPN 147
urine 25
see also hypernatraemia; hyponatraemia
solvents, organic, poisoning 291
Southern blotting 270–3
specimen collection 295–7
    requesting and interpreting tests 3
spermatogenesis control 230
statistical variation 4–5
Stein–Leventhal syndrome 239
steroid contraceptives, gonadal function, female
        239
steroids
    pregnancy 239–40
    synthesis and secretion 217
stomach, gastrointestinal disease 124–6
succinylcholine, apnoea 104–5
sulphaemoglobin 183, 184
surgical patients, fluid balance disorders 30
Synacthen test 213–15
syndrome of inappropriate secretion of ADH
        (SIADH) 22, 32
    defined 226

tacrolimus 287
terminal ileal function 131
testosterone, transport and metabolism 230–1
tests
    diagnostic
        predictive value, positive/negative results 8–10
        sensitivity 10
    discretionary/selective 1
    near-patient 3
    normal ranges 7
    positive diagnostic 9
    reference ranges 6
    requesting and interpreting 1–14
    screening 2–3
        diseases in elderly patients 258–9
        neonates 12
        rare diseases 11–12
    variations in results 4–5
        between-individual 6
        biological causes 5
        blunders 5
        distribution of results in reference population
            6–7
        Gaussian distribution 4
        within-individual 5–6
    see also screening tests
theophylline, therapeutic drug monitoring 285, 288
thiamin 141, 143
thrombolytic therapy, myocardial infarction 105
thyroid disease
    autoantibodies 200
    geriatrics 260
    hyperthyroidism 197, 200, 203
    hypothyroidism 199–200, 204
    medullary carcinoma 201
    paediatrics and neonate 197

secondary disorders 197–8
tests affected by thyroid dysfunction 201
thyroglobulin 200–1
thyroid antibodies 200
thyroid enzymes 201
thyroid function 191–204
  drugs affecting 198
  regulation 192
  status 192–4
  tests
    abnormal plasma in euthyroid patients 195
    abnormal serum TSH 196
    cases 202–4
    interpreting results 195–204
    selective use 194–5
thyroid hormones
  measurements, abnormal results 198–9
  reference ranges 247
  T4, T3 and rT3 191–5
    formulae 192
    synthesis 191–5
  thyroid status 192–3
thyroid-stimulating hormone (TSH)
  abnormal
    pregnancy 197
    thyroid function tests 196
  measurement 193
    geriatrics 260
  misleading TSH results 197–8
  reference range 247
  TSH-receptor antibodies 200
thyroliberin see thyrotrophin releasing hormone
  (TRH)
thyrotrophin see thyroid-stimulating hormone (TSH)
thyrotrophin releasing hormone (TRH), TRH test
  221–6
thyroxine see thyroid hormones
tobramycin, therapeutic drug monitoring 285
tonicity, defined 16
total parenteral nutrition (TPN)
  'big bag' composition 146
  indications 146
trace elements, nutrition 138–40
transferrin 178–9
  carbohydrate-deficient 119
trauma, metabolic response 30–1
triglycerides 137–8, 165, 170
  breath test 129
  metabolism 168
trophoblastic tumours, hCG 239
troponins 107
tryptophan 130, 144
  carcinoid syndrome 132–3
tubular function tests, renal disease 55–8
tumour markers 95–7

uraemia, prerenal/postrenal 53–4
urate
  defective elimination 190

gout 189
overproduction 190
plasma 186–9
urea, abnormal, renal disease 54–5
urinary indican 130
urine
  acidification tests 57–8
  electrophoresis, protein separation 87, 94–5
  failure to concentrate 56
  near-patient tests 298–9
  osmolality 16, 25, 55–6
  output 60
  polyuria 25
  sodium 25
  specimen collection 296–7
urobilinogen measurements 115, 299

vasoactive intestinal peptide (VIP), Verner–Morrison
  syndrome 133
vasopressin 226
  DDAVP test 57
  fluid deprivation test 56–7
  secretion 16–18
Verner–Morrison syndrome 133
virilism, gonadal function, female 238–9
vitamin A 141, 142
vitamin C 141, 145
vitamin D 71–3, 78–80, 141
  defective metabolism 82
vitamin E 141, 142
vitamin K 113, 141, 143
vitamins, principal functions and RDAs 140–5
vomiting, metabolic alkalosis 7–8, 27–8, 41
von Gierke's disease 159

Waldenström's macroglobulinaemia 93–4
water balance 15–19
  depletion and excess 20
  disorders 19–26
  intake and output 17
  intoxication 25–6, 30–1, 32
  sodium homeostasis disorders 19
water retention, acute/chronic 22
Wilson's disease
  ceruloplasmin 91, 98, 119
  Kayser–Fleischer rings 98, 119

xanthine, oxalate and cystine excretion, renal
  disease 64
xanthine oxidase 188
xanthochromia 282–3
xylose absorption tests 128, 130–1

zinc 138, 139–40
Zollinger–Ellison syndrome, gastrinoma 125,
  134